Frontiers of Medi

Frontiers of Medicine

Being the Third Edition of
Lectures in Medicine

C. W. H. HAVARD
MA, DM(Oxon), FRCP(Lond)
Consultant Physician,
Royal Free Hospital and Royal Northern Hospital

WILLIAM HEINEMANN MEDICAL BOOKS LTD
LONDON

FIRST PUBLISHED 1967 BY STAPLES PRESS
SECOND EDITION 1969
THIRD EDITION PUBLISHED BY WILLIAM HEINEMANN
MEDICAL BOOKS LTD 1973

ISBN 0 433 13370 8

PRINTED IN GREAT BRITAIN BY
REDWOOD PRESS LIMITED
TROWBRIDGE, WILTSHIRE

TO MARK, JOHN, SUKIE & MARY

CONTENTS

PREFACE TO THE FIRST EDITION

This book is based on a series of lectures given to clinical students in their final undergraduate year. Most of the chapters are concerned with recent advances in the investigation or management of disease or current concepts of the nature of disease. The topics were chosen because they constituted gaps in the clinical teaching or because the subjects were not readily available for study in the standard textbooks. The book is not intended for the scholar but rather for the student, practitioner and general physician, whose practice must cover the whole of general medicine and for whom keeping pace with the spate of current medical advances provides an insoluble problem. The three final chapters of the book are concerned with subjects on which I am not qualified to write and I am grateful to my colleagues Dr J. E. Stark, Mr M. P. Curwen and Dr L. C. Payne for their contributions on 'Viruses and Disease', 'Statistics in Medicine' and 'Computers in Medicine' respectively. References are not quoted as they discourage the general reader and interrupt the text but a selected bibliography for further reading is given at the end of the book.

I am grateful to many colleagues for helpful advice and in particular to Miss Joan MacAlister, Mr Michael Curwen, Dr Douglas A. Chamberlain, Dr P. J. Lawther, Dr A. M. Dawson, and Dr C. M. B. Pare. I thank Dr A. W. Spence for his constant help and encouragement.

I hope this book will provide an opportunity for those whose time is limited to review some recent concepts of the nature of disease and some advances in the practical management of sick patients.

PREFACE TO THE THIRD EDITION

The aim of this book is to review recent advances in Medicine and modern concepts of the nature of disease in a manner readily intelligible to those not actively engaged in the particular field under discussion. In addition subjects are chosen because they are not readily available for study in standard text-books.

The first edition appeared in 1967 under the title of 'Lectures in Medicine' and a second edition followed two years later. With a change of publisher a fresh caption seemed appropiate for the third edition and the title offered in a review of a previous edition has been selected.

Four chapters of the second edition have been excluded to make way for new topics. Two chapters have been completly rewritten and major additions and alterations have been made to others. I am grateful to my colleagues Tim Chard and John Landon for the chapter on 'Radio-immunoassay' and to Jack Hirsh for the chapter on 'Bleeding Disorders and Fibrinolysis', which are two of the new contributions included in this edition.

I hope that a third edition within five years is evidence that the challenge to the student, practitioner and general physician to keep abreast of current advances has been accepted and that in some small way this book has helped.

C.W.H.H. 1972

LIST OF ILLUSTRATIONS

INVITED CONTRIBUTORS

T. CHARD, M.D., M.R.C.O.G.
Senior Lecturer in Reproduction Physiology,
Hon. Consultant in Clinical Measurement,
St. Bartholomew's Hospital Medical College, London.

JACK HIRSH, M.D., F.R.A.C.P.
Professor of Pathology, MacMaster University, Hamilton, Ontario.

JOHN LANDON, M.D.
Professor of Chemical Pathology,
St. Bartholomew's Hospital Medical College, London.

M. H. LESSOF, M.D., F.R.C.P.
Professor of Medicine, Guy's Hospital Medical School, London.

L. C. PAYNE, Ph.D.
Automation Consultant

PAUL TURNER, M.D., B.Sc., M.R.C.P.
Professor of Clinical Pharmacology,
St. Bartholomew's Hospital Medical College, London.

I

Inborn Errors of Metabolism

INTRODUCTION

The inborn errors of metabolism are the inherited metabolic diseases of childhood although sometimes if the disease is not severe it may not be detected until adult life. Some of these disorders are, however, the cause of severe illness which may be fatal within a few weeks. All genetically determined diseases are basically inborn errors of metabolism although in some, such as Huntington's chorea or the hereditary ataxias, the metabolic error awaits demonstration. Some drug idiosyncrasies have been shown to be the result of inborn metabolic errors and it is likely that many more will be proven to have a similar basis. The inborn errors of metabolism are becoming more important as they are becoming more common and are being more commonly diagnosed. Furthermore, as other diseases such as infections are ceasing to be major causes of death the importance of these conditions is enhanced.

It is of fundamental importance to realize that biochemical as well as morphological diseases can be inherited. All biochemical processes in the body are under genetic control. These processes can be resolved into a series of individual chemical reactions and each reaction is dependent upon a specific enzyme and hence is under the control of a different gene. An enzyme is a protein which functions as a catalyst in a biochemical reaction. Mutation of a gene may result in a structural change in the enzyme constitution or indeed in a failure of its synthesis and either will be associated with an inability to carry out the specific biochemical reaction. As all enzymes are proteins it is probable that most inborn errors of metabolism are due to an inherited alteration in the amino acid constitution of the relevant enzyme protein with a consequent loss of its catalytic activity. It makes little difference to the body whether the change in the enzyme is qualitative or quantitative, because it is the activity of the enzyme that is important. Thus, if the enzyme is completely deficient the biochemical reaction for which it is responsible cannot take place. Similarly if the enzyme constitution is altered by as little as one amino acid in the molecule it is likely that it will be ineffective as a catalyst. Hence, the position as regards the chemical reaction is the same as if the enzyme was absent. In evaluating enzyme function it is the chemical activity of the enzyme that the biochemist evaluates and not its chemical structure. Therefore in most errors of metabolism it is not known whether the mutation is one which alters the structure of the enzyme or prevents its formation.

Furthermore genes not only determine the structure of proteins but also regulate their synthesis. Some mutations produce their effects by altering the rate of synthesis of the specific protein without necessarily altering the structure. An abnormal gene can thus cause a defect in enzyme activity in a number of ways.

1. By the synthesis of a structurally altered protein with defective catalytic activities.
2. By the synthesis of a structurally altered protein whose catalytic activity is unaffected, but whose stability is impaired so that it is more rapidly denatured. The increased destruction of the enzyme would mean that the amount present at any given time was reduced and hence the level of activity would be less.
3. By causing a true failure in synthesis. In this situation the enzyme protein would not be formed at all.

Inborn errors of metabolism like any other inherited characteristic may be transmitted by recessive or dominant genes which may be sex linked or carried on the autosomes. If the metabolic error is transmitted by a dominant gene the affected enzyme is either completely normal if the gene is absent or completely abnormal if the gene is present. The disease is then an 'all or none' phenomenon. More commonly, however, the errors of metabolism are transmitted by recessive genes and there is a further possibility that the heterozygote, who carries the gene in only a single dose, may have a partial defect of enzyme function. Appropriate biochemical tests can identify the heterozygote for phenylketonuria and galactosaemia, and female carriers of the gene for nephrogenic diabetes insipidus, which is a sex linked recessive characteristic, have some impairment of urine concentration. Tissue culture characteristics of the skin of carriers of fibrocystic disease permit their identification. The mode of inheritance of most inborn errors of metabolism is recessive so that the enzyme deficiency is due to the presence in double dose of a rare gene. Two outwardly normal carriers of the gene marry with the result that one in four of their children will carry a double dose of the gene and suffer from the disease. The metabolic block may affect protein, fat, carbohydrate, nucleic acid, porphyrin or pigment metabolism.

Not all enzyme defects are concerned with intermediary metabolism. In cystinuria the excessive excretion of cystine and other amino acids is not due to a defect in the metabolism of cystine but a failure of the renal tubule to reabsorb it. The transport of metabolites across the renal tubular cell is an active and specific process and is controlled by enzymes. If the enzyme is deficient in quantity or quality the relevant metabolite will not be reabsorbed and such conditions as renal glycosuria, renal tubular acidosis, Fanconi syndrome, cystinuria, nephrogenic diabetes insipidus and vitamin D resistant rickets may result.

Whilst all enzymes are protein not all proteins are enzymes so that inborn differences in the formation of circulating plasma proteins, which do not function as enzymes, may also occur. The disorders of haemoglobin formation known as the haemoglobinopathies and the disorders of plasma protein synthesis are familiar examples. The former include sickle cell disease and thalassaemia in which there is inability to form normal adult haemoglobin and the latter include hypogammaglobulinaemia and haemophilia.

THE CONCEPT OF INBORN ERRORS OF METABOLISM

Errors affecting intermediary metabolism

To understand the concept of the inborn metabolic block and its resulting biochemical disturbances let us consider the metabolic fate of phenylalanine and tyrosine illustrated in Diagram 1.

Diagram 1

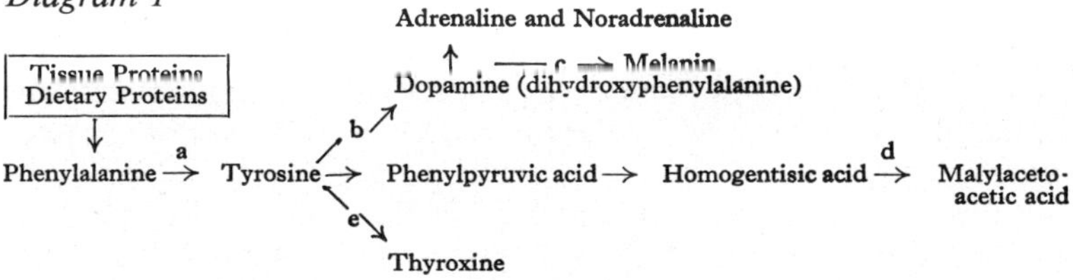

In phenylketonuria enzyme 'a' (phenylalanine hydroxylase) is deficient. This enzyme catalyses the conversion of phenylalanine to tyrosine. Phenylalanine is continuously supplied in dietary protein and from the breakdown of tissue protein and it therefore accumulates in considerable quantities, giving rise to the clinical features of the disease. The failure to form tyrosine is of little consequence as adequate amounts of this amino acid are obtained from the diet. It is of interest that heterozygotes for this gene, that is persons who possess the gene in a single dose, show a similar qualitative disturbance in metabolism but it is quantitatively less. Blood phenylalanine levels are one and a half times higher than normal compared with a twentyfold increase in those who have the disease because of a double dose of the gene. Phenylketonuria occurs in 1 in 40,000 births and the incidence of the heterozygote state is estimated as 1 in 100.

If enzyme 'd' (homogentisic oxidase), which catalyses the conversion of homogentisic acid to maleylacetoacetic acid, is deficient alkaptonuria results. Homogentisic acid accumulates in the blood and is excreted in the urine in increased amounts. This turns the urine black on standing, giving rise to the characteristic feature of the disease. Apart from a predisposition to degenerative joint disease and ochronosis (staining of cartilage black) the affected individual remains healthy. If one gives such a patient homogentisic acid by mouth it is all excreted in the urine, whilst if one gives a normal person homogentisic acid by mouth it is readily metabolized.

In albinism melanocytes fail to synthesize the enzyme tyrosinase which catalyzes both reactions b and c. This is necessary for the conversion of tyrosine to melanin through dihydroxyphenylalanine (dopamine), the same enzyme being involved in both chemical reactions. Tyrosine is hydroxylated to dopamine in the adrenal gland through another pathway, which does not require the enzyme tyrosinase, so that albinos do not show any deficiency of adrenaline and noradrenaline.

If enzyme 'e' is lacking the child will be a cretin with a goitre because thyroxine cannot be formed. Excessive stimulation of the gland by thyrotrophic hormone from the pituitary causes the goitre. This is, of course, a rare form of cretinism, iodine deficiency and congenital thyroid agenesis being more frequent causes. Iodine is ingested as inorganic iodide and the small amounts circulating in the blood are trapped by the thyroid gland. This trapping mechanism depends on a thyroid enzyme, which can be inhibited by perchlorate. The iodide concentrated in the gland is then oxidised to free iodine which combines with tyrosine to form mono-iodotryrosine and di-iodotyrosine. Conjugation of two molecules of di-iodotyrosine leads to the formation of thyroxine. Deficiencies of the enzyme concerned with the trapping of the small amounts of circulating iodine or those required for the synthesis of thyroxine may occur and are genetically determined. The common end result is a goitre with associated cretinism.

Thus inborn metabolic defects are the result of the congenital defect or deficiency of a specific enzyme which results in a block at some particular point in the normal course of metabolism. The substrate may accumulate either within the cells as in glycogen storage diseases, Gaucher's and Niemann-Pick disease and in the mucopolysaccharide deposition characteristic of gargoylism or it may accumulate in the plasma as in phenylketonuria. The enzyme may be deficient throughout the whole body as in galactosaemia, where the defect is in the enzyme which converts galactose phosphate to glucose phosphate. As a result the blood galactose level rises and galactose accumulates in the tissues; this causes severe liver damage, cataract, mental impairment and retardation of growth. The child is usually listless and refuses to take feeds within the first week of life and this is soon followed by vomiting, loss of weight, jaundice, diarrhoea and hypoglycaemia. The diagnosis is suggested by the detection in the urine of a reducing substance with a negative test with glucose oxidase. Galactose can then be identified chromatographically. If galactose can be excluded from the diet the child will develop normally. The dietary management of these patients is not easy as galactose in the form of the disaccharide lactose is the main carbohydrate of milk. Alternatively enzymes may be deficient in only one of several tissues in which they are normally found. Two sorts of glycogen storage disease occur due to deficiency of the enzyme glucose–6–phosphatase or of amyloglucosidase both of which are concerned with the conversion of glycogen to glucose. In the latter form the deficiency affects the liver and muscle and intracellular deposition of glycogen occurs in both. In the former, as the enzyme under normal circumstances only occurs in liver and kidney, deficiency disease does not affect muscle. As a result of the inability to make glucose, hypoglycaemia tends to occur on fasting. In red cell pyruvate kinase deficiency, which is responsible for certain congenital non-spherocytic haemolytic anaemias of childhood, the enzyme deficiency occurs in the red cells but not in the white cells.

In glucose–6–phosphate dehydrogenase deficiency the situation is somewhat different. In this disorder, which is not uncommon in Negroes, the defect is due to a gene located on the X chromosome. In affected males the level of this enzyme in the red cells is only about 15 per cent of the normal. These individuals are healthy but develop an acute haemolytic anaemia when they eat fava beans or receive certain drugs such as anti-malarial compounds and sulphonamides. There is an alteration in the molecular structure of the enzyme but no abnormality in its enzyme activity occurs. However because of the alteration in molecular structure the enzyme is broken down at an increased rate. This means that the level of activity of the enzyme in the red cells is lower than normal. Young red cells have a normal level of activity but this decreases rapidly with advancing age of the red cells. Thus in this condition the enzyme deficiency is due to excessive destruction of the enzyme and not to any alteration in its catalytic activity.

The enzyme defects giving rise to inborn errors of metabolism occur in a variety of organs and examples involving liver, kidney, muscle and thyroid have received comment. The small intestine may also be involved and there is now convincing evidence that coeliac disease of childhood and idiopathic steatorrhoea in the adult are the result of an enzyme deficiency in the mucosal cell of the small intestine, which renders such individuals susceptible to the toxic effects of wheat gluten.

Errors affecting plasma proteins

Inherited abnormalities resulting in the failure to synthesize plasma proteins in adequate amounts account for the clinical conditions of hypogammaglobulinaemia, afibrinogenaemia and hepato-lenticular degeneration (Wilson's disease). Hypogammaglobulinaemia presents with recurrent bacterial infections, particularly of the respiratory tract and the skin, on account of the inability to form circulating antibodies to foreign bacteria. In hepato-lenticular degeneration, or Wilson's disease, there is a metabolic error in the production of caeruloplasmin, the copper-carrying plasma protein. Copper metabolism and transport are disturbed and the defect is associated with both an enhanced absorption of copper from the gut and deposition of the metal in the brain and liver. This results in a nodular cirrhosis of the liver and cavitation of the lenticular nuclei in the brain. The patient, who is usually a child, presents with ascites or jaundice if the major damage occurs in the liver, or dysarthria and tremor if brain damage is dominant.

Alternatively, the inherited anomaly may result not in the failure to form a specific protein but in the formation of a protein similar in most respects to the normal but differing in some fine detail, which is however sufficient to render that protein incapable of performing its function. Sickle cell disease provides the best example of this state of affairs. This condition is due to the inheritance of an abnormal haemoglobin, which differs in only one of several hundred of the amino acid residues, which make up the globin protein molecule, and yet the end product is so inadequate that the disease is rapidly fatal. The mere substitution of a glutamic acid by a valine residue in the beta polypeptide chain of normal haemoglobin profoundly reduces the stability of the pigment when it is deoxygenated. As a result the red cells become deformed and assume the characteristic sickle-cell shape when the oxygen tension is low, as on the venous side of the circulation. This change in red cell shape is associated with increased fragility and an exaggerated viscosity of the blood, which results in the multiple scattered infarcts, characteristic of the disease. In a similar way variations in the structure of the enzyme serum cholinesterase render certain individuals unduly sensitive to the muscle relaxant suxamethonium. Serum cholinesterase normally breaks down suxamethonium. In certain individuals the serum level may be normal and yet they are unable to break down suxamethonium because the chemical structure of their enzyme differs slightly from the normal enzyme protein and hence lacks the catalytic properties of the normal enzyme.

Undefined errors of metabolism

In many errors of metabolism the precise metabolic error is unknown. In haemochromatosis, for example, there is a metabolic error in the intestinal cell which is responsible for the increased iron absorption characteristic of the disease. High serum concentrations of iron and deposition of iron in the tissues result. Iron is normally attached to transferrin, the beta globulin by which it is carried in the serum, within the intestinal cell. The metabolic error responsible for the increased and uncontrolled transfer of iron to the carrier protein has not, however, been defined.

In gout there is a disturbance of purine metabolism which results in an increased production of uric acid. Uric acid is the end product from the degradation of the nucleic acid constituent of nucleoprotein. Hyperuricaemia may be anticipated in any condition where there is an increased turnover of nucleoprotein as occurs in polycythaemia rubra vera or leukaemia and 'secondary gout' may occur in such situations. In primary gout there is evidence that increased synthesis of the nucleoprotein is the cause of the hyperuricaemia. The metabolic reason for this is not known and furthermore the relationship between the blood level of uric acid and the clinical manifestations of gout is not precise so that other factors are certainly involved.

Knowledge of the metabolic errors in the porphyrias is also incomplete. The porphyrins take part in many important cellular functions particularly those involving the respiration of the cell. In man they form haem by combination with iron, whilst in the plant chlorophyll is a porphyrin magnesium complex.

In man the red cells require haem for haemoglobin and other cells require haem for synthesis of myoglobin, cytochromes and catalase. The inborn errors of porphyrin metabolism are classified into, (1) erythropoietic, or (2) hepatic, according to the organ involved. The characteristic abnormality is the excretion of large amounts of uroporphyrin or porphobilinogen or both. In the erythropoietic variety the excessive porphyrin production occurs in the bone marrow and the metabolic block is known. It consists of an inability of about half the marrow normoblasts to form uroporphyrinogen from porphobilinogen. The metabolic pathway through uroporphyrinogen I to uroporphyrin is not affected but the end-products of this reaction are pigments of no use to the body. The red cell progeny do not survive normally and a mild haemolytic anaemia results.

Porphobilinogen thus changes spontaneously into uroporphyrin (and other pigments) especially in acid solution so that the main urinary pigment in this condition is uroporphyrin. The accumulation of the pigment uroporphyrin in the blood causes photosensitivity and characteristic cutaneous lesions and its appearance in the urine gives it a burgundy-red colour. This variety of porphyria is very rare.

In the hepatic porphyrias no metabolic block has been demonstrated and the over production of porphyrin precursors by the liver is the cause of the disease. The metabolic reasons for this are obscure. The increased production of the pigment uroporphyrin may cause light sensitive cutaneous lesions, as in the erythropoietic porphyrias but the explanation of the other manifestations of the disease is uncertain. There is no real evidence that a circulating toxic factor present in the blood causes the symptoms of porphyria. Porphyrins themselves and their precursors are non-toxic. Symptoms are probably caused by some underlying biochemical disorder associated with the hepatic defect in acute types of porphyria. The clinical symptoms include:

(a) Visceral symptoms of abdominal pain and vomiting.

(b) Neurological symptoms of peripheral neuritis which may lead to quadriplegia and respiratory failure.

(c) Mental symptoms of confusion and even psychosis.

One of the difficulties in the diagnosis of this condition is that porphobilinogen is colourless so that if this is the porphyrin being produced in excessive amounts the urine will not be red. The clinical syndromes will depend upon the particular porphyrin being produced in excess and the hepatic porphyrias are therefore subdivided into: 1. acute intermittent porphyria, 2. chronic cutaneous porphyria, 3. mixed porphyria. All varieties are aggravated and precipitated by barbituates and sulphonamides and each variety is usually associated with an inappropriate secretion of anti-diuretic hormone producing a dilution hyponatraemia which may aggravate the symptoms. Drugs that are contraindicated in porphyria include barbiturates, sulphonamides, oestrogens, oral contraceptives, chloroquine, griseofulvin, methyl dopa and dichloralphenazone (Welldorm).

CAUSE OF DISEASE IN INBORN ERRORS OF METABOLISM

1. Diseases resulting from the deficiency of a specific enzyme. These may be due to:

(i) The failure to form the products of the reaction which it normally catalyses.

e.g. (a) familial goitre.
(b) congenital adrenal hyperplasia.
(c) albinism.

(ii) The accumulation of the precursor of the blocked reaction.

e.g. (a) phenylketonuria.
(b) galactosaemia.
(c) glycogen storage disease.
(d) alkaptonuria.
(e) oxaluria.
(f) hyperbilirubinaemia.
(g) Gaucher's disease.
(h) Niemann-Pick disease.

(iii) Impaired transport of substances across the renal tubule. The absence of such enzymes concerned with renal tubular transport mechanisms may lead to:

e.g. (a) renal glycosuria.
(b) renal tubular acidosis.
(c) Fanconi syndrome.
(d) vitamin D resistant rickets.
(e) cystinuria.
(f) nephrogenic diabetes insipidus.

2. Impaired formation of a plasma protein which is not an enzyme.

   e.g. (a) hypogammaglobulinaemia.
   (b) afibrinogenaemia.
   (c) hepatolenticular degeneration.
   (d) haemophilia.
   (e) Christmas disease.

3. Formation of an abnormal protein which is not an enzyme.

   e.g. (a) sickle cell disease.
   (b) thalassaemia.

The result for the patient will depend on the nature and significance of the biochemical reaction involved, and whether the substances concerned can be derived from other sources. In many cases the accumulation of the substrate is of little importance because it can be metabolized through other pathways. Even the formation of the end-product may not be vital as it may itself be obtainable from the diet. Hence, in phenylketonuria the failure to form tyrosine is of little importance as this can be obtained from the diet, and the disease results from the accumulation of phenylalanine. Phenylalanine cannot be metabolized through other pathways so that it accumulates in the blood and poisons the brain. Occasionally the accumulating substrate has no toxic effect but because it is relatively insoluble it tends to precipitate in the urinary tract giving rise to calculi. This is the situation in xanthinuria or oxaluria. Sometimes the accumulating substrate is harmless, such as in pentosuria. In alkaptonuria the accumulating substrate is relatively harmless, though by its deposition in cartilage it gives the ears a black colour and predisposes to degenerative disease of joints. In galactosaemia, where the enzyme converting galactose phosphate to glucose phosphate is deficient, the disease is primarily due to the intracellular accumulation of galactose phosphate although a deficiency of circulating glucose predisposes to hypoglycaemia.

Failure to form the end product results in such conditions as goitrous cretinism (familial goitre) where one of the enzymes required for the synthesis of thyroxine is lacking. Similarly in congenital adrenal hyperplasia one of the enzymes concerned with the synthesis of hydrocortisone is affected so that not only is there a deficiency of hydrocortisone but, as the result of stimulation of the adrenal cortex by pituitary ACTH precursor substances, which are androgenic, accumulate and cause the virilization characteristic of the disease.

Enzymes also act as carriers in renal tubular transport. Every membrane is in a sense a diffusion barrier and certain substances can only enter a cell under enzyme control. If the enzyme concerned with the transport of cystine or sugar across the renal tubule is deficient cystinuria or renal glycosuria will result.

Thus, these inherited metabolic diseases may be considered under the errors of metabolism or deviations of metabolism and Diagram 2 diagrammatically represents these disorders. Deviations of metabolism are the result of a renal leak. The presence of amino-aciduria or glycosuria may either be the result of an overflow through the kidney due to high plasma levels or may be 'renal' due to some defect in renal tubular reabsorption. Such defects in renal tubular transport may be the result of renal disease as well as a consequence of deviations of metabolism.

Diagram 2

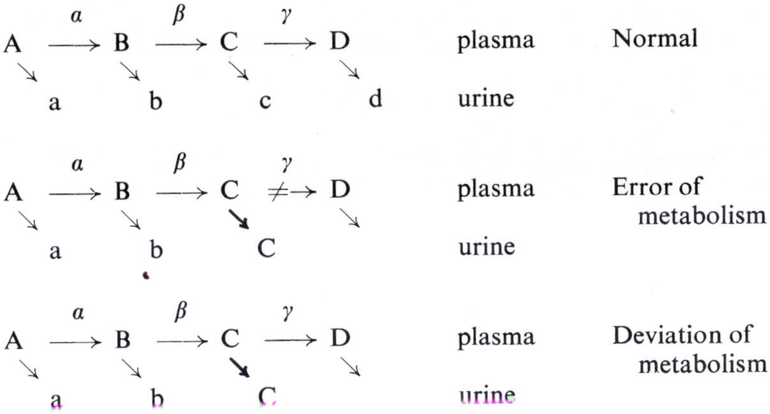

→ = enzyme
↘ = excretion route.

Some of the inborn errors of metabolism are benign conditions and both pentosuria and fructosuria are without symptoms and harmless. Others are more serious such as phenylketonuria but are amenable to treatment. A few are rapidly fatal and the best example is Maple syrup disease in which a severe neurological disturbance and mental retardation are associated with the accumulation in the blood of the amino acids valine, leucine and isoleucine. The numbers of inborn errors of metabolism now known are very numerous. The rapid increase in knowledge is largely due to the introduction of chemical methods for detecting small quantities of urinary constituents. Sir Archibald Garrod, who originally described inborn errors of metabolism, required gramme quantities of metabolities in the urine before chemical analysis could be performed. Thirty years later micro-methods were introduced and then milligramme quantities could be detected. More recently, with the introduction of chromatography microgramme quantities of urinary constituents can be detected.

CLASSIFICATION

The biochemical investigations are of paramount importance in demonstrating the common defect and classifying the various disorders as the clinical picture in any one disease may be variable. Patients with inherited renal tubular acidosis for example may present with either renal stones, osteomalacia or even periodic paralysis secondary to potassium depletion. The following classification of inherited metabolic disorders is generally accepted:

1. Disorders of carbohydrate metabolism.

   (a) *diabetes mellitus.*
   (b) *pentosuria.*
   (c) *fructosuria.*
   (d) *glycogen storage diseases.*
   (e) *galactosaemia.*
   (f) *hyperbilirubinaemia.*

2. Disorders of amino acid metabolism.

   (a) *Familial goitre.*
   (b) *Phenylketonuria.*
   (c) *Alkaptonuria.*
   (d) *Albinism.*
   (e) *Primary hyperoxaluria and oxalosis.*
   (f) Maple syrup urine disease.
   (g) Tyrosinosis.

3. Abnormal lipid metabolism (lipoidoses).

   (a) *Essential familial hyperlipidaemia and* hypercholesterolaemia.
   (b) *Infantile amaurotic familial idiocy.* (Tay Sach's disease).
   (c) *Niemann-Pick disease* (sphingomyelinosis).
   (d) *Gaucher's disease* (cerebrosidosis).

4. Disorders of steroid metabolism.
    (a) *Congenital adrenal hyperplasia.*

5. Disorders of purine and pyrimidine metabolism.
    (a) *Gout.*
    (b) Xanthinuria.

6. Abnormalities in metal or electrolyte metabolism
    (a) *Wilson's disease* (hepatolenticular degeneration).
    (b) *Haemochromatosis.*
    (c) *Periodic paralysis.*
    (d) Pseudo-hypoparathyroidism.

7. Diseases of porphyrin metabolism.
    (a) *The porphyrias.*

8. Disorders of mucopolysaccharide metabolism.
    (a) Gargoylism.

9. Diseases manifest primarily in the blood and blood-forming tissues.
    (a) *Hereditary spherocytosis.*
    (b) *Drug induced haemolytic anaemia* (glucose phosphate dehydrogenase deficiency).
    (c) *Haemoglobinopathies* and *thalassaemia.*
    (d) *Defects in blood coagulation*
        (i) Haemophilia,
        (ii) Christmas disease,
        (iii) Afibrinogenaemia,
        (iv) Von Willebrand's disease.

10. Diseases manifest primarily in the renal tubule.
    (a) *Fanconi syndrome* (osteomalacia, renal glycosuria aminoaciduria and hyperphosphaturia).
    (b) *Renal glycosuria.*
    (c) *Renal tubular acidosis.*
    (d) Nephrogenic diabetes insipidus.
    (e) Vitamin D resistant rickets (familial hypophosphataemia).
    (f) Cystinuria.
    (g) Hartnup disease.

11. Diseases involving a deficiency of circulating enzymes or plasma proteins.
    (a) *Hypogammaglobulinaemia.*
    (b) Analbuminaemia.
    (c) Acatalasia.

TREATMENT OF INBORN ERRORS OF METABOLISM

Treatment of these disorders will obviously depend on whether the accumulation of the substrate or the deficiency of the metabolite is responsible for the disease but the main lines of therapy will include:

1. *Limiting the intake of the substrate.* Hence the successful treatment of phenylketonuria depends on a diet low in phenylalanine, and that of galactosaemia on the exclusion of galactose. Low purine diets used to be advised for the treatment of gout but these have been abandoned since the advent of uricosuric agents which promote the increased excretion of uric acid and xanthine oxidase inhibitors which restrain the final oxidation in its synthesis.
2. *Supplying the missing metabolite.* Treatment of familial goitrous cretins and of congenital adrenal hyperplasia is straightforward. Thyroxine and cortisone respectively should be administered in physiological amounts.
3. *Avoiding precipitating factors where these are relevant.* In patients with cholinesterase deficiency, the muscle relaxant drugs used in anaesthesia should be avoided. In porphyria barbiturates and sulphonamides are contra-indicated, as these drugs both precipitate and aggravate the disease.
4. *Increasing elimination of stored substances.* In hepatolenticular-degeneration (Wilson's disease) copper excretion can be enhanced by chelating agents such as penicillamine, versene and B.A.L. In haemochromatosis venesection and the administration of the chelating agent desferrioxamine will enhance the excretion of iron. Probenecid and other uricosuric agents will increase uric acid excretion in gout.

Many of the inborn errors of metabolism are rare and of little importance. They will not therefore all be discussed but a few will be considered because they illustrate physiological facts which help in the understanding of a wider variety of diseases or because they illustrate new concepts in the understanding of the pathogenesis of old diseases.

LIPOIDOSES

Traditionally the lipoidoses have been regarded as reticuloses. In that the reticuloses include a 'group of diseases of reticulum in which proliferation is followed by differentiation into one or several of the possible cell progeny', such a label is not incorrect. However, it is misleading in that the primary defect may be wrongly assumed to be a malignant proliferative disorder akin to Hodgkin's disease or reticulum cell sarcoma. In hypercholesterolaemic xanthomatosis the histiocytic proliferation is clearly secondary to the extra-cellular perversion of metabolism and in Gaucher's and Niemann-Pick's disease the disorder is one of intracellular lipid metabolism and the infiltration of the bone marrow and other tissues with cells laden with lipoid material is secondary to the inborn error of lipid metabolism.

The inborn errors of lipid metabolism can be subdivided into two groups.

1. Those in which the excess lipid is in the blood.
2. Those in which the excess lipid is in the cells (intra-cellular).

Group 1 includes essential familial hyperlipaemia and essential familial hypercholesterolaemia and group 2 includes Gaucher's disease, Niemann-Pick's disease and amaurotic familial idiocy. The precise biochemical defect in these conditions remains uncertain.

RENAL TUBULAR TRANSPORT DEFECTS

In this group of diseases the defect is due to a failure of tubular absorption and not to any defect in intermediate metabolism. In renal glycosuria the disorder is one of reduced capacity of the renal tubule to reabsorb glucose and is not due to any defect in carbohydrate metabolism resulting in filtration through the glomerulus of increased quantities of glucose. Similarly in cystinuria the increased cystine (and other amino acids) is due to a reduced ability to absorb them across the renal tubule and not to any disturbance in the metabolic breakdown of cystine. Transport of metabolites across the renal tubular cells is an active process, which is dependent on enzymes, and if there is an inborn deficiency of one of these enzymes defects in renal tubular transport mechanisms will result. One enzyme may be responsible for the reabsorption of several substances, particularly when these are amino acids. Amino acids appear in normal urine but only in minute quantities and glycine is the main amino acid present. By methods of urine chromatography about seven amino acids can be seen in the normal chromatograph.

Different people have slightly different patterns of amino acid excretion (just as they have different finger prints) although the plasma levels are the same. Because amino acids are common breakdown products of individual proteins one enzyme may be responsible for the absorption of several amino acids, and if this enzyme is deficient multiple aminoaciduria will result. Examples of the renal tubular transport defects include:

1. *Renal glycosuria.* This is the result of the excretion of glucose in the urine at normal concentrations of blood glucose. It is not associated with any clinical abnormality and is inherited as a Mendelian dominant characteristic.

2. *Renal tubular acidosis.* This results from a defect of acidification of the urine despite the presence of systemic acidosis and is due to an inability of the renal tubule to excrete hydrogen ions. As a result blood acidosis develops but the urine remains alkaline as hydrogen ions cannot be secreted adequately. In their place other cations, in particular calcium and potassium, are lost and this may result in osteomalacia or nephrocalcinosis with the former and hypokalaemia with the latter. A similar inability to secrete hydrogen ions in the presence of systemic acidosis may occur in acquired disease such as pyelonephritis or, of course, during administration of carbonic anhydrase inhibitors such as acetazolamide (Diamox).

3. *Cystinuria.* Four amino acids, cystine, lysine, arginine and ornithine are excreted in excess in this condition. The only amino acid of clinical importance here is cystine as it is insoluble and leads to stone formation.

4. *The Fanconi syndrome.* This comprises renal glycosuria, acidosis, hyperphosphaturia and amino-aciduria and so is a combination of 1, 2, 6 and amino-aciduria. The loss of amino acids does not in itself cause symptoms, but cystine being insoluble, may precipitate and cause renal stones.

5. *Nephrogenic diabetes insipidus.* Here the renal tubule is insensitive to the action of vasopressin so that diabetes insipidus results despite the presence of a normal hypothalamic-hypophyseal system. This condition is a sex-linked recessive characteristic. The women who carry the disease can usually be identified as their water concentrating capacity is reduced.

6. *Vitamin D resistant rickets or familial hypophosphataemia.* This results from a deficiency in the reabsorption of inorganic

phosphate from the renal tubule and is inherited as a sex-linked dominant characteristic. This defect may occur alone or it may be associated with multiple deficiencies in tubular reabsorption such as occur in the Fanconi syndrome. The osteomalacia that results does not respond to the usual therapeutic doses of vitamin D but can be corrected by massive doses. It is also possible to produce improvement by the oral administration of large amounts of phosphate.

7. *Hartnup disease.* In this disease a pellagra-like rash occurs due to an inability to convert tryptophane to nicotinic acid. These patients are usually asymptomatic until exposed to the sun when they develop a typical skin rash. The massive amino-aciduria characteristic of the disease is renal in origin but is not responsible for the symptoms.

CONGENITAL ADRENAL HYPERPLASIA

This disease is a result of inherited inborn defects in the hydroxylating enzymes of the adrenal gland which normally convert progesterone into hydrocortisone, corticosterone and aldosterone. The defects, of which there are several, result in the accumulation of androgenic precursors which cause virilization, accelerated growth and epiphyseal ossification. As the secretion of the adrenal androgens is controlled by ACTH the enhanced pituitary stimulation, which arises because of the low serum levels of hydrocortisone, further increases androgen production. Two hydroxylations are involved in the synthesis of hydrocortisone from 17-hydroxyprogesterone and each requires a specific enzyme. The more important varieties of congenital hyperplasia result from defects of the 21-hydroxylase and 11-hydroxylase enzymes (Fig. 1). A third less common type has been described in which a block occurs preventing the formation of progesterone.

If there is a partial block of the 21 hydroxylase system the plasma hydrocortisone level may be maintained by the increased secretion of ACTH. However, despite the increase in ACTH the hydrocortisone level may be below normal and children with this defect are unlikely to be able to survive stress. They are also liable to salt loss as there is in addition an abnormality in the synthesis of aldosterone. Lack of the enzyme 11-hydroxylase stops synthesis of hydrocortisone at the stage of compound S and also prevents the formation of corticosterone from 11-deoxycorticosterone. The accumulation of deoxycorticosterone leads to hypertension and the inability to form hydrocortisone to adrenal insufficiency.

Progressive virilization is the most conspicuous manifestation of this disease and is due to the excessive production of androgens. The rapid growth, increased musculature and accelerated epiphyseal

Progesterone —(hydroxylation at C.17)→ 17-hydroxyprogesterone —(hydroxylation at C.21)→

11-Deoxyhydrocortisone (compound S) —(hydroxylation at C.11)→ Hydrocortisone

FIG. 1 The hydroxylation of progesterone to cortisol

growth are due to the protein anabolic action of the androgen. In the female virilization of the external genitalia takes place and the infant is readily mistaken for a male with undescended testes.

HAEMOGLOBINOPATHIES

Haemoglobin is a pigment composed of an iron protoporphyrin complex combined with a protein globin. It is the globin portion which varies in the different types of haemoglobin. Impairment of adult haemoglobin formation is the characteristic abnormality of the haemoglobinopathies, which are hereditary haemolytic anaemias, genetically determined and related to race. The haemoglobin may be abnormal because: (1) there is a defect in the synthesis of normal adult haemoglobin and this occurs in thalassaemia when there may be an absence of one or both of the polypeptide chains characteristic of normal adult haemoglobin, or (2) an abnormal form of haemoglobin such as haemoglobin S (that of sickle cell disease) is formed instead of adult haemoglobin. This abnormality may involve as little as one amino acid of the 300 in the haemoglobin molecule. In sickle cell haemoglobin one single amino acid molecule (that of glutamic acid) is replaced by another (valine) and this results in such a deficient end product that the ensuing disease is rapidly fatal. In haemoglobin C one single amino acid, again that of glutamic acid, is replaced by another, this time lysine.

Haemoglobin A is the normal pigment of adults and consists of two fractions. A1 is the major part comprising 98 per cent and A2 the minor part comprising the remaining 2 per cent. At birth foetal haemoglobin (haemoglobin F) predominates and 80 per cent of the haemoglobin of the foetus is haemoglobin F. It usually disappears in the first six months of life unless the child suffers from some chronic anaemia, in which case it may persist. Each haemoglobin is under independent genetic control and the globin fraction is made up of a series of polypeptide chains. The complete amino acid sequence of four of these chains is known and the four chains are called alpha, beta, gamma and delta. Haemoglobin A molecule is composed of two alpha and two beta chains and is therefore labelled $\alpha_2\beta_2$, that of haemoglobin A2 is composed of two alpha and two delta chains and is therefore called $\alpha_2\delta_2$, and haemoglobin F comprises two alpha and two gamma chains, $\alpha_2\gamma_2$. The haemoglobin of normal individuals is thus under the control of four genes each responsible for the synthesis of one of the four polypeptide chains. If the gene concerned with the production of alpha polypeptide chains is abnormal there will be defective production of haemoglobin A, A2 and F because they all contain alpha chains and this is the situation in alpha thalassaemia. In the fatal hydrops foetalis of homozygous alpha thalassaemia the foetus is unable to produce the alpha chains to link up with the gamma chains it can produce, and so form foetal haemoglobin. Instead the free gamma chains form a tetramer called Haemoglobin Barts. This haemoglobin is useless because it lacks the ability to surrender oxygen at low oxygen tensions. Hence the infant dies of anoxia with mild anaemia. In beta thalassaemia it is the gene controlling production of beta chains that is abnormal and hence although haemoglobin A cannot be formed haemoglobin A2 and haemoglobin F production will not be impaired and hence these haemoglobins will exist in increased proportion.

In sickle cell disease the defect is in the constitution of one of the polypeptide chains. Haemoglobin S of sickle cell anaemia differs from normal adult haemoglobin by the substitution of one amino acid for another in a certain position of the beta chain. Although more than 30 differing forms of haemoglobin have been described, in each the abnormality is due to a single aminoacid substitution in the beta polypeptide chain. Some of these substitutions result in a marked functional abnormality of the haemoglobin, some make the pigment unstable without affecting its activity so that it is destroyed too rapidly, whilst others seem to produce little abnormality at all. Haemoglobinopathy resulting from the inheritance of the abnormal haemoglobins C, D, E are examples of the non-thalassaemic, non-sickling diseases. Haemoglobin Hammersmith, Genoa, Köhn and New York are more recently discovered variants. The large number of structural variants of the haemoglobin molecule has raised the possibility of similar variations occurring in other body proteins. In other haemoglobinopathies the polypeptide chain may be of normal amino acid constitution but present in an abnormal arrangement. For example, haemoglobin H is composed of 4 beta chains.

The haemoglobinopathies have characteristic racial distributions. The sickle cell trait is common among the Negro population in Africa and the U.S.A. It is inherited as a simple Mendelian dominant. Sixty per cent of the haemoglobin is normal and 40 per cent is haemoglobin S. The gene for haemoglobin S produces the trait when present on one of the pair of chromosomes and causes sickle cell anaemia when present on both chromosomes. The trait has a frequency of 20 per cent in several East Africa populations and 4 per cent of new-born children will be homozygous and die of sickle cell anaemia in infancy. Sickling can be demonstrated if the blood is examined under reduced oxygen tension both in patients with the trait and those with the complete disease. The sickling is due to the physical state of the haemoglobin in the erythrocytes.

In thalassaemia or Cooley's anaemia there is no abnormal haemoglobin but there is impaired synthesis of adult haemoglobin. The failure in synthesis may effect the alpha or the beta chain of the haemoglobin molecule but any alpha or beta peptide that is synthesized is normal in composition. This is probably a defect in the controller gene (p. 2) which regulates the rate of peptide synthesis. The heterozygous state is benign but when there is a double dose of the gene a severe hypochromic microcytic anaemia results which is associated with early death. It is found commonly in the population around the Mediterranean. Combinations of thalassaemia and sickle cell anaemia exist, part of the haemoglobin of such patients being haemoglobin S, and this condition is less severe than that caused by a double dose of the gene for haemoglobin S which occurs in sickle cell anaemia.

Heterozygous states with haemoglobin C, D and E also exist and the disorders are known as sickle cell haemoglobin C disease, sickle cell haemoglobin D disease and sickle cell haemoglobin E disease.

Selected Bibliography

HARRIS, H. (1959) *Human Biochemical Genetics.* Cambridge University Press.

HARRIS, H. (1970) Genetical Theory and the Inborn Errors of Metabolism. *Brit. Med. J.* 1, 321.

STANBURY, J. B., WYNGAARDEN, J. B. and FREDRICKSON, D. S. (1972) *Metabolic Basis of Inherited Disease.* 3rd Ed. McGraw-Hill, New York.

II

Chromosome Abnormalities and Disease

INTRODUCTION

A human being originates in the union of two gametes, the ovum and the sperm. These two cells contain all that the new individual can inherit from his parents. The hereditary elements or genes are carried on the chromosomes, which are present in the cell nucleus. Man has 46 chromosomes, comprising two sex chromosomes and 44 autosomes. The autosomes, which are the somatic or non-sex chromosomes, can be matched according to their size and shape and arranged in 22 homologous pairs. (PLATE 1.) In the female the pair of sex chromosomes are equal in size and are called XX. In the male the pair are unequal and are called XY. Every somatic cell of the male contains 44 autosomes and one X and one Y chromosome and every somatic cell of the female contains 44 autosomes and two X chromosomes. The hereditary elements themselves are the genes and are arranged in a linear manner along the length of the chromosomes. The chromosomes are long filaments, which during division become coiled and interwoven like spiral springs. Genes are responsible for the protein synthesis of the cell. They instruct the cell how to make a particular polypeptide chain for a particular protein.

Genes carry in coded form the detailed specifications for the thousands of kinds of protein molecules the cell requires for its existence, for its enzymes, for its repair work and for its reproduction. These proteins are synthesised from the twenty natural aminoacids, which are uniform throughout nature, and which exist in the cell cytoplasm as part of the metabolic pool. The protein molecule consists of aminoacids joined end to end to form long polypeptide chains. An average chain contains 100 to 300 aminoacids. The sequence of bases in the nucleic acid chain of the gene corresponds in some fundamental way to the sequence of amino-acids in the protein molecule, and hence it determines the structure of the particular protein. This is the genetic code. Deoxyribonucleic acid (DNA) is the bearer of this genetic information.

DNA has a long backbone made up of repeating groups of phosphate and the sugar deoxyribose. To this backbone four bases are attached as side groups at regular intervals. These four bases are the four letters used to spell out the genetic message. They are adenine, thymine, guanine and cystosine (A, T, G and C in Figure 2). The molecule of DNA is made up of two chains coiled round a common axis to form what is called a double helix. The two chains are held together by hydrogen bonds between pairs of bases. Since adenine only pairs with thymine and guanine only with cystosine, the sequences of bases in one chain fixes the sequence in the other. Several hundred bases would be contained in the length of DNA of a typical gene. If the message of the DNA base sequence is a continuous succession of thymine, the ribosome will link together a series of the aminoacid phenylalanine. If the base sequence is a succession of cystosine the ribosome will link up a series of prolines. Thus each aminoacid has its own particular code of bases. In fact each aminoacid is coded by a word consisting of three adjacent bases. In addition to carrying genetic information, DNA is able to synthesise or replicate itself and so pass this information on to daughter cells.

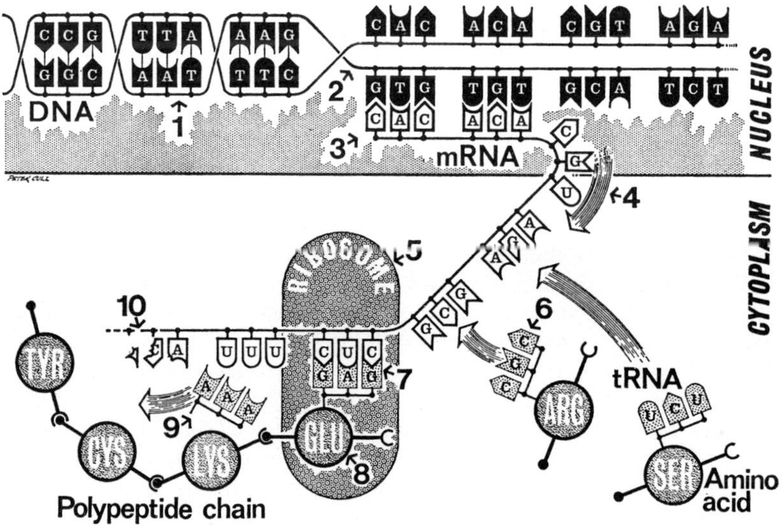

FIG. 2 The transfer of genetic information

Legend of Figure 2

1. Double chain of DNA lies in nucleus.
2. DNA uncoils in preparation for activity as a template of the code.
3. Messenger (m) RNA forms the coded template of the single chain of DNA.
4. m–RNA, carrying the code, moves out into the cell cytoplasm.
5. Ribosome moves along the chain of m–RNA.
6. Transfer (t) RNA carries its individual aminoacid to the correct position in the chain of m–RNA.
7. t–RNA has locked into position on the chain of m–RNA which is lying on the ribosome.
8. The aminoacid is carried by t–RNA and linked into its proper position in the developing polypeptide chain.
9. t–RNA having deposited its aminoacid moves off.
10. The short-lived m–RNA disperses.

All DNA is part of the chromosome and so it remains confined to the nucleus. Proteins are synthesised by the ribosomes which are in the cytoplasm. DNA achieves control over protein production in the cytoplasm by directing the synthesis of ribonucleic acid (RNA). Most of the DNA in a cell is inactive, otherwise the cell would synthesise simultaneously every protein that the individual was capable of forming. When part of the DNA structure becomes 'active' it acts as a template for the ribonucleic acid (RNA) which itself acts as a template for protein synthesis *when* it becomes attached to the ribosome (Fig. 2). Ribonucleic acid exists in three forms. First 'messenger RNA' carries the necessary 'message' for the synthesis of a specific protein, from the nucleus to the ribosomes. Secondly, 'transfer RNA' collects the individual aminoacids, which exist in the cytoplasm as part of the metabolic pool, and carries them to the ribosome. Thirdly, there is RNA in the ribosome itself.

RNA has a similar structure to DNA, but the sugar is ribose instead of deoxyribose, and uracil replaces the base thymine. Before the ribosome can produce the proteins, the aminoacids must be lined up in their correct sequence on the messenger RNA template. This alignment is carried out by transfer RNA, of which there is a specific form for each individual aminoacid. Transfer RNA can not only recognize its specific aminoacid but also identify the position it is required to occupy on the messenger RNA template. This is because each transfer RNA has its own sequence of bases and recognizes its site on the messenger RNA by pairing bases with it

(Fig. 2). The ribosome then travels along the chain of messenger RNA and links the aminoacids, which have thus been arranged in the requisite order, by peptide bonds and the protein is released.

Proteins are important for two main reasons. Firstly, all the enzymes of living cells are made of protein. One gene is responsible for one enzyme. Genes thus control all the biochemical processes of the body and are responsible for the inborn difference between human beings. Secondly, proteins also fulfil a structural role in the cell so that genes controlling the synthesis of structural proteins are responsible for morphological differences between human beings.

During ordinary somatic or mitotic division each chromosome divides longitudinally, duplicating itself with an exact copy of all the genes it bears. When the cell divides each double chromosome separates, one half passing to each of the two daughter cells, so that the two daughter cells contain exact replicas of the 23 pairs of chromosomes of the mother cell. In the formation of the gametes (ovum and sperm) a special kind of cell division takes place, called meiosis or reduction division, in which two divisions of the nucleus occur and only one division of the chromosomes so that the number of chromosomes in the gametes is half that of the somatic cells. The gamete thus receives only one member of each pair of chromosomes from the parent cell.

It was not until 1956 that the number of chromosomes in the human cell was established as 46. The morphology of the human chromosomes has only been appreciated since the discovery that colchicine has the property of stopping mitosis at the stage of the metaphase, when the chromosomes assume their most visible form. Tissue culture provides a source of dividing cells, whose mitoses may be arrested by colchicine. The cells used are white blood cells which are incubated in their plasma with an added synthetic culture medium. There is as yet no known way of producing meiosis artificially. Chromosomes can be seen quite clearly under a microscope and arranged in order of decreasing size. Variations in size, the position of the centromere and specific characteristics of shape enable the 22 pairs of autosomes to be identified and numbered from 1–22. The paired sex chromosomes are of equal length in the female (XX) but of unequal length in the male (XY). The longest chromosome is 7–8 microns in length and the shortest about 1·5 microns.

In 1949 it was discovered that cells of females had a nucleolar satellite, which stains readily with certain dyes, whereas no such body could be detected in the cells from males. This is because the two X chromosomes in the female contain more chromatin than the XY pair in the male and are therefore more visible when stained. It is believed that one X chromosome remains condensed and physiologically inactive when the cell is not dividing and this forms the sex chromatin characteristic of female cell nuclei. The sex chromatin is not a complete index of sexual genetic make-up. All that can be inferred is whether an individual does or does not carry two X chromosomes. It does not indicate whether the normal Y chromosome is present. This sex chromatin body can be identified in 30 to 60 per cent of cells in the female. Buccal smears and biopsies of skin are the most favoured sources of cells as these have an open nucleus, though polymorphonuclear granulocytes can also be used. As the chromatin body (or drumstick of the polymorph) is formed from part of the X chromosome of the female cell it is not present in cells, which carry only one X chromosome, such as those of normal males or patients with Turner's syndrome (XO). If a cell carries three X chromosomes two chromatin bodies will be visible in the cells.

Recently it has become possible to identify the Y chromosome. The anti-malarial drug quinacrine has been shown to be extremely useful for staining chromosomes with a fluorescence that is clearly visible through an ultraviolet microscope. The Y chromosome fluoresces intensely and this fluorescence is even visible in non-dividing (interphase) cells. Quinacrine is thus a reliable way of sexing human cells whether they are resting or dividing.

CHROMOSOME ABNORMALITIES

Chromosome abnormalities may consist of alterations in the number of chromosomes or structural abnormalities of the chromosome itself. Alterations in the number can be accurately detected but structural abnormalities must be gross before they can be recognized by present microscopic methods. It may be possible to recognize a loss of half a micron in certain chromosomes although larger losses may not be detectable in others. The amount of genetic material involved is enormous for it has been estimated that 100,000 genes are carried on each chromosome. There is thus no chance of recognizing the gene mutations responsible for the inborn errors of metabolism considered in Chapter 1 for these could involve the misplacement of only a single base in the deoxyribonucleic acid (DNA) chain of the gene. The astonishing fact is that the loss of genetic material involved in the recognizable structural abnormalities of chromosomes is compatible with life at all.

Most chromosome abnormalities are too large to permit survival of the bearer or too small to be identified and for this reason few diseases secondary to abnormalities of chromosomes are recognized. This is particularly true of the autosomes. Abnormalities of the sex chromosomes are better tolerated and a few of these are compatible with normal survival. This is probably because the sex chromosomes contain relatively little genetic material for their size. It has been mentioned that in the female only one of the X chromosomes is physiologically active when the cell is not dividing and that the inactive 'X' chromosome condenses to form the nucleolar satellite, characteristic of the sex chromatin of the female. In some cell lines the active X chromosome will be maternal in origin and in others it will be paternal. This is the so-called X-chromosome inactivation hypothesis or Lyon hypothesis and it helps to account for the relatively slight differences between male and females, when one considers the enormous differences that result from the additional nuclear material arising from an extra autosome. The inactivation of the X-chromosome is a random phenomenon except when it is abnormal, in which case the anomalous chromosome usually forms the sex chromatin. The formation of the gonads is under the control of genes located on the sex chromosomes. A double dose of some genes on the X chromosomes is required to initiate feminization, whilst the genes on the Y chromosome, in the presence of a single X chromosome, initiate the development of the male gonad. The gonads once formed control further differentiation.

CELL DIVISION

The chromosome anomalies arise because of abnormalities of cell division. It is therefore necessary to understand the normal processes involved in mitosis and meiosis before these anomalies can be appreciated.

Mitosis

This is the process of cell division for somatic cells and for the ovum after fertilization. Each chromosome becomes doubled by splitting lengthwise and forming two chromatids, which remain held together by the centromere. These chromatids are exact copies of the original chromsomes and contain duplicates of all the genes they bear. When cell division takes place the pull of the spindle splits the centromere and each doubled chromatid separates, one passing to one pole of the nucleus and the other to the opposite pole. The nucleus and the cell itself then also divide forming two new daughter cells, containing precisely the same 23 pairs of chromosomes and carrying exactly the same complement of genes as did the mother cell. In this form of cell division the chromatids are held together only for a short time by the centromere and the position of the centromere is constant for any given chromosome.

Meiosis

Meiosis or reduction division is the form of cell division that only occurs in the gonads, that is the testis and ovary, to give rise to the germ cells (the sperms and ova). Two types of sperm cells are produced: the one contains 22 autosomes and a Y sex chromosome and the other contains 22 autosomes and an X sex chromosome. All the ova, however, produced by normal meiosis have 22 autosomes and an X sex chromosome. Two divisions of the nucleus occur and only one division of the chromosomes so

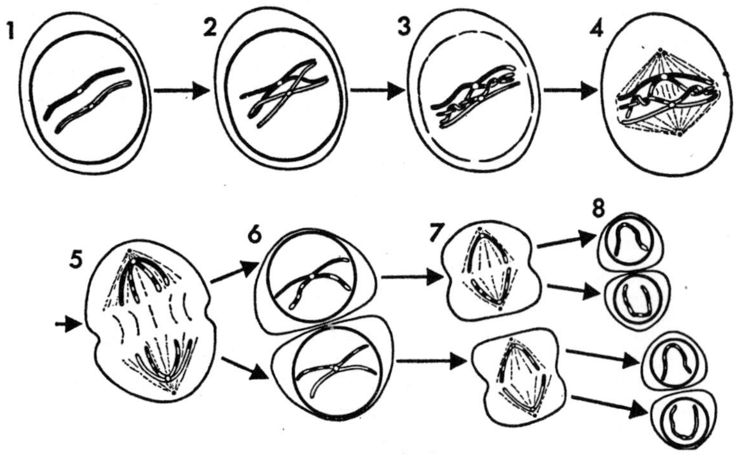

FIG. 3 Meiosis

that the number of chromosomes in the ova and sperms is half that of somatic cells. Each chromosome pair divides so that the gamete receives only one member of each pair. The number of chromosomes is restored to full complement at fertilization so that the zygote has a complete set, each chromosome from the nucleus of the sperm pairing up with its corresponding partner from the ovum. The first stage of meiosis involves the pairing of homologous chromosomes which join together and synapse lengthwise. (Fig. 3.) The chromosomes then become doubled by splitting along their length and the chromatids so formed are held together by centromeres. As the homologous chromosomes, one of which has come from the mother and the other from the father, are lying together genetic interchange can take place between the chromatids and in this way new combinations of genes arise. All four chromatids are closely interwoven and re-combination may take place between any maternal and any paternal chromatids. This process is known as crossing over or re-combination. After this period of interchange homologous chromosomes then move apart, one to the one pole and the other to the opposite pole of the nucleus, though the chromatids are held together by chiasmata, which are considered to be the positions where cross-overs have occurred. The cell then divides and the nucleus of each new cell now contains 23 and not 46 chromosomes. The second meiotic division then occurs, the centromeres divide and the chromatids move apart to opposite poles of the nucleus so that there are still 23 chromosomes in each of the daughter nuclei so formed. The cell divides again so that there are 4 gametes, each containing a half number (haploid) set of chromosomes. However, owing to the re-combination or crossing over, the genetic material is not identical with either parent or with other spermatozoa.

INHERITED DISEASES

Dominant genes

A dominant characteristic is an effect which is produced whenever the gene is present. If a disease is due to a dominant gene those affected are heterozygous, that is they only carry the gene on one of the pair of chromosomes concerned. Affected persons married to normal individuals transmit the gene directly to one half of the children. (Fig. 4a.) In the ABO blood group system A and B are dominant over O. Huntington's chorea is due to the inheritance of a dominant gene, as is neurofibromatosis. Another dominantly inherited condition is multiple polyposis of the colon. As the chance of such polyps becoming malignant is great, total colectomy is indicated and it is therefore important to identify these cases early. Haemolytic disease of the newborn, due to Rhesus (Rh) incompatibility, is the commonest genetically determined disease in this country. The Rh antigen is a dominant characteristic which in haemolytic disease of the newborn is inherited from the father. The mother, being Rh negative, may develop antibodies against antigen present on the foetal red cells if they enter the maternal circulation and these antibodies may give rise to the disease in the foetus.

Achondroplasia is an example of a dominant mutation, for the majority of affected persons have normal parents and siblings. However the chances of the children of a patient with achondroplasia being affected are one in two as with any other dominant characteristic. Other diseases inherited as dominant characteristics include, spherocytosis, haemorrhagic telangiectasia and polycystic kidney. Further examples are listed in Table 1.

TABLE 1

Examples of Diseases Transmitted by Dominant Recessive and Sex-linked Recessive Genes

Dominant	*Recessive*	*Sex-linked*
Spherocytosis	Fibrocystic disease of the pancreas	Haemophilia
Achondroplasia	Phenylketonuria	Christmas disease
Huntington's chorea	Alkaptonuria	Duchenne muscular dystrophy
Multiple polyposis of the colon	Congenital adrenal hyperplasia	Glucose phosphate dehydrogenase deficiency
Facioscapulohumeral muscular dystrophy	Albinism	Congenital hypo-gammaglobulinaemia
Haemorrhagic telangiectasia	Galactosaemia	Nephrogenic diabetes insipidus
Polycystic kidney	Glycogen storage diseases	Colour blindness
Dystrophia myotonica	Gargoylism	Vitamin D resistant rickets
Idiopathic diabetes insipidus	Hepatolenticular degeneration	
Elliptocytosis	Sickle cell anaemia	
Osteogenesis imperfecta	Thalassaemia major	
Peroneal muscular atrophy	Retinitis pigmentosa	
	Niemann-Pick disease	
	Friedreich's ataxia	
Periodic paralysis	Cystinuria	
	Cystinosis	

Recessive Genes

If a disease is due to a recessive gene, those affected must have the gene on both members of the chromosome pair (i.e. be homozygous). The possession of a single recessive gene does not result in overt disease and the bearer usually carries this potentially unfavourable gene without knowing. If he marries another carrier of this recessive gene there is a one in four chance that their children will receive the gene in double dose and so have the disease. (Fig. 4b.)

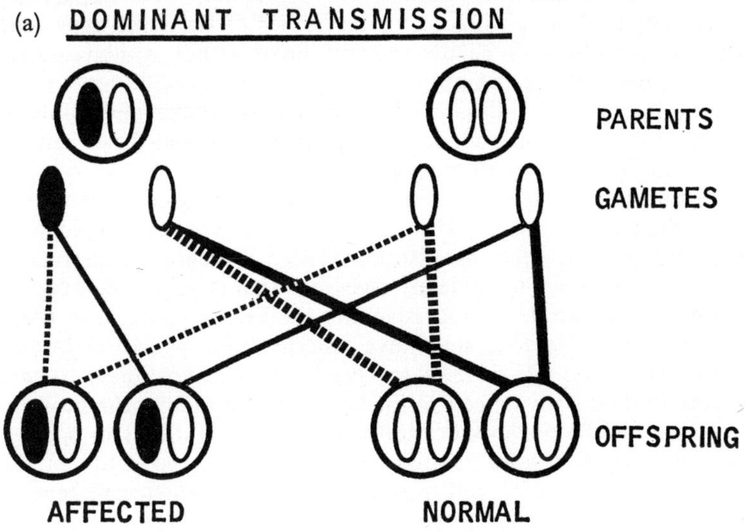

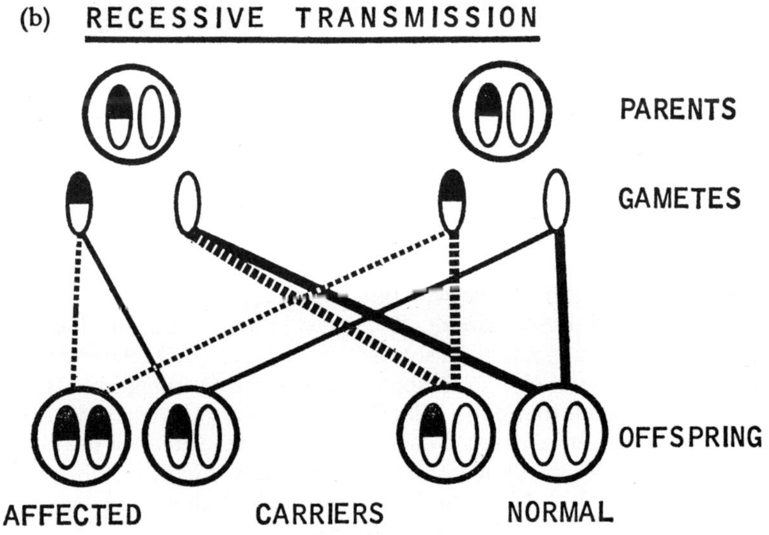

FIG. 4 Inheritance of characteristics
(*a*) dominant (*b*) recessive

If an individual sufferer from a recessive disease marries an apparently normal person, though heterozygous carrier of the same gene, one half of the children will be affected and the other half will be carriers of the disease. The commonest of such recessive conditions in this country is fibrocystic disease of the pancreas, which affects about one child in two thousand. It can be calculated that 5 per cent of the population must carry the gene.

Most of the inborn errors of metabolism, such as phenylketonuria, galactosaemia and congenital adrenal hyperplasia are due to recessive genes. Further examples are listed in Table 1. There are characteristics which may be incompletely recessive, that is neither completely dominant nor completely recessive and the heterozygote, who bears the gene in a single dose, may have a slight defect whilst the homozygote, with a double dose of the gene, has a severe illness. There are certain mild bony defects in the heterozygote such as the shortening of the middle phalanx of the second fingers and toes in brachyphalangia which results in gross deformity of the skeleton in the homozygote. The sickle cell trait is a result of the sickle cell gene in single dose and sickle cell anaemia is the consequence of a double dose. Thalassaemia minor and major demonstrate a similar incompletely recessive characteristic.

Sex-linked genes

If a condition is sex linked affected males are homozygous for the mutated gene as they carry it on their single X chromosome. The X chromosome carries many genes whilst the Y chromosome bears few genes, if any, other than those concerned with determining masculinity. The genes on the X chromosome of the male are thus not matched by corresponding genes on the Y chromosome. There is thus no chance of the Y chromosome neutralizing any recessive trait on the X chromosome. A recessive gene can therefore produce disease since it will not be suppressed by the normal gene of the homologous chromosome. The same recessive gene on the X chromosome of the female will be suppressed by the normal gene on the other X chromosome. Such sex-linked conditions include haemophilia, Christmas disease, the severe form of Duchenne type of muscular dystrophy and nephrogenic diabetes insipidus. (See Table 1.) If the mother of an affected child has another male relative affected she is a heterozygote carrier and half her sons will have the disease and half her daughters will be carriers. (See Fig. 5b.) The sister of a haemophiliac thus has a 50 per cent chance of being a carrier. An affected male cannot transmit the gene to his son because the X chromosome of a son must come from the mother: all his daughters however will be carriers as the X chromosome of the

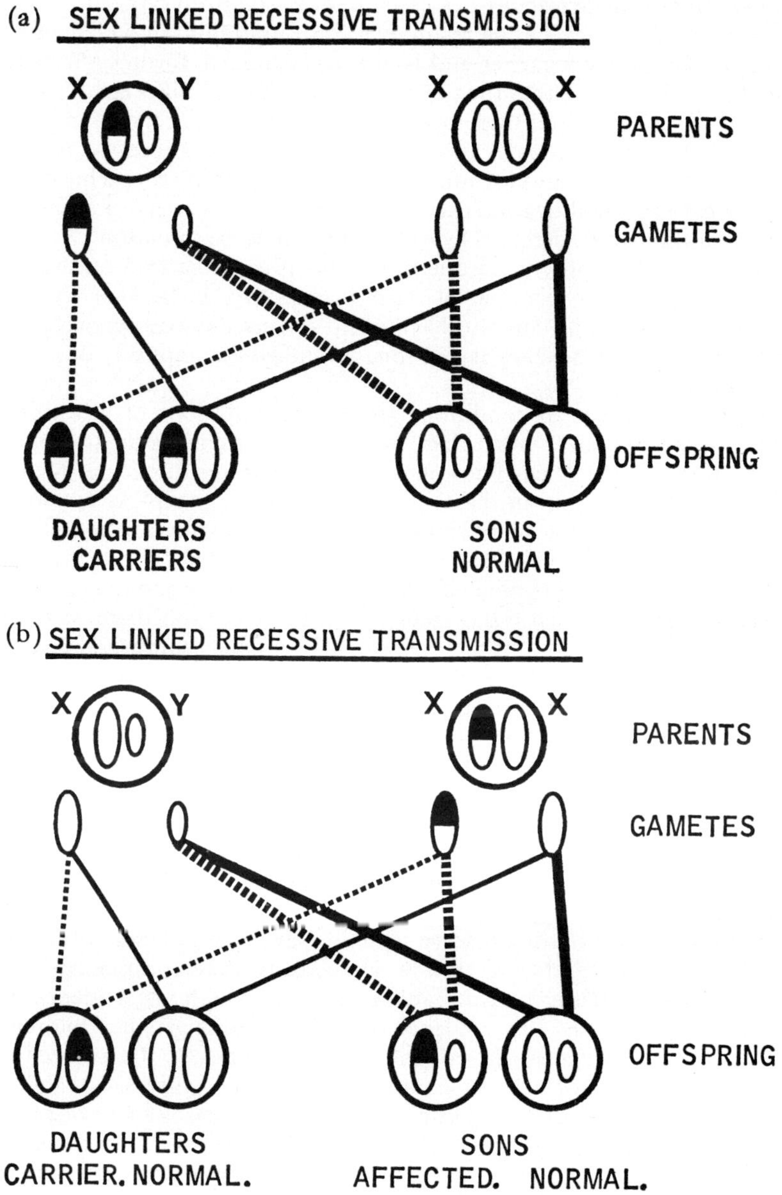

FIG. 5 Inheritance of sex-linked recessive characteristics

father must be transmitted to all his daughters. (Fig. 5a.) Hence sex-linked recessive characteristics cannot be passed from father to son. Sporadic cases may be the result of a fresh mutation, in which case the mother is not a carrier and is not likely to have further affected children. It is probable that one-third of haemophiliacs arise as a result of mutation and these patients will be the first in their families to be affected. Sometimes the carrier of a sex-linked recessive gene can be identified. A proportion of haemophilia carriers reveal haematological abnormalities and carriers of the sex-lined variety of retinitis pigmentosa can be detected by ophthalmoscopic examination.

A few rare disorders are due to dominant genes carried on the X chromosome. An example of such a condition is familial hypophosphataemia with vitamin D resistant rickets. Glucose phosphate dehydrogenase deficiency is due to a sex-linked incompletely dominant gene.

Many hundreds of conditions are due to mutations of genes on the autosomes and more than sixty conditions are due to gene mutations on the X chromosomes. Gene mutations duplicate themselves at cell division in the same way as normal genes. As a result of these mutations a number of alternative forms for a given gene exist and these are called allenes. In many inherited conditions the disease is due to the combined action of several genes and the genetic element is then called multi-factorial. In this situation there will be an increased incidence of the disease in the families concerned but it will not follow the Mendelian ratio. The greater the number of independent genes involved in determining a certain disease, the more complicated will be the pattern of inheritance. Furthermore, many inherited disorders are the result of a combination of genetic and environmental influences. Diabetes mellitus is the most familiar example of such multifactorial inheritance. The predisposition to develop diabetes is an inherited recessive character although the gene is not always able to express itself and this is called incomplete penetrance. Whether or not the individual with the genetic predisposition towards the disease actually develops diabetes will also depend on environmental factors. Diabetes is more common in the relatives of diabetic patients and even more so amongst identical twins. However, as the incidence of diabetes amongst the children of marriages between diabetic patients is well below 100 per cent, the gene does not receive complete functional expression. Non-genetic factors which are of importance in precipitating overt disease are obesity, excessive intake of carbohydrate foods and pregnancy. The influence of diet was made apparent during the two world wars when the mortality rates for diabetes mellitus showed a fall throughout Europe.

Schizophrenia is another example of the combined effects of genetic and environmental influences in precipitating disease. The risk of schizophrenia in a child, one of whose parents has the disease, is one in ten but this figure is modified by the early environment of the child.

The capacity of genes for replication has recently been explained in terms of the structure of the deoxyribonucleic acid (DNA) molecule, which consists of a long double spiral with thousands of mononucleotides, each containing sugar, phosphoric acid and bases. A single change in the base sequence causes a permanent change in genetic information and provides a chemical explanation of mutations. Genes control the production of specific proteins. These proteins are either structural proteins in the cell and thus a definitive product of the gene or they act as enzymes and are thus a link in a biochemical reaction in the body.

CHROMOSOME ABNORMALITIES AS A CAUSE OF DISEASE

As the correct number of human chromosomes was established less than a decade ago it is only recently that chromosome abnormalities have been associated with clinical diseases. Chromosomes may be lost or duplicated or abnormalities in the structure of individual chromosomes may occur. These changes are arbitrarily distinguished from changes at individual gene loci known as mutations, which are not, or ever likely to be, visible. Indeed alterations from the normal in such a complex process as nuclear division are not unexpected. The surprising fact is the infrequency of such errors. About one in 200 liveborn babies has an abnormality of development caused by a chromosome anomaly, and two-thirds of these involve the sex chromosomes. There is little doubt that the frequency of these abnormalities in the early embryo is much higher but because of the serious nature of the defect early spontaneous abortion occurs. Chromosome studies on such early abortions show that one half has chromosome abnormalities with errors of autosomes being three times as common as sex chromosome anomalies. Two of the most common abnormalities in such foetuses are triploidy with 69 chromosomes and trisomy of chromosome 16. These two anomalies almost always cause spontaneous abortion. It has been estimated that 1 in 40 conceptions results in a severe chromosome abnormality.

Abnormalities of chromosome structure may arise because of:

1. *Deletion;* where a segment of a chromosome is lost.
2. *Inversion;* where a segment of a chromosome becomes detached and re-attached the other way round. Genes will then appear

in the wrong order and thus will not correspond with their opposite numbers on homologous chromosomes.

3. *Duplication;* where a segment of a chromosome is included twice over. One chromosome will have too little nuclear material and one too much. The individual inheriting too little may be non-viable and the one with too much may be abnormal.

4. *Translocation;* where chromosomes of different pairs exchange segments.

5. *Errors in division of centromere.* Sometimes the centromere divides transversely instead of longitudinally. If the centromere is not central, one of the daughter chromosomes will arise from the two short arms of the parent chromosome and the other from the two long arms. These abnormal daughter chromosomes are called isochromosomes.

These changes have important bearings on heredity as the effect of a gene depends not only on its nature but on its position on the chromosome with reference to other genes. Genes do not act in isolation but against the background of other genes. Each gene normally has its own position on the chromosome and this corresponds precisely with the position of its allene on the homologous chromosome of the pair. Each member of a pair of chromosomes will normally carry precisely the same number of genes in exactly the same order. Characteristic clinical syndromes, due to abnormalities of chromosome structure, are less constant than those due to the loss or gain of a complete chromosome. This is because the degree of deletion, inversion and duplication is inconstant. However, translocation between chromosomes 15 and 21 of the parent is associated with a familial form of mongolism in the offspring (p.46), and deletion of part of an X chromosome may result in Turner's syndrome (p. 41).

Non-Disjunction

Whilst alternations in the structure of chromosomes arise as a result of deletion or translocation, alterations in the number of chromosomes usually arise as a result of non-disjunction, occurring during maturation of the parental gametes. The two chromosomes of each pair (homologous chromosomes) may fail to come together at the beginning of meiosis and continue to lie free. If one chromosome then passes to each pole of the spindle, normal gametes may result but if both chromosomes pass to one pole and neither to the other, two kinds of abnormal gametes will be produced. One kind of gamete will contain both chromosomes of the pair and the other gamete will contain neither. Whilst this results in serious disease when the autosomes are involved the loss or gain of sex chromosomes seems to be well tolerated. The loss of an autosome is incompatible with life and the amount of malformation produced by a gain of an autosome is proportional to the size of the extra chromosome carried.

Only a few instances of a gain of an autosome are known. An additional chromosome 21 (one of the smallest autosomes) results in mongolism and trisomy of chromosome 13 and 18 are associated with severe mental, skeletal and congenital cardiac defects (p. 46). Diseases resulting from the gain of a sex chromosome are not as severe. A normal ovum contains 22 autosomes and an X sex chromosome. A normal sperm contains 22 autosomes and either an X or a Y sex chromosome. Thus as a result of non-disjunction of the 'X' chromosomes at the first meiotic division during the formation of female gametes the ovum may contain two 'X' chromosomes or none at all, whilst in the male the sperm may contain both X and Y chromosomes (XY) or none at all. (Fig. 6.)

The various permutations and combinations of a normal ovum being fertilized by an abnormal sperm or an abnormal ovum being fertilized by a normal sperm will produce a variety of sex chromosome constitutions of the zygote, namely XXY, XO, XXX and YO. XXY results in the Klinefelter syndrome, XO in Turner's syndrome, XXX in the triple X syndrome (p. 44). An individual with YO constitution has not been described and therefore it is presumably not compatible with life. The X sex chromosome is virtually an autosome because it carries many genes that are not connected with sex development. The Y chromosome bears few genes apart from those concerned with determining masculinity. It is, therefore, not surprising that YO zygotes are not viable. If there is no X chromosome there can be no clotting mechanism as the gene for factor VIII is located there.

TABLE II

Normal ovum	*Abnormal sperm*	*Zygote*	*Disease*
X	XY	XXY	Klinefelter's syndrome
X	O	XO	Turner's syndrome

Abnormal ovum	*Normal sperm*	*Zygote*	*Disease*
XX	X	XXX	Triple X syndrome
XX	Y	XXY	Klinefelter's syndrome
O	X	XO	Turner's syndrome
O	Y	YO	Non-viable

Thus Klinefelter's syndrome (XXY) may arise because the X chromosomes of the developing ovum fail to separate from each other at meiosis and both go to the same end of the spindle. One

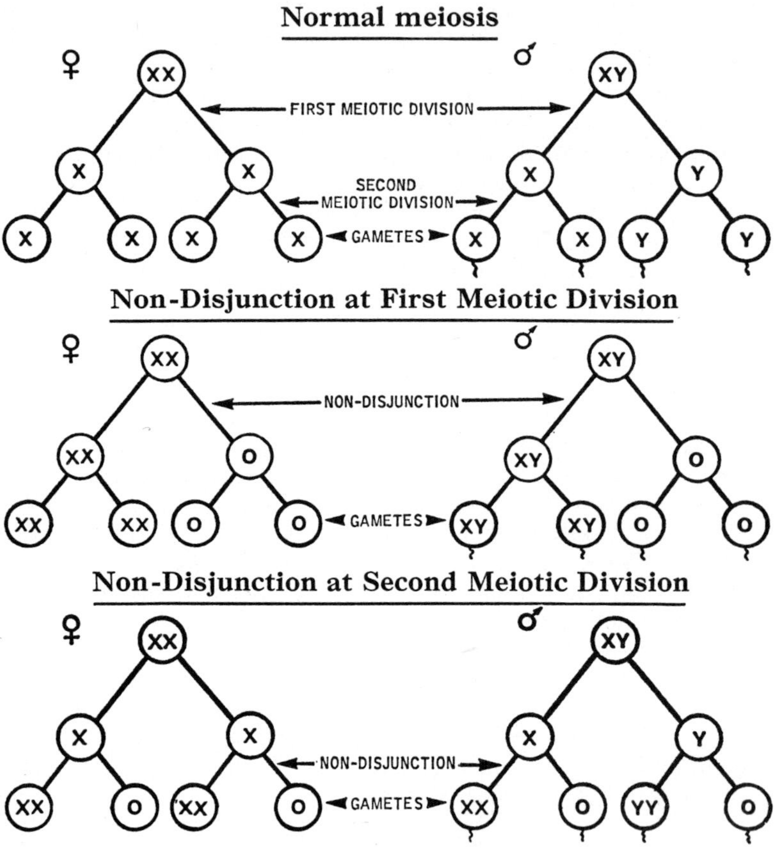

FIG. 6 The formation of gametes

(*a*) normal meiosis

(*b*) non-disjunction at first meiotic division

(*c*) non-disjunction at second meiotic division

ovum therefore receives two X chromosomes and the other none. If the double X ovum is fertilized by a Y bearing sperm, Klinefelter's syndrome results whereas if it is fertilized by an X bearing sperm a triple X individual results. The ovum with no X chromosome would result in Turner's syndrome if fertilized by an X bearing sperm, and a

YO zygote if fertilized by a Y bearing sperm. This latter combination is presumably lethal as no individual has ever been described with this chromosome constitution.

Both Klinefelter's and Turner's syndromes could also result from non-disjunction occurring during the formation of the spermatozoa. As a result of both X and Y chromosomes going to one pole of the spindle and none to the other, one sperm will contain both X and Y chromosomes and the other no sex chromosome. If a normal ovum is fertilized by a sperm of the former constitution Klinefelter's syndrome will result and if by one of the latter, Turner's syndrome will develop. The gamete receiving the extra chromosome is called trisomic whilst its counterpart, which is a chromosome short, is called monosomic.

Similarly a failure to separate at meiotic cell division may involve the autosomes. Thus, as a result of non-disjunction of chromosome 21 the oocyte of the mother will produce one ovum with two chromosome 21's and another with none at all. When an ovum with two chromosome 21's is fertilized by a normal sperm with its single chromosome 21 the resulting zygote will have three chromosome 21's and will develop into a mongol child.

Non-disjunction may also occur at the second meiotic division (Fig. 6.) If this occurs another type of abnormal gamete may result, namely, a sperm with a sex-chromosome constitution YY. If this fertilizes a normal ovum a zygote with a chromosome constitution of XYY will result. Individuals with this abnormal constitution and delinquent behaviour have been described (p. 45). If the YY sperm fertilizes an XX ovum the zygote will have the sex-chromosome constitution of XXYY and this has been recorded in rare cases of Klinefelter's syndrome. If an abnormal XX sperm fertilizes an abnormal XX ovum the zygote will have a sex-chromosome constitution of XXXX. This constitution has been described in some normal females with mental retardation. It is also possible that non-disjunction may occur during both the first and second meiotic divisions, and if this happens gametes with even more bizarre sex-chromosome constitutions may occur.

DISEASES DUE TO VARIATION IN NUMBER OF SEX CHROMOSOMES

Some of the diseases due to variations in the number of sex chromosomes are disorders of sexual development. It would, therefore, be profitable to review the pattern of normal development to permit a better understanding of its anomalies. There are four stages of sexual development, (I) gonadal differentiation, (II) development of internal genitalia, (III) external genital differentiation, (IV) puberty.

The testis and ovary both develop from the undifferentiated gonad which appears in the fourth week of gestation. This indifferent gonad has a cortex and a medulla. In the presence of a Y chromosome the medulla of this structure evolves into a testis and the cortex regresses. In the presence of two X chromosomes the cortex differentiates into an ovary and the medulla regresses. (Fig. 7.)

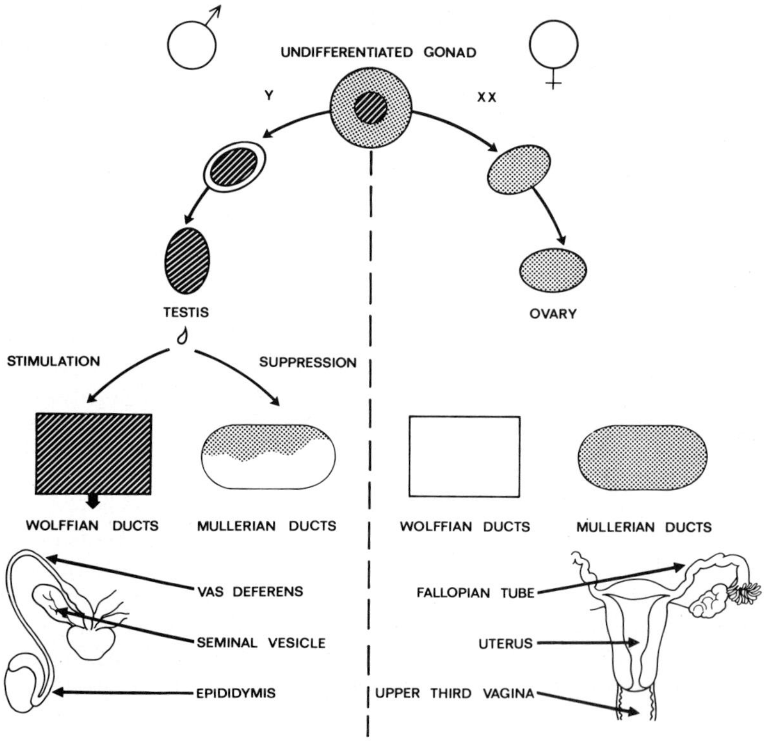

FIG. 7 Gonadal development

The internal genitalia also develop from separate primitive structures that transiently co-exist in embryos of both sexes. In the male the Wolffian ducts give rise to the vas deferens, the seminal vesicles and the epididymis and the Müllerian ducts regress (the prostatic utricle is a remnant). In the female the Müllerian ducts fuse to produce the fallopian tubes, the uterus and the upper vagina and the Wolffian ducts regress. The development of the Wolffian ducts and the suppression of the Müllerian ducts requires the presence of a functioning foetal testis from which an 'inducer' diffuses locally to both suppress the Müllerian ducts and stimulate the development of the Wolffian ducts. This inducer is not androgen which is unable to suppress the Müllerian ducts. In the absence of this substance the duct system differentiates along feminine lines irrespective of the genetic sex. Thus if there is no gonad, as in gonadal agenesis, the ducts will develop along female lines. Jost showed in 1947 that surgical castration of the animal foetus before the time of sexual differentiation prevented masculinization and all the litters grew up as apparent females. The developing testis was thus essential for masculinity but the ovary was not essential for feminity. The female form both internal and external was that of the neuter sex. The third stage of sexual development namely the differentiation of the external genitalia, also involves development from primitive structures common to both sexes. In the female the genital folds become the labia minora, the genital swellings the labia majora and the genital tubercule the clitoris, whilst in the male under the influence of androgens the shaft of the penis, the glans penis and the scrotum are respectively developed. Failure of the genital folds to fuse correctly in the male results in hypospadias. Thus both in the development of the internal genitalia and the external genitalia differentiation to the male form requires a positive influence, otherwise development follows the female pattern. The final stage of sexual development is puberty when pituitary gonadotrophin production increases to adult levels, and secondary sex characteristics appear.

Turner's Syndrome

This is the condition of ovarian dysgenesis. The gonad is represented by a ridge on the broad ligament in the normal position of the ovary, and it is composed of connective tissue without follicles. It is of interest that the XO gonad has follicles at birth though in only 20 per cent of the normal quantity. The second X-chromosome seems necessary to maintain the ovary. There is thus primary amenorrhoea and no development of the breasts or sexual hair occurs. (PLATE II.) In the syndrome described by Turner these features of ovarian dysfunction were associated with shortness of stature, webbing of the neck and cubitus valgus and there was no impairment of intelligence. Although the development of the ovary is influenced to a varying degree, most patients with this syndrome are of short stature and rarely reach a height of more than 5 ft. A number of congenital defects, additional to those originally described by Turner, may be associated with the condition and coarctation of the aorta, deafness and mental deficiency are well recognized. Most women with this condition have only 45 instead of the normal 46 chromosomes and this is due to non-disjunction of the sex chromosomes occurring during meiosis. Their sex chromosome constitution is XO instead of XX. (PLATE III.) These patients are thus chromatin negative on nuclear sexing, because, as has been mentioned, the chromatin body of the cell is due to the second X chromosome normally present in the female cell. However, one-quarter of these patients have 46 chromosomes and are chromatin positive. These patients tend to have a less severe form of the syndrome and only rarely show the skeletal malformations although they are often short in stature. They have the normal number of chromosomes but one of the X chromosomes is structurally abnormal (an isochromosome) and it is believed to arise out of an error in the division of the centromere, when it divides transversely instead of longitudinally. As the centromere is not central this will result in one daughter chromosome arising from the two short arms of the parent chromosome and the other daughter chromosome from the two long arms. Sometimes deletion of part of an X chromosome occurs so that this chromosome will then appear smaller than normal. Although these patients have 46 chromosomes one of the X chromosomes is abnormal and this may result in Turner's syndrome. The other cause of Turner's syndrome with a normal number of chromosomes is the result of what is called mosaicism. In this condition some of the cells have 46 chromosomes and others have 45 and this is due to non-disjunction occurring after fertilization during one of the early divisions of the zygote. The patient's tissues thus have two populations of cells. Such patients may have normal stature and some secondary sex development due to the presence of the XX cell line, and may indeed even appear quite normal.

The XO constitution of most cases of Turner's syndrome explains why, though they are female in appearance, they have the high frequency of red/green colour blindness characteristic of males (8 per cent) as the gene for this is a sex-linked recessive located on the X chromosome. In the colour-blind male there is no normal allene to mask it and nor will there be a normal allene to mask it in patients with only a single X chromosome (XO).

Thus Turner's syndrome is a condition of ovarian infantilism occurring in a patient, who is an apparent girl. It is the only disorder, so far described, in which there is a deficiency of an entire chromosome. It is however uncommon and, when associated with an XO sex chromosome constitution, is probably of the order of 1 in 3,000 females. This number of XO births is the residue of a much larger number of XO zygotes for 90 per cent of XO foetuses miscarry. Less severe forms of the disease due to mosaics and abnormalities of the structure of the X chromosome occur and if these are included the incidence is greater. The frequency of the XO chromosome anomaly in early spontaneous abortion is high, probably about one in 15, but because of the serious nature of the disorder few of such embryos reach maturity

Absence of the short arm of an X chromosome leads to primary amenorrhoea and streak ovaries without the other stigmata of Turner's syndrome. All patients with classical Turner's syndrome have in common a deficiency of the short arm of an X chromosome. The commonest abnormality is an XO constitution but less commonly there is an isochromosome of the long arm or just deletion of the short arm of an X chromosome. The anatomical and clinical features of a patient with Turner's syndrome are largely determined by the precise abnormality in the chromosome composition. Features of masculinization may occur when the pattern is XO/XY.

Klinefelter's Syndrome

The original syndrome described by Klinefelter consisted of gynaecomastia, testicular atrophy and infertility. Intelligence was unimpaired. Cases have been described with associated mental defects and striking tallness of stature but the only constant feature of the syndrome is testicular atrophy with resulting azoospermia and infertility. The strophy of the testis is the result of a peritubular fibrosis, which begins to appear in childhood and progresses until all the seminiferous tubules are replaced by fibrous tissue. Gynaecomastia, mental retardation and eunuchoidism may be associated (PLATE IV), but the former is inconstant and the latter are infrequent. However, it is generally considered that the presence of the additional X chromosome limits the intelligence quotient so that it is reduced below what it would have been if the sex chromosome complement had been normal. Furthermore, abnormalities in the electroencephalogram are frequent in patients with XXY chromosome constitution. Klinefelter's syndrome is much more common than Turner's syndrome and occurs in 1 in 300 of the male population. Most patients with Klinefelter's syndrome have 47 chromosomes instead of the normal 46. They are chromatin positive because they have an extra X chromosome, the sex chromosome constitution being XXY instead of XY.

Patients with this syndrome show that the Y chromosome is strongly sex determining and can no longer be regarded as functionless, for the patient who has an XXY constitution may have the appearance of a normal male and the only incapacity be infertility.

However, the loss of a Y chromosome leads to the development of a bodily form which is essentially feminine (XO Turner's syndrome). Most patients with Klinefelter's syndrome have the chromosome pattern or genotype XXY. A few are mosaics and some of their cells contain 46 chromosomes with a normal XY constitution and others contain 47 chromosomes with the abnormal constitution XXY. Such patients will have less severe forms of the disease. Mosaics have also been described in which some body cells contain the normal female constitution of XX and 44 autosomes and the remainder 44 autosomes and an XY sex chromosome pattern. A few rarer and more severely affected variations of the syndrome have been described with 48 chromosomes and an XXXY genotype and even 49 chromosomes and an XXXXY genotype.

Triple X syndrome

In 1 in 1,000 female births the chromosome constitution of the patient is XXX, that is they have an extra chromosome so that their number is 47 instead of 46 and the extra chromosome is an X sex chromosome. This is known as trisomy X, the super-female or the triple X syndrome. The name super female gives a misleading picture of an extra endowment of all that makes a female female. The patients are, however, outwardly normal and usually mentally deficient. They are often fertile and usually produce normal offspring. They are chromatin positive but the sex chromatin bodies are duplicated because of the extra X chromosome carried. Variants of this syndrome, in which the cells contain four X chromosomes, have been described. The abnormalities in these patients are usually greater than with the simple XXX constitution and on nuclear sexing the chromatin bodies increase in number, the number of chromatin bodies being one less than the number of X chromosomes in the cell.

Thus chromosome abnormalities involving the sex chromosomes tend to reflect conditions of abnormal sex development, whilst abnormalities of the autosomes are associated with defects in somatic growth and development. There is much overlap as patients with Turner's syndrome often have somatic defects in addition. It must be realized that not all intersexual conditions are due to abnormal sex chromosomes. Congenital adrenal hyperplasia is due to an inborn defect in the synthesis of hydrocortisone in a patient with a normal female chromosome constitution; excessive androgen production results in virilization. True hermaphrodites usually have an XX constitution though mosaics may also occur with some cells of XX and others of XY constitution. A small proportion have an XY chromosome pattern. True hermaphrodites have both testicular and ovarian tissue in their gonad (ovo-testis) or an ovary on one side and a testis on the other. If an individual has a testis a Y chromosome should be present (p. 40). And yet true hermaphrodites are usually XX and one in 60,000 apparently normal males has an XX chromosome constitution. The explanation of this apparent contradiction lies in the fact that the effective testis determining genes are not absent but have become translocated onto one of the X chromosomes.

XYY Syndrome

The chromosome constitution XYY occurs in 1 in 500 male births which makes it the most common form of aneuploidy in human beings. It is found with increased frequency in men with violent and criminal propensities. The incidence of this chromosome abnormality in apparently healthy men with criminal records of violence has been estimated at 5 per cent. These men may be mentally subnormal. No associated physical abnormality has been described apart from tallness of stature. The mean height of patients with XYY chromosome constitution is 73·1 inches compared with 67 inches in normal males. There is, however, a tendency to sterility as the seminiferous tubules degenerate. In XYY patients two thirds of the spermatozoa have a single Y chromosome and only 5 per cent are XY. One per cent of sperms carry 2 Y chromosomes and yet XYY births are less than 1 in 500. There is no evidence that spontaneous abortions are frequent in the XYY syndrome and it seems probable, therefore, that there is sperm selection in the female genital tract.

DISEASES DUE TO ABNORMALITIES OF AUTOSOMES

The loss of an autosome is always fatal and no condition has been described with a deficiency of an autosome. A number of instances of the gain of an autosome have been reported and the defects are usually severe, the child either having mongolism or gross skeletal and congenital cardiac lesions. The mechanism for the loss or gain of a chromosome, whether it is an autosome or a sex chromosome, is the process of non-disjunction. The most commonly affected autosome is chromosome 21 and trisomy 21 results in mongolism. (PLATE V.) In certain mongols, however, the additional chromatin may come, not from an extra chromosome but from a segment breaking away from one chromosome and becoming attached to another. This process is called translocation. Mongolism has been found associated with Klinefelter's syndrome. In this case the number of chromosomes was 48 instead of a normal 46, one of the extra chromosomes being the chromosome number 21 associated with mongolism and the other being an additional X sex chromosome, giving the XXY sex chromosome complement of Klinefelter's syndrome.

Mongolism

The incidence of mongolism is one in six hundred births. There is a striking correlation between the incidence of this anomaly and the maternal age, being 1 in 2,000 for mothers below the age of 30, 1 in 300 between the ages of 35 and 39 and 1 in 50 above the age of 45 years. It is most frequently due to non-disjunction, resulting in an extra chromosome 21, and the relationship with maternal age suggests that the non-disjunction occurs on the female side. A few mongols have the normal chromosome constitution of 46 chromosomes but the extra chromsome 21 in these cases has been translocated on to another chromosome. In this situation the extra chromosome is present but has become attached to another chromosome. A few cases of mongolism, especially when the mother is young, are the result of a chromosome translocation in one of the parents and here there is a high risk (1 in 3) of a further mongol being born in subsequent pregnancies. The parents of mongols, due to this cause, have a detectable chromosome abnormality, which is due to a translocation between chromosome 15 and 21. In itself the translocation does not cause disease and may be transmitted through several generations. However, occasionally it affects meiosis in such a way that an extra chromosome 21 is transmitted to the gamete, producing a rare form of familial mongolism. Chromosome mosaics may occur in mongols and these patients tend to have the syndrome in an incomplete form.

The extra chromosome 21, characteristic of mongolism, is present in all the cells and this includes the leucocytes. Chromosome abnormalities of leucocytes occur in leukaemia and it is of interest therefore that there is an enhanced incidence of leukaemia in Mongols.

Other anomalies

An extra chromosome 18 may result from non-disjunction of chromosome number 18 (Trisomy E) and this is associated with severe somatic defects which cause early death. These include mental defect, congenital cardiac malformations and abnormalities of the ears and jaw. An extra chromosome 13 (Trisomy D) may also occur and this results in eye defects, hair lip, cleft palate and congenital cardiac abnormalities. This too causes early death.

The incidence of E trisomy (Edwards syndrome) is 1 in 5,000 live births, and that of D trisomy (Patau's syndrome) 1 in 9,000 live births. A syndrome due to a structural anomaly involving deletion of the short arm of chromosome 5 has also been described. This syndrome is called the cri-du-chat syndrome.

Mutations

These are changes at single gene loci and can occur during mitosis or meiosis or even during the resting stage. When this happens during meiosis, that is during the formation of ova or sperms, the condition will be inherited as the zygote resulting from a gamete bearing the mutation will carry the mutation. Mutations occurring in somatic cells are not inherited. When this occurs only some of the cells of the individual are affected, though if somatic mutation occurs soon after the formation of the zygote the number of cells affected will be large and the result will be a mosaic. Many mutations are limited because they are harmful and associated with death of the foetus.

Mosaicism

If non-disjunction occurs after the formation of a zygote, that is during a mitotic cell division and not a meiotic cell division, some of the cells will have one chromosome constitution and others another. The term mosaicism describes a condition, in which a substantial minority of cells differ from the majority in their chromosome content. How substantial this minority is will depend on how early during cleavage the zygote undergoes non-disjunction. Some women have an XO/XXX chromosome constitution of their cells, due to non-disjunction occurring during an early mitotic division in a zygote of a normal XX constitution; three X chromosomes pass to one daughter cell and one X chromosome to the other. These two cells give rise to daughter cells of similar chromosome constitution and so perpetuate their kind. Such women are likely to be abnormal and suffer from ovarian dysgenesis giving rise to primary amenorrhoea and deficient breast development.

Chromosomes of cancer cells

The cells of malignant tumours and leucocytes in leukaemia frequently have detectable abnormalities of their chromosomes. These chromosome abnormalities are acquired. They are confined to the malignant cells and do not occur in other body cells. They may comprise alterations in the number of chromosomes or in the morphology of individual chromosomes. The Philadelphia chromosome is a constant feature in the cultures of leucocytes and bone marrow cells from patients with chronic myeloid leukaemia and it consists of a deletion of part of chromosome 21. This is the first recorded instance in which a specific chromosome anomaly is associated with a specific type of neoplastic disease. Cells with the Philadelphia chromosome are present in the bone marrow some time before the clinical manifestions of leukaemia develop and it would seem that deletion of part of chromosome 21 confers on the cell leukaemic properties or, at any rate, a pre-disposition towards leukaemia. It is of interest that radiotherapy to the spine for such conditions as ankylosing spondylitis will induce chromosome abnormalities in the patients' blood cells and it is known that there is an increased incidence of leukaemia in patients thus treated. Similarly the treatment of polycythaemia rubra vera with radioactive phosphorus is also associated with induced changes in the chromosomes of the blood cells. These include alterations in number as well as in morphology. These changes occur soon after treatment and are usually present several months later. There is also an increased incidence of leukaemia in patients with polycythaemia rubra vera treated with radioactive phosphorus. It should not be assumed therefore that these forms of treatment should not be used for radioactive phosphorus has increased the mean survival of patients with polycythaemia rubra vera from 3 years to 11 years. Although there is an undoubted increase in the incidence of leukaemia in these patients the benefits of treatment are great.

The chromosome abnormalities associated with cancer are variable and no characteristic pattern is associated with any specific type of neoplastic cell. It does appear, however, from animal experients that cells with abnormal chromosome patterns are predisposed towards malignant change. The high incidence of acute leukaemia in mongolism is believed to be a consequence of the genetic abnormality, and the high incidence of ovarian tumours in patients with gonadal dystenesis and an XO chromosome pattern may have a similar relationship.

Selected Bibliography

CLARKE, C. A. (1964) *Genetics for the Clinician.* 2nd Ed. Blackwell, Oxford.

FRASER ROBERTS, J. A. (1970) *An Introduction to Medical Genetics.* 5th Ed. Oxford University Press, London.

LENNOX, B. (1961) Chromosomes for Beginners. *The Lancet* 1, 1046.

POLANI, P. E. (1964) *Chromosomology in Symposium of Advanced Medicine.* Ed. COMPSTON, N. Pitman, p. 284.

III

Drug-Induced Disease

It is not surprising that the introduction of so many potent and toxic chemicals into clinical use has been accompanied by an alarming increase in drug-induced disease. We now live in an era of safe surgery and dangerous medicine. The admonition of the ancients 'at least do no harm' requires reaffirmation today. An appreciation of the potential hazards of drug therapy will breed an attitude of caution and thoughtful consideration of the indications and the risks before prescribing. The craze for drugs is an alarming phenomenon of our generation: many people depend on them for the relief of insomnia, fear, anxiety, excitability, depression and lethargy. The clinician is responsible for giving these drugs to patients, and must therefore be alert to the signs of toxicity, hypersensitivity and possible impending disaster.

Before a new drug is submitted to clinical trial in this country the Department of Health Committee on the Safety of Drugs reviews and assesses the evidence on the basis of which the manufacturers have concluded that it is reasonably safe to initiate such trials. The toxic effects of a drug will be recorded in any clinical trial but unless these effects occur with considerable frequency they are unlikely to be encountered in the limited number of patients included in such a trial. It is in the subsequent use of the drug in general practice that the real value and potential hazards of the drug will be revealed.

Only seldom can the occurrence of side-effects be predicted on the basis of the structural formula of a drug; many of the more serious effects that may result when a drug is given to man cannot be anticipated from observation in animals. It is only in the long run that many undesirable side-effects can be recognized as such. It took 80 years to learn that aspirin can give rise to gastro-intestinal haemorrhage and nearly as long before it was realized that amidopyrine caused agranulocytosis.

The blessings of modern therapeutics carry an increased responsibility to resist wanton therapy and to give careful attention to the indication and complications of treatment. Whilst there is little doubt about the justification for chloramphenicol therapy in typhoid fever, it should never be used for trivial upper respiratory infections. Although chloramphenicol aplasia of the bone marrow is rare, it is nevertheless true that in the majority of fatal cases the patient would not have died if he had not received the drug. The importance of questioning patients about possible drug sensitivity cannot be overstressed and the warnings of drug-induced urticaria or dermatitis should not be discounted lightly. A clear distinction must be drawn between the patient's 'wants' and what the physician thinks he needs, and the reckless administration of drugs for the sole purpose of pleasing the patient and saving the doctor time and trouble must be avoided. The situation is aggravated by the advertizement of useless remedies. A recent index of ethical compounds available for prescription in Great Britain includes 25 preparations for the treatment of obesity, and over 5 million prescriptions are written annually for stimulants and appetite suppressants in England and Wales. These drugs are not without adverse effects and in some there is a danger of addiction. They are all derived by modification of the amphetamine molecule and they all give rise to psychomotor activation when given in large doses. Chronic abuse of these drugs can lead to psychosis. It is, alas, so much easier to be convinced by the hypnotism of advertizement than face the fact that dietary restriction is the only useful measure to combat obesity and self-discipline and willpower the best weapons with which to defeat the appetite. The hazards of drug therapy could once be discussed under skin rashes and blood dyscrasias, but are now the subject of books on diseases of medical progress.

It is difficult to place the hazards of drug therapy in correct perspective but the Department of Health Committee on the Safety of Drugs, by collecting and analyzing the data on various adverse reactions to drugs, is undoubtedly proving to be of great value. Adverse reactions range from minor symptoms such as dry mouth or drowsiness up to potentially fatal damage to the liver or bone marrow. Drug reactions have been reported in from 10 to 18 per cent of patients receiving treatment. Fortunately most of these reactions are not serious, and a majority are caused by a relatively small number of drugs. Digitalis and antibiotics head the list though this probably reflects in part the frequency of administration. The incidence of adverse reactions rises with the number of different drugs prescribed to each patient and the combination of digitalis and diuretics is a potent source of reaction. Some idea of the problem can be gleaned by the recent estimate that 5 per cent of beds in a general hospital are occupied by the complications of drug treatment. It has also been reported that in nearly 10 per cent of patients admitted to hospital with jaundice a drug is to blame, and 40 per cent of patients with severe hepatic necrosis have received drugs known to damage the liver. Although there is no diagnostic test to differentiate hepato-toxic drug jaundice from virus hepatitis the association in these cases between taking the drug and the onset of jaundice makes a casual relationship probable.

A recent analysis of deaths from therapeutic misadventure showed that corticosteroids were responsible for 16 per cent of these disasters. Anticoagulants, phenylbutazone and chloramphenicol were the next most frequent causes of drug-induced death. Six deaths from renal disease following the administration of phenacetin were reported and for the first time the contraceptive pill enters the list as a cause of death. Nevertheless the hazards of taking drugs must be kept in perspective. They are small in comparison with the risks of smoking. Only 146 deaths from adverse reactions to drugs were reported in 1967. Although this is certainly an under-estimate of the true incidence, it remains a small proportion of patients receiving treatment. The death rate for patients taking chloramphenicol or monoamine oxidase inhibitors is 1 in 10,000 to 1 in 100,000 and each year the chance of being killed in a car accident is greater than 1 in 10,000. Furthermore the risks of not using the drug must be considered.

Drugs may precipitate crises in symptomless inborn errors of metabolism. Porphyria variegata, the South African variant of porphyria, provides an example of what is almost entirely a drug-induced disease. The metabolic disorder is widespread and can be detected by the presence of porphyrin in the stools, but under natural conditions it is often without symptoms and usually does no harm. The advent of barbiturates has, however, rendered acute episodes of the disease commonplace and these cries may terminate in paralysis and death.

No attempt will be made to list all the toxic effects of commonly used drugs, but rather to stress the wide variety of mechanisms involved in untoward reactions to drugs with the serious and even fatal nature of many.

The reactions to drugs may be considered under:

1. Overdosage (a) absolute, (b) relative
2. Intolerance
3. Side-effects

4. Idiosyncrasy
5. Secondary effects
6. Hypersensitivity and allergic reactions.

OVERDOSAGE

With overdosage toxic effects occur in direct relation to the total amount of the drug in the body, and they are therefore likely to occur in any patient provided a certain blood level is exceeded. These effects may result from absolute overdosage or as a result of accumulation of the drug within the body. In renal failure, drugs normally excreted in the urine may accumulate in the blood and cause their toxic effects in doses which, under normal circumstances, would be excreted without difficulty. Drugs that are eliminated or inactivated slowly tend to accumulate in the body and toxic levels may develop more readily. Digitalis overdosage results from accumulation; since the advent of the thiazide diuretics, hypokalaemia has become more of a clinical problem and this increases the sensitivity of the heart to digitalis so that toxicity occurs more readily. Digitalis is capable of producing or aggravating congestive cardiac failure, and the classical electrocardiographic signs may be absent in a large proportion of patients. The margin between thereapeutic and toxic levels is narrow and becomes even narrower in the elderly patient and in those with advanced heart disease. A recent analysis of hospital patients on digitalis showed electrocardiographic evidence of overdosage in 12 per cent. Atrioventricular block, paroxysmal atrial tachycardia, ventricular tachycardia or premature ventricular contractions (coupling) may result. If the drug is continued in excessive dosage mortality will be high. Traditionally the symptoms of nausea and vomiting and the physical sign of bradycardia were taught as classical evidence of digitalis intoxication. Nowadays the purified glycosides, such as digoxin, are less irritant to the gastro-intestinal mucosa and cardiac arrhythmias are a more frequent sign of overdosage. Tachycardia may be a feature of digitalis intoxication rather than bradycardia and this may lead to an aggravation of heart failure. The various neuropsychiatric manifestations such as visual disturbance, confusion, hallucination and depression are easily overlooked, especially in the elderly.

Toxicity is encountered in the epileptic child who becomes mentally retarded and clumsy as a result of overdosage with anticonvulsant drugs. Patients with Parkinsonism are often treated with increasing doses of drugs intended to control the muscular rigidity. Sometimes they fail and if the dose is increased mental confusion and depression appear as manifestations of overdosage. Over-enthusiastic self-administration of vitamin D has produced hyper-calcaemia and renal failure. It is not generally appreciated that a number of drugs listed in official publications are toxic. Strychnine and arsenic for example are perhaps better known for their poisonous effects than for any therapeutic benefit.

Chlorpromazine agranulocytosis is the result of cumulative toxicity. Large doses given consecutively over a period of days produce this effect, and the reaction can be reproduced in the same person by giving a comparable dose again after recovery. A small dose, however, has no effect, and this excludes an immunological mechanism. It has been estimated that the incidence of chlorpormazine agranulocytosis is as high as 0·3 per cent. If recognized promptly patients usually recover completely about ten days after the drug has been stopped.

The use of reserpine, chlorpromazine and the more recent phenothiazine derivatives has been associated with a wide variety of neurological effects, but Parkinsonism and epilepsy are the most frequent: these drug-induced neurological syndromes are directly related to dosage. Depression and psychosis may follow the administration of corticosteroids, reserpine, chlorpromazine and isoniazid.

Carbon tetrachloride, DDT and chloroform cause hepatic necrosis by direct poisoning of hepatic cells if the dose is sufficient. Methyl-testosterone and the nortestosterone derivatives (which are used as anabolic agents) cause an obstructive jaundice if given in excess dosage. Frank jaundice or abnormalities in bromsulphthalein excretion will develop in anyone who receives sufficient drug for long enough. This is an overdosage phenomenon and must be distinguished from drug jaundice due to idiosyncrasy which will be considered later.

INTOLERANCE

Intolerance is a lowered threshold to the normal pharmacological action of a drug. It is often merely a manifestation of the normal variation found in all biological phenomena. The characteristic effect of the drug is thus produced by an unusually small dose. The varying effect of alcohol on different subjects in similar dose is well known, and likewise some subjects develop cinchonism on small doses of quinine. It may be the result of variations in intenstinal absorption, metabolism, excretion or susceptibility to the drug. These variations may be genetic in origin, the patient inheriting an enzymatic defect which prevents normal detoxification of a drug. However, there are many acquired diseases that alter the rate of absorption, utilization and excretion of drugs. Chronic renal failure and liver disease are especially relevant. No sedative drug is really safe for the patient with liver disease and the more potent drugs can produce prolonged narcosis. The effects of corticosteroids and oestrogens are enhanced in patients with liver disease because they are broken down in the liver. Drugs excreted by glomerular filtration, such as streptomycin, will be retained in patients with chronic renal failure. The urine pH affects the excretion of many drugs. Blood levels following a single dose of catecholamines may persist for 24 hours if the urine is alkaline.

Damage to the eighth cranial nerve may follow the administration of the antibiotics streptomycin, dihydrostreptomycin, neomycin and kanamycin, the blood level being of decisive importance. Streptomycin affects predominantly the vestibular branch of the nerve, whilst with the others injury is confined to the auditory branch. The deafness produced is permanent. Many patients with vestibular damage due to streptomycin received only a few grammes. Parenteral administration of these drugs should therefore be restricted to the treatment of serious infections, and it is now rarely necessary for them to be used in the management of urinary tract infections. Kanamycin and neomycin are particularly ototoxic and the indications for their parenteral use are rare. Careful observation for signs of damage to the eighth nerve must be undertaken in all patients receiving this group of antibiotics: it is, however, an inadequate safeguard, because a latent period of up to several weeks may elapse before the toxic effect of these antibiotics becomes manifest. As these drugs are excreted through the kidney, even a minor degree of impaired renal function becomes a major hazard. This is probably the reason why elderly patients are particularly liable to toxic effects.

Of the potentially retinotoxic drugs, chloroquine and certain phenothiazine derivatives, such as thioridazine (Melleril) are the most widely prescribed. As central vision only fails after extensive retinal damage has occurred, expert examination of the fundus should be undertaken at intervals in patients receiving these compounds over long periods. The established lesion is irreversible, so that early detection is important. Corneal changes though less serious are more common and a recent survey has shown that 30 per cent of patients treated with anti-malarial drugs developed corneal changes which regressed when treatment was withdrawn. The characteristic symptom of haloes around naked lights should suggest drug-induced corneal changes.

It must be remembered that drugs are administered not only to normal adults, but to the very old, the very young and to unborn children, and the dose tolerated may vary. The thalidomide disaster reminded us that drugs may pass through the placental barrier and reach the foetus in sufficient concentration to damage the cerebral cortex or impair normal development. The sensitivity of older patients to drugs such as barbiturates is perhaps simply the result of accumulation as a consequence of inability of the aged to eliminate the drug adequately. Barbiturates often increase restlessness and confusion in the elderly, and when given in large doses expose the patient to the risk of respiratory tract infection, incontinence and pressure sores. Furthermore, hypotension as a complication of drug therapy is a special hazard in the old patient. The lowering of body temperature produced by the phenothiazine compounds and imipramine is of particular importance in the elderly for there is little doubt that hypothermia causes more deaths than is generally realized.

Intolerance is also likely to be a result of constitutional differences in the synthesis of specific enzymes involved in the mode of action, metabolism or excretion of a drug. The genetically determined enzyme defect has recently been established in a few instances of drug intolerance and it seems probable that more will follow. An increased liability to the side effects of isoniazid, for example, depends on an inherited inability to acetylate this substance. The rate at which isoniazid can be acetylated and hence degraded depends on an enzyme, which is absent in a significant proportion of the population. If the enzyme is absent, isoniazid can only be inactivated slowly and this is associated with high blood levels of the drug and a greater tendency to develop peripheral neuritis as the result of treatment. 'Slow inactivation' is inherited as a recessive characteristic and there is a marked racial difference in the gene frequency. Fifty per cent of Indians and Negroes are slow inactivators of isoniazid and 10 per cent of the population of Japan.

Prolonged apnoea is an alarming reaction which is seen following the administration of the muscle relaxant suxamethonium to certain patients. It occurs in subjects who show a familial deficiency or abnormality of the enzyme pseudo-cholinesterase in the serum, suxamethonium being normally destroyed by plasma pseudocholinesterase. About one in two thousand persons in this country is affected and the condition is without symptoms until the patient is given suxamethonium. The action of the cholinesterase inhibitors physostigmine and neostigmine will be enhanced in such patients due to decreased cholinesterase activity.

For drugs like the anti-depressants that are not excreted unchanged by the kidney, the concentration reached in the plasma is determined by the rate of metabolism in the liver. The endoplasmic reticulum of the liver cell changes the lipid-soluble drug into a water-soluble metabolite by a process of hydroxylation, and the water-soluble metabolite can then be excreted by the kidney. Changes in the rate of metabolism of a drug are more important in determining the plasma level than alterations in intestinal absorption. The factors influencing the rate of metabolism of any drug are both genetic and environmental. The most important environmental factor is the coincident administration of another drug that stimulates the process of hydroxylation. The barbiturates, for example, will increase the rate of breakdown by inducing the formation of drug-metabolizing enzymes in the microsomes of liver cells (p. 70). Individual differences in both the therapeutic and toxic effects of many drugs depend on their rate of metabolism. It has been shown that the administration of the same dose of the anti-depressant amitriptyline to different patients results in a thirty-fold variation in the plasma level attained. The patients with the higher blood levels have a higher incidence of toxic effects.

Premature children lack some normal enzymes and therefore may have greater difficulty in detoxifying certain drugs. This accounts for their intolerance of phenacetin, vitamin K, sulphonamides and other compounds.

It should be remembered that the pH of the urine is important in determining the rate of excretion and hence the duration of activity of acidic and basic drugs and that variations in pH may give rise to intolerance. Sixty per cent of a dose of mecamylamine, which is a weak base, is excreted in 24 hours if the urine is strongly acid but only 20 per cent if it is alkaline. Other basic drugs will be similarly affected and some of these in common usage include amphetamine, procaine, pethidine and quinine. Acidic drugs likewise will be excreted more rapidly in an alkaline urine and phenobarbitone, phenylbutazone and nitrofurantoin are examples.

SIDE-EFFECTS

The term side-effects should be reserved for therapeutically undesirable but unavoidable effects of drugs. Many of these are specific, the undesired effect being a normal pharmacological action of the drug. In these circumstances the dose has to be adjusted so as to produce the therapeutic effect with the minimum of side-effects. Side-effects limit the use of many effective thereapeutic drugs. It is unfortunate that the term side-effect has come to mean little more than a drug action not sought at the moment and fails to convey the serious implications that it may have for the patient.

The ganglion-blocking drugs such as hexamethonium and mecamylamine block nerve conduction through autonomic ganglia; as a result of sympathetic block, the blood pressure is effectively lowered, but as a consequence of parasympathetic block dry mouth, impotence, and constipation result. Even with pure adrenegic nerve inhibitors such as guanethidine and bethanidine failure of ejaculation without impotence is common and may cause great concern to the patient.

The hypnotic effect of many antihistamines limits their dosage. Anticoagulant therapy may be associated with haemorrhage into the pericardium and even spontaneous subdural haematomata; numerous reports of ileus due to intra-mural intestinal haemorrhage have recently appeared. Furthermore, if these drugs are stopped too rapidly, there may be a period of rebound hypercoagulability with possible recurrence of thrombosis.

A side-effect of chlorpromazine is peripheral vasodilatation, which almost invariably follows its parenteral administration: the consequent hypotension may be considerable and this is of particular importance in chronic renal failure, in which recurrent vomiting is frequently and effectively treated with chlorpormazine. The fall in blood pressure, however, may aggravate renal failure with disastrous consequences.

The development of thyroid hypofunction in some patients receiving phenylbutazone (Butazolidin) or para-amino salicylic acid (PAS) is a side-effect, which results from interference with the iodine-trapping mechanism of the thyroid through suppression of the enzyme tyrosine iodinase.

The side-effects of the corticosteroid compounds are many and serious: they include a decreased resistance to infection, peptic ulceration, increased catabolism of protein, osteoporosis and many others. Peptic ulceration is also a side-effect of phenylbutazone, cincophen and colchicine.

Megaloblastic anaemia may follow the treatment of epilepsy with phenytoin (Epanutin, Dilantin) or primidone (Mysoline). It results from inhibition of the action of folic acid, but there is no absolute deficiency of the vitamin. Phenytoin and primidone interfere with enzyme systems concerned with folic acid metabolism, and no patient treated with folic acid has failed to respond. Serum vitamin B_{12} concentrations in these patients are usually normal, and treatment with this vitamin alone is frequently ineffective.

Hypokalaemia is a frequent side-effect of diuretic therapy and this is especially common when the thiazide diuretics are used, and in conditions of secondary hyperaldosteronism, such as hepatic cirrhosis.

Steatorrhoea may be a side-effect of neomycin, para-amino salicyclic acid or phenindione administration. This is presumably due to local irritant action which impairs the integrity of the mucosal cells of the small intestine.

Damage to the bone marrow is a side-effect of treating malignant diseases with cytotoxic drugs. Ionizing radiation, alkylating agents such as nitrogen mustard preparations, cyclophosphamide, chlorambucil, uramustine, urethane and the purine (6 mercaptopurine) and folic acid (methotrexate) antagonists all suppress bone marrow function. In the usual therapeutic doses the depression of bone marrow function is reversible but permanent damage may result from overdosage.

Salicylates regularly cause gastro-intestinal bleeding, probably on account of a local irritant action on the gastric mucosa. Usually the blood loss is minimal. Less frequently hypochromic anaemia develops and occasionally there is overt gastro-intestinal haemorrhage. Other drug-induced small gut lesions include annular ulceration of the small intestine which may result from a combination of thiazide with enteric coated potassium. Although abdominal discomfort often follows the ingestion of these tablets the diagnosis is not usually made until intestinal obstruction develops. The potassium chloride is the offending substance due to the speed with which it is sometimes released from enteric-coated tablets.

Subacute combined degeneration of the cord frequently follows treatment of vitamin B_{12} deficiency with folic acid and reports of undiagnosed patients with pernicious anemia developing this condition after treatment with oral vitamin preparations containing folic acid continue to appear. When patients with pernicious anemia are given folic acid the anaemia usually improves but the central nervous system damage proceeds at an enhanced rate.

IDIOSYNCRASY

True idiosyncrasy implies an inherent abnormal qualitative reaction to a drug and it is primarily the result of a constitutional defect in the patient. The abnormal sensitivity of patients with porphyria to barbiturates and sulphonamides is an example. Hereditary biochemical defects of erythrocytes are responsible for many drug-induced haemolytic anaemias and for favism. Drug-sensitive red cells are deficient in the enzyme glucose–6–phosphate dehydrogenase, which plays an important part in the metabolism of glucose and is necessary for the continued integrity of the cell. This defect is inherited as a sex-linked incomplete dominant trait, and the red cells of patients with this abnormality have a normal life span until challenged by certain drugs, when the older cells are rapidly destroyed, resulting in haemolytic anaemia. Fourteen per cent of American Negroes are affected and 60 per cent of Yemenite Jews in Israel. The perpetuation of the gene is due to the greater resistance against malaria that it carries. Severe and even fatal haemolysis has followed the administration of the antimalarial compounds pamaquine and primaquine in sensitive individuals. These red cells are sensitive not only to fava beans and primaquine, but also to sulphonamides, acetanilide, phenacetin, para-aminosalicyclic acid, nitrofurantoin, probenecid and vitamin K analogues.

When patients with porphyria are given certain drugs, particularly barbiturates and sulphonamides, they are liable to develop acute neurological episodes with peripheral and respiratory paralysis, which may result in death. Porphyria variegata, the South African variety of porphyria, is an example of an inborn error of metabolism which was without serious symptoms until the advent of barbiturate drugs. Taking these drugs can precipitate total paralysis and death. The metabolic error is inherited as a dominant characteristic and there are now 8,000 affected persons in South Africa, all of whom can be traced to a single couple who married in the seventeenth century.

The factors determining the bone marrow aplasia which may follow the administration of chloramphenicol are largely unknown. Temporary depression of the bone marrow occurs regularly with plasma chloramphenicol levels of 25 mcg./100 ml. and this toxic effect is a pharmacological property of the drug. In one controlled trial the toxic bone marrow depression developed in two out of 20 patients on 2 g. a day of chloramphenicol, and in 18 of the 21 patients on 6 g. daily there was progressive erythrocyte depression, mild thrombocytopenia and evidence of disturbed granulocyte production. These changes all disappeared on stopping the drug and reappeared when the drug was readministered in a large dose but not in a small dose. This is suggestive of an overdosage effect. However, the more familiar bone marrow aplasia is generally regarded as either due to idiosyncrasy or possibly a hypersensitivity reaction induced by previous or prolonged usage. There is a one in 60,000 risk of developing aplastic anaemia from chloramphenicol but there is no way of recognizing which patient will react unfavourably to the drug. Whilst a high dose and repeated courses appear to be more likely to cause damage, single courses of less than 10 g. can cause fatal aplasia. In micro-organisms it is known that chloramphenical inhibits the synthesis of DNA and RNA, and this probably accounts for its bacteristatic effect. It seems probable therefore that the sensitive patient may be unable to excrete the drug normally or he may have a biochemical defect of bone marrow cells. This is supported by the fact that multiple vaculoes are found in the early erythroblasts of patients receiving chloramphenicol and these are the marrow cells with the largest amount of RNA. In a survey by the U.S. Food and Drug Administration in 1952, 139 cases of aplastic anaemia following chloramphenicol administration were reported and 96 of these were fatal. In Britain 30 deaths in four years following chloramphenicol have been reported to the Ministry of Health Committee on the Safety of Drugs. The only effective treatment is blood transfusion: hope of recovery must never be lost, for remissions of bone marrow failure have occurred after several years of transfusion existence. Only in one-quarter of patients with aplastic anaemia is it possible to attribute the condition to a drug or other chemical substance.

Drug Jaundice

Drug jaundice may be due to idiosyncrasy or overdosage. Some drugs cause damage to hepatic cells with resulting necrosis. Others cause an obstructive type of jaundice by impeding the flow of bile within the canaliculi and this is called cholestatic jaundice. Others cause jaundice through haemolysis of red cells. Each of these varieties of jaundice may be an overdosage effect of a drug and the toxicity is then directly related to the dosage and duration of treatment. For example, carbon tetrachloride, chloroform and tannic acid cause necrosis of liver cells when a certain dose is exceeded. Methyltestosterone (but not testosterone propionate) and other nortestosterone derivatives which are used in therapeutics as anabolic agents (norethandrolone and methandienone) may all cause an obstructive jaundice due to biliary stasis if the dose is large enough and the duration of treatment long enough, and the impairment of bromsulphthalein excretion parallels the dose. Phenacetin and acetanilide will cause haemolysis of the red cells in anyone if the dose is large enough. These are examples of overdosage.

Certain drugs, however, precipitate the same types of jaundice as a result of idiosyncrasy. Then only a small percentage of the patients receiving the drug will develop jaundice and the size of the dose and the duration of treatment will not be relevant. Furthermore, these drugs will not cause damage to the liver in experimental animals because the jaundice is due to a constitutional defect in the patient. Haemolytic anaemia resulting from a variety of drugs in patients with glucose phosphate dehydrogenase deficiency has been considered. Hepatocellular jaundice as a result of idiosyncrasy of the patient has been produced by a variety of drugs, the most important of which are the monoamine oxidase inhibitors used in the treatment of depression. More rarely the sulphonamides, phenylbutazone and thiosemicarbasone may be responsible. Recently the anaesthetic fluothane (Halothane) has been associated with hepatocellular jaundice. It appears that multiple exposures to fluothane are usually required and a pyrexia after the initial exposure is a premonitory sign. The mechanism of production of drug-induced hepatitis is unknown. Iproniazid (Marsilid) was the first monoamine oxidase inhibitor to be associated with this variety of jaundice. It occurred in about 1·4 per cent of patients taking the drug and the mortality of those affected was 25 per cent. The severity of the disease reulted in withdrawal of the drug and although other members of this group of drugs are not immune the risk is less. Hepatocellular jaundice has been recorded following pheniprazine, isocarboxazid, phenelzine and phenoxypropazine. An obstructive jaundice due to intra-hepatic biliary stasis not uncommonly occurs as a result of idiosyncrasy to drugs of the phenothiazine group and to certain of the oral hypoglycaemic agents. It occurs in 1–2 per cent of patients treated with chlorpromazine (Largactil) and is unrelated to the dosage. Cholestasis has also been reported following promazine (Sparine), chlorpropamide (Diabinese) and tolbutamide and also after the antibiotics erythromycin estolate and PAS. The obstructive jaundice may persist for five months or more but ultimate recovery is the rule and parenchymatous liver cell damage is minimal. The cause is not known though excessive permeability of cholangioles causing increased viscosity of the bile has been suggested.

The cholestatic jaundice complicating oral contraceptive therapy is related to idiosyncrasy. It is of interest to note that the only large series of patients with cholestatic jaundice associated with oral contraceptives have come from Scandinavia and Chile. It is from these countries that the cholestatic jaundice of the last trimester of pregnancy has been most commonly described. Indeed half the patients who are sensitive to the contraceptive have suffered from this condition. It would seem, therefore, that these patients have a constitutional defect which renders them sensitive to some steroid in the contraceptive pill, which is also produced during pregnancy.

SECONDARY EFFECTS

Secondary effects are the indirect consequence of the primary action of a drug. They are in no way the pharmacological result of drug administration, but occur because of some effect the drug has produced. The vitamin deficiency and secondary infection with monilia or resistant staphylococci that may occur when the normal bacterial flora of the gut has been altered by antibiotics are examples. Most cases of staphylococcal enterocolitis, which is a serious and frequently fatal condition, seem to be related to the administration of prophylactic antibiotics, particularly the broad-spectrum varieties such as the tetracyclines. Staphylococcal pneumonia may similarly complicate the antibiotic treatment of virus pneumonia. It seems that when the normal flora of the body is altered by treatment with broad-spectrum antibiotics, especially chloramphenicol and tetracycline, there is a liability to super-infection with antibiotic-resistant micro-organisms. Apart from staphylococci and candida albicans, drug-resistant strains of proteus and pycocyanea may occur. Monilia infections are usually confined to the upper and lower end of the gastro-intestinal tract, producing soreness of the mouth and oesophagus or pruritus ani. Infection of the intestines themselves may occur leading to diarrhoea. Infection by such micro-organisms, which have limited pathogenic capacity under normal circumstances, has been called 'opportunistic infection'. Corticosteroids, by their anti-inflammatory effect, may lead to reactivation of a tuberculous focus or diffuse spread of a purulent infection which would otherwise have been localized.

Uric acid calculi and gout may complicate the treatment of polycythaemia rubra vera and leukaemia. Hyperuricaemia may be a feature of these conditions before treatment and indeed the serum uric acid concentrations often exceed the levels found in gout. When the myeloproliferative disorder is treated, with consequent cell destruction and release of nucleoprotein, the serum uric acid levels rise further and the high concentrations in the urine precipitate as urinary gravel. Patients should therefore be advised to drink plenty of fluid and take alkalis to prevent the formation of uric acid acid calculi.

The thrombo-embolic complications of the oral contraceptives are examples of secondary effects. Oestrogen therapy has been known to be associated with an increased incidence of thrombophlebitis for many years, both when given to women for the purpose of suppressing lactation and to men with prostatic cancer. There is also a small but definite risk of thrombo-embolic disease in women on the pill. One in every 2,000 women on the pill is admitted to hospital with venous thrombosis compared with one in 20,000 women not on oral contraceptives. There is also an increased risk of developing cerebral arterial thrombosis which is of the same order as that for venous thrombo-embolism. The contraceptive pills with higher oestrogen content are more likely to cause thrombosis than those with a lower proportion of oestrogen, and most of the high oestrogen preparations have now been withdrawn.

Drug addiction may be considered as a secondary effect, for it is an indirect consequence of a drug action. The opening of new centres in Britain for the treatment of drug addiction is a measure of the increasing problem of addiction to drugs in this country. The official figure of 2,782 for the number of heroin users in Britain in 1968 is almost certainly an underestimate. In addition to the true addicts there are a number of generally stable and integrated individuals who obtain diamorphine for weekend use and have earned themselves the label of 'chippers'. In addition to diamorphine there has always existed a core of addicts to alcohol, morphine and its derivatives, to cocaine and in small numbers to chloral and paraldehyde. In 1968 there were 4,243 convictions in the courts for offences involving drugs controlled under the 1965 Dangerous Drugs Act, an increase of 40 per cent over 1967. Pethidine, phenmetrazine, barbiturate and amphetamine addiction have recently become a real danger and occasional addicts to levorphanol (dromoran), methadone (physeptone) and methylpentynol (Oblivon) occur. It is well to remember that death has followed the withdrawal of barbiturates and meprobamate in those who have been addicted. This is relevant to the management of drug addicts admitted to hospital because of septicaemic pneumonia or other serious illness. Morphine derivatives can be stopped with little hazard to the patient but it may be dangerous to discontinue barbiturates suddenly. Physical dependence on barbiturates is thus not only more severe and dangerous than opiate dependence but more easily overlooked.

HYPERSENSITIVITY AND ALLERGIC REACTIONS

Hypersensitivity may be defined as a drug reaction in which clinical symptoms are conditioned by previous exposure and sensitiztion to the drug. They are mediated by an antigen-antibody reaction. If the drug is a protein it can act by itself as an antigen. Otherwise it may combine with a plasma protein or tissue protein to form an antigenic combination. The lympho-follicular system then forms free or cell-borne antibodies which attach themselves to the antigen that is wrongly recognized as foreign. Antigen-antibody reactions can affect any system in the body and type 1 hypersensitivity reactions are associated with the liberation of histamine or histamine-like substances so that oedema, urticaria or anaphylactic shock are common features. The great majority of drug reactions and many of the most important and serious ones are due to hypersensitivity. However, it is important to realize that a drug may induce an immunological response as evidenced by the formation of circulating antibodies without the production of any clinical manifestations of hypersensitivity. In most individuals who have received penicillin it is possible to detect circulating antibodies but only a few develop hypersensitivity reactions following a further dose.

Fever is a common manifestation of drug allergy and many drugs can cause fever with or without any other features of hypersensitivity. Drug hypersensitivity may be associated with either humoral antibody or with delayed type hypersensitivity.

Hypersensitivity reactions include:

1. Urticarial rashes and angioneurotic oedema
2. Asthma
3. Anaphylactic shock
4. Serum sickness
5. Dermatitis
6. Thrombocytopenic purpura
7. Leucopenia
8. Haemolytic anaemia
9. Arteritis.

Immediate Reaction

The first three of these hypersensitivity reactions tend to occur in persons with a history of allergy and the response is immediate. Drugs which may produce this type of reaction include aspirin, organic arsenicals, penicillin and streptomycin. These reactions are due to type I hypersensitivity, and histamine or a closely related substance is released. It is fallacious to assume that negative skin tests are a safeguard against any of these constitutional reactions. Hypersensitivity reactions to vaccines may also occur and the child with eczema is especially susceptible.

Urticaria is associated with the release of histamine and focal capillary damage. If the process becomes generalized, a large volume of plasma may be diverted from the intravascular compartment into the extracellular tissues with resulting anaphylactic shock. Urticaria is one of the commonest drug reactions, and it is usually associated with intense itching. The eyelids, lips and face are the commonly affected areas. It responds to treatment with adrenaline, ephedrine or antihistamine compounds, and the more severe cases will require short-term corticosteroid therapy, especially if such vital areas as the larynx are involved.

Anaphylactic shock usually occurs within one hour of taking the offending drug, or even earlier if it is given intravenously. It has been associated with a wide variety of drugs, but penicillin, horse serum, arsphenamine and salicylates are probably the most important. Thirty cases of penicillin anaphylaxis in 5 years were recorded in New York City and each year 300 deaths attributable to penicillin occur in the United States of America alone. Oral penicillin has caused fatal anaphylaxis and even topical penicillin has produced a violent anaphylactic reaction. The treatment is urgent and subcutaneous adrenaline, 1 ml. (1:1,000), intravenous hydrocortisone sodium succinate (100 mg. or more) and an intramuscular antihistamine should be given without delay. Nevertheless, serum sickness remains the commonest type of penicillin reaction. Prevention is better than cure, and although these reactions cannot always be prevented, the warning of a patient claiming to be sensitive to a drug must be given the greatest respect.

Delayed Reaction

These include serum sickness, dermatitis, purpura, leucopenia haemolytic anaemia and arteritis. The latent interval between exposure to the antigen and the hypersensitivity reaction varies from a couple of days to many weeks, but it is usually 5–14 days. Drugs causing this type of reaction are usually organic compounds.

There is now little doubt that various forms of vasculitis may be the result of drug hypersensitivity. The rising incidence of polyarteritis nodosa in the years following the introduction of sulphonamides has been attributed to the contribution of cases of arteritis caused by these drugs. Arteritis is probably a better term than periarteritis, as all layers of the artery are involved and the term nodosa is confusing as nodules occur infrequently. 'Hypersensitivity angiitis' covers the wide range of vasculitis induced by drugs. Capillary dilatation with minimal exudation occurs in drug erythema; capillary damage with increased permeability and exudation characterizes urticaria; more severe capillary injury results in rupture with purpuric haemorrhages. These manifestations of capillary injury occur in the viscera as well as in the skin and when the capillaries of renal glomeruli suffer the picture of drug-induced gomerulonephritis is produced. Common clinical manifestations include petechial skin lesions, haematuria and renal failure, often associated with fever, arthralgia, oedema and myositis. This variety of vasculitis is an example of immune-complex disease because it is due to antigen-antibody complexes settling in the small blood vessels and activating complement (p. 84).

The small arteries are a favoured site of drug hypersensitivity reactions and frequently this has serious consequences, for apart from the symptoms produced by the necrotizing arterial lesions, thrombosis of the lumen may occur and tissue necrosis result from ischaemia. Severe hypertension is a familiar result of narrowing of the renal arteries by this process. The most important suspects amongst the drugs believed to cause arteritis are the sulphonamides, but cases have also been reported following phenytoin, arsenicals, thiouracil, phenobarbitone, chlorpromazine, aspirin, gold salts and antibiotics. The Stevens-Johnson syndrome, which comprises erythema multiforme, ulceration of the oral mucosa and urethritis, and which has a vascular basis may be associated with treatment with the long-acting sulphonamides. Three fatal cases attributable to this drug have recently been reported.

Procaine amide is an ester of para-amino benzoic acid with a similar chemical constitution to sulphonamides. Recent evidence suggests that it may occasionally precipitate systemic lupus erythematosus. Arthralgia, cutaneous lesions and positive LE preparations occur and remission usually follows withdrawal of the drug. The antinuclear factor is present in the serum of 44 per cent of patients who have received procaine amide for four months or more. The titre of antinuclear factor, however, bears no relationship to the presence of symptoms. This drug-induced SLE closely resembles the spontaneously occurring disease with the exception that the lung manifestations are much more common in the syndrome caused by procaine amide, whereas renal manifestations are extremely rare. Drug-induced lupus syndromes have also been reported after isoniazid and after a number of chemically dissimilar anti-convulsant drugs. The hydrallazine syndrome is now more of historical interest than clinical importance. When this drug was in frequent use for the treatment of hypertension, nearly 10 per cent of the patients receiving it developed a disease which closely mimicked systemic lupus erythematosus. However, despite the similarity in clinical picture, LE cells were infrequently demonstrated in the peripheral blood and recovery on stopping the drug was the rule.

Serum sickness is a type III hypersensitivity reaction due to circulating antigen-antibody complexes. By definition it is a manifestation of sensitivity to serum but the same clinical and pathological picture can occur 1–3 weeks after the administration of drugs such as penicillin, streptomycin, thiouracils and sulphonamides. In the few fatal cases that have occurred, visceral lesions similar to those of hypersensitivity arteritis have been demonstrated, and the enlarged lymph glands show a cellular proliferation essentially similar to that occuring in the spleen after intense antigenic stimulation.

An increasing number of drugs are known to be associated with hypersensitivity reactions manifested by eosinophilia and transient pulmonary infiltration. Para-aminosalicyclic acid, penicillin, mephensin and nitrofurantoin (Furadantin) have all caused pulmonary eosinophilia.

Thrombocytopenic purpura has been shown to result from the administration of a large number of drugs but apronal (Sedormid) and quinine are the most familiar. The serum of these patients contains an abnormal substance, the antibody, which destroys platelets only in the presence of the drug concerned, thus causing thrombocytopenia. The drug may be taken for days or weeks without untoward symptoms and then suddenly, perhaps following a single dose, purpura develops. Frequently the first attack is mild and ignored, but sometimes it is severe and fatal. Rapid recovery may follow the early withdrawal of the drug and the importance of prompt recognition of these hypersensitivity reactions is of the utmost importance to the health and, indeed, the survival of the patient.

With apronal (Sedormid) lesions of the capillaries may occur independently for purpura appears occasionally in the presence of normal numbers of platelets, and it seems probable that both thrombocytopenia and capillary damage may result from the action of the same antibody. Other drugs which may cause thrombocytopenia include sulphonamides, ergot, digitoxin, antithyroid drugs, barbiturates, sodium aurothiosulphate (Sanocrysin), phenazone derivatives and amidopyrine.

Leucopenia of immunological origin is not uncommonly a reaction to drugs. The mechanism is similar to that found when viral substances lead to the formation of auto-antibodies against leucocytes in such conditions as virus pneumonia and infective mononucleosis. Primary damage to the bone marrow does, of course, occur as a toxic reaction, but in these cases granulopoiesis is rarely affected alone, both erythropoiesis and platelet production also being impaired. Over 200 compounds have been recorded as causing leucopenia, but amidopyrine, organic mercurials, sulphonamides, thiouracils, phenylbutazone, gold, antihistamines, hydantoins and phenacetin are the most important: in many of these circumstances anti-leucocyte agglutinins have been demonstrated to account for the leucopenia. The clinical picture is dominated by the infection the agranulocytosis. The clinical picture is dominated by the infection to which the leucopenia predisposes.

Drug-induced immune haemolytic anaemia is produced by mechanisms similar to those responsible for thrombocytopenia. Red cell antibodies occur much more frequently than frank haemolysis. For example 20 per cent of patients on prolonged methyl dopa therapy develop a positive antiglobulin test but only 1 per cent develop an auto-immune haemolytic anaemia. Other drugs producing haemolytic anaemia include quinine, phenacetin, digitoxin, PAS, antazoline, phenothiazines, salicylazosulphapyridine, nitrofurantoin and vitamin K substitutes.

DRUGS IN COMBINATION

Drugs in combination may cause serious toxic effects from which each individual drug in similar dosage is free when given separately.

Two or more drugs may be prescribed by the same doctor or they may be prescribed by separate doctors each unaware of the other's treatment. Patients also are not forthcoming about treatments obtained from other sources. Nor is communication between general practitioner and hospital out-patient clinic as free as desirable. Dangerous combinations of drugs cannot be avoided by the sheer act of cataloguing and memorizing. (Some examples of drug interactions are, however, given in the table at the end of the chapter.) Multiple prescribing should therefore be avoided whenever possible.

Little is known about the interaction between drugs but it can occur in a variety of ways.

1. One compound may have a direct effect on another, as for example the inactivation of heparin by protamine. One antibiotic may antagonize another: if a bactericidal drug is combined with an antibiotic that is only bacteristatic its effect may be reduced for many bactericidal drugs (such as penicillin) only kill rapidly dividing cells. Tetracycline may thus interfere with the action of bactericidal drugs such as penicillin, streptomycin and particularly methicillin.

2. One drug may alter the intestinal absorption of another. Drugs may react in the gut to form insoluble complexes which are not absorbed: calcium lactate reacts with phytic acid from vegetables, tetracyclines chelate calcium and aluminium. Desferrioxamine chelates iron and prevents its absorption. Aluminium hydroxide decreases the absorption of phosphate. Liquid paraffin may trap fat soluble vitamins and decrease their absorption. More important is the enhanced absorption of alcohol produced by certain drugs such as the phenothiazines which combine a sedative action with an anticholinergic effect. These drugs increase the efficiency of alcohol absorption.

3. Within the circulation one drug may displace another from the plasma protein to which it is bound. Drugs are bound mainly to the albumin fraction and the binding is readily reversible. The unbound fraction of the drug is the biologically active form and so release from plasma binding increases its pharmacological activity. Hence hypoglycaemia results when patients on tolbutamide are given sulphonamides and bleeding may occur when patients on warfarin are given phenylbutazone or clofibrate. The folic acid antagonist methotrexate is displaced from its bond with plasma albumin by such drugs as salicylates and sulphonamides. Toxic manifestations of methotrexate may therefore be precipitated by combined treatment with these drugs. In premature babies, who have relatively small quantities of plasma albumin, sulphonamides may produce toxic effects by displacing bilirubin from its bond with

albumin, enabling unbound bilirubin to diffuse into the brain and cause kernicterus. The pyrazolone compounds such as phenylbutazone, oxyphenbutazone and sulphinpyrazone and the salicylates will displace the following drugs from their binding protein, thereby increasing their biological activity.

(i) Coumarin anticoagulants
(ii) Oral hypoglycaemic drugs of the sulphonylurea series
(iii) Methotrexate
(iv) Long acting sulphonamides.

4. One drug may displace another at its receptor site. Atropine, for example, has no pharmacological activity of its own but, because its structure is sufficiently similar to acetylcholine, it is taken up by the receptor site at the parasympathetic nerve endings and it prevents acetylcholine having its normal effect. Tubocurarine behaves in a similar way at the motor end-plate. Hexamethonium displaces acetylcholine at autonomic ganglia. Spironolactone is a competitive antagonist to aldosterone on the renal tubule. Salicylates antagonize the uricosuric effects of probenecid by competition at renal tubular level.

5. One drug may accelerate or retard the metabolism of another drug. Monoamine oxidase inhibitors block the metabolism of pethidine and certain sympathomimetic amines. Severe reactions may follow when pethidine, morphine, amphetamine or imipramine (Tofranil) is given in addition. Excitement, coma and hyperthermia may occur and sudden respiratory collapse resulting in death has been reported. Phenelzine (Nardil), isocarboxazid (Marplan), nialamide (Niamid) and tranylcypromine (Parnate) demand particular respect in this situation. The dose of each drug alone may be quite safe, but their combination lethal. Alarming hypertensive episodes have been provoked in patients receiving monoamine oxidase inhibitors by taking amphetamine, and dangerous potentiation may occur with ephedrine, adrenaline and noradrenaline. Ephedrine, it should be remembered, is present in many proprietary remedies for dysmenorrhoea, bronchitis and nasal congestion. Some cheeses contain a high content of pressor amines such as tyramine, which may not be inactivated if the enzyme monoamine oxidase is inhibited. Imipramine (Tofranil) may cause sweating, salivation, excitement, coma and hyperthermia in patients taking monoamine oxidase inhibitors. The enzyme monoamine oxidase normally inactivates such drugs as pethidine and the sympathomimetic drugs, so that the effects of these drugs are grossly exaggerated if the enzyme is inhibited. It has been suggested that patients receiving these drugs

should always carry a card stating the compound and dose, just as diabetics and patients receiving corticosteroids should do.

The enzyme systems in the liver concerned with the metabolism and detoxification of drugs are often affected by previous administration of other drugs. Thus treatment with one drug may increase the activity of the enzyme system concerned with detoxifying that drug so that a similarly related compound will be metabolized at an increased rate. This is called enzyme induction. Thus barbiturates accelerate the break-down of coumarin anticoagulants and reduce their pharmacological effect. They also stimulate the enzymes metabolizing griseofulvin, phenylbutazone and phenytoin and so reduce their half life. Drug metabolism can be stimulated by drugs other than barbiturates; the antihistamines, the oral hypoglycaemic agents and the uricosuric agents are examples. On the other hand, one drug may inhibit the enzyme system concerned with the degradation of another so that the effect of the second drug is enhanced. Hence clofibrate may increase the action of anticoagulants. Pheno thiazine tranquillizers potentiate the cerebral depressant effects of hypnotics, alcohol, reserpine and pethidine. Alcohol and hypnotics may also produce true potentiation and many deaths have resulted from this combination. There is always a risk that phenothiazines and antidepressants will potentiate other substances which have pharmacological effects on the nervous system. The pyrazolone drugs inhibit phenytoin metabolism and so potentiate the effects of phenytoin. Similarly allopurinol, by inhibiting the enzyme xanthine oxidase, reduces the degradation of mercaptopurine and hence potentiates its effects.

6. One drug may accelerate or reduce the excretion of another. Probenecid prevents the excretion of penicillin by a direct action on the renal tubules. In addition drugs may alter the renal excretion of other drugs by changing the urine pH. The excretion of weak bases such as mecamylamine, amphetamine and pethidine is accelerated by making the urine acid and there are risks of accumulation when the urine becomes alkaline. Weak acids such as salicylates and phenobarbitone are more rapidly excreted in alkaline urine.

DRUGS IN PREGNANCY

Unnecessary drugs during pregnancy should be avoided because of the adverse effects of some drugs on the foetus in doses which have no harmful effect on the mother. Unnecessary is the operative word because serious disease in the mother will require treatment whether she is pregnant or not and, indeed, untreated disease in the mother may predispose to harmful effects on the foetus. These adverse reactions can be considered under two headings.

Effects due to enhanced pharmacological action

Drugs may pass through the placenta and harm the foetus because their pharmacological effects are enhanced as the enzyme systems responsible for degradation of the drug are undeveloped. Thus, if the drug can pass through the placenta the pharmacological effect on the foetus may be great whilst that on the mother minimal. Anticoagulants may thus induce foetal haemorrhage, ganglion blocking agents produce intestinal ileus in the foetus, and antepartum administration of thiazides produce thrombocytopenia in the new-born. Many progestogens have androgenic side-effects and their administration to mothers for the purpose of preventing recurrent abortion may produce marked virilization of the female foetus. Antithyroid drugs administered in excessive dosage to pregnant women who are thyrotoxic may cause goitres in the foetus and even depress its thyroid function in addition. Bilateral nerve deafness may result in children whose mothers have received streptomycin during pregnancy. The number of cases of otoxicity in children due to this cause is, however, small and the administration of this antibiotic to a pregnant mother should not be withheld when it is clearly indicated. Tetracycline administered during the last trimester commonly stains the deciduous teeth of the child yellow. Whilst the quality of the stained teeth may be affected to some degree this has not been shown to be serious. The second teeth will not be affected unless the child receives subsequent and frequent courses of tetracycline between the ages of 6 months to 5 years. It is important to remember that substances cross the placental barrier just as they cross cell walls or penetrate the blood brain barrier. There is evidence that placental permeability may be altered by changes in the maternal and foetal blood flow, by maternal infection and by haemorrhage. Once the drug has passed the placental barrier its effect will depend on the ability of the foetal tissues to metabolize or detoxify the substance.

Teratogenic effects

It is understandable that a drug may interfere with a mechanism essential for growth and result in arrested or distorted development of the foetus and yet cause no disturbance in the adult, in whom these growth processes have ceased to be relevant. Thus the effect of a drug upon a foetus may differ qualitatively as well as quantitatively from its effect on the mother. The susceptibility of the embryo will depend on the stage of development it has reached when the drug is given. The age of early differentiation, that is from the beginning of the third week to the end of the tenth week of pregnancy is the time of greatest susceptibility. After this time the likelihood of congenital malformation resulting from drug treatment is less, although the death of the foetus can occur at any time as a result of drugs crossing the placental barrier or as a result of their effect on the placental circulation. There is an increased risk to the foetus, due to a failure of placental function, amongst mothers receiving corticosteroid therapy throughout their pregnancy.

It is important to remember that there is no satisfactory test on animals that will clear a drug of the possibility of producing congenital malformation in man. Indeed, many drugs such as aspirin, caffeine, insulin and thyroxine cause foetal abnormalities in some animal species but there is no evidence that they do so in man. Furthermore, the problem must be kept in perspective and it should be appreciated that only 1 per cent of congenital malformations are the result of environmental factors, which include not only drugs but infections such as german measles and irradiation. The risk that any random pregnancy will end in some serious malformation is about 1 in 40.

Circumstantial evidence suggests that the alkylating agents and antimetabolites used in the treatment of reticuloses and leukaemia are teratogenic. There is some evidence that the oral hypoglycaemic agents and antihistamine preparations may also be responsible for a few congenital malformations. It is not surprising that drugs which are specifically designed to kill cells, whether these are neoplastic cells, bacterial cells, fungi or protozoa, should have harmful effects on the undifferentiated and rapidly multiplying cells of the foetus. Drugs which inhibit mitosis have their greatest effect on cells which are dividing most rapidly and these must include the cells of the early embryo. Antibiotics are designed to kill bacterial cells and they should therefore be used with caution in early pregnancy. Chloramphenicol inhibits the normal multiplication of bone marrow cells constantly once a certain blood level is exceeded, and this antibiotic is contra-indicated during pregnancy. Nevertheless, if a pregnant woman develops an infection which requires treatment with antibiotics there is at present insufficient evidence to withhold them.

A drug is unlikely to be teratogenic if it has no other toxic effects in man. However the adverse effects of any drug are not fully appreciated until the drug has been in use for two years and so it is inadvisable to prescribe new compounds to women who might be pregnant. It is always difficult to be certain whether a drug is responsible for a foetal abnormality. This is especially so when the drug is seldom given to mothers at the critical time and when the effect is observed in only a small proportion of foetuses. There is, however, suggestive evidence that the following drugs may be responsible for foetal abnormalities.

1. *Thalidomide*. The relation of thalidomide to foetal abnormalities is well established and approaches 100 per cent when the drug is given from the thirty-fourth to the forty-fifth day of pregnancy. Some 4,500 children in West Germany alone were deformed by this drug.

2. *Cancer chemotherapeutic agents*. There is good evidence that methotrexate causes foetal abnormalities and it seems probable that other drugs that damage rapidly dividing cells, such as busulphan and mercaptopurine, are likely to have harmful effects on the developing foetus. There were 34 abortions in one series of 52 patients given methotrexate during the first trimester. Ten of the 12 foetuses examined had malformations.

3. *Androgenic steroids*. Virilization of the female foetus may occur when the mother is given androgenic steroids. If they are used before the twelfth week fusion of the corpora may occur. Natural progesterone has little androgenic activity but many of the synthetic nortestosterone derivatives are androgenic. The administration of oestrogen does not counteract these androgenic properties.

4. *Corticosteroids*. There is evidence that patients on corticosteroid therapy have a small risk of producing children with cleft palate. There is also evidence that corticosteroids diminish the placental circulation, and in this way provide an increased risk to the foetus.

5. *Phenmetrazine* (*Preludin*). Foetal malformations in two separate pregnancies in a patient taking this drug in the first trimester have been recorded. Although this evidence is not conclusive the possibility of a relationship must be considered.

6. *Tolbutamide*. Both normal and abnormal infants have been born to mothers receiving tolbutamide in early pregnancy. In the experimental animal malformed foetuses have been produced when pregnant animals received tolbutamide. The drug should be avoided in pregnancy, especially as insulin is a more effective treatment for patients with diabetes.

7. *Vitamin D*. The syndrome of aortic stenosis, mental subnormality and hypercalcaemia has recently been reported in association with excessive amounts of vitamin D consumed by the mother.

Conclusion

The first step required to halt the rising incidence of drug-induced diseases is to recognize the fact that ill health is frequently due to drugs. It is therefore of paramount importance to ascertain in detail what drugs have been taken by the patient over the previous months. This must now be an important part of the clinical history of every patient. The labelling of containers with the name of the drug is an essential measure to enable this vital information to be known. Every drug carries a hazard for somebody and a calculated risk is taken every time a drug is administered. It is only safe when its potential benefits outweight its potential side-effects. There are six ways in which we can reduce the morbidity and mortality that results;

1. By recognizing that ill health may be due to drugs.

2. By avoiding the use of drugs for purely placebo effects.

3. By avoiding the use of potentially hazardous drugs for trivial infections and diseases.

4. By watching for hypersensitivity drug reactions as keenly as for direct toxic effects: premonitory symptoms such as fever, rashes, slight haemorrhages, nausea, vomiting, headache, and dyspnoea occur in a significant proportion of patients who are destined to develop serious drug reactions. A routine blood count or test of liver function is no adequate guide or warning of impending disaster and a negative skin test is no guarantee against a hypersensitivity reaction.

5. By knowing the effects and complications of the drugs used. The intelligent administration of a few familiar compounds is far preferable to the random use of a large number of drugs, the virtues of which may depend largely on advertizement.

6. Human understanding and sympathy are two powerful therapeutic remedies, the value of which tends to be neglected in this scientific age. Their place in the management of the functional disorders is of paramount importance and their increased application would obviate the use of many tranquillizers, sedatives and antispasmodics.

Selected Bibliography

MOSER, R. H. (1969) *Diseases of Medical Progress*. 3rd Ed. Thomas, Springfield, III.

Leading Article (1970) Metabolism of Drugs, *Brit. Med. J.* 1, 767.

WITTS, L. J. (1965) Adverse Reactions to Drugs. *Brit. Med. J.* 2, 1081.

Drug	*In conjunction with*	*Effect*
Alcohol	Antihistamine, barbiturates, hypnotics	Enhanced depressant effects on central nervous system
Amphetamines (including appetite suppressants and other cerebral stimulants)	(a) Hypotensive agents (b) Monoamine oxidase inhibitors	(a) Antagonism of hypotensive effects (b) Risk of hypertensive crisis
Anticoagulants	Anabolic agents Clofibrate Phenylbutazone Salicylates	Enhanced anticoagulant effect
Oral hypoglycaemic agents	Monoamine oxidase inhibitors Propranolol Phenylbutazone Salicylates Sulphonamides	Enhanced hypoglycaemic effect
Digitalis	Thiazides	Increased risk of toxicity due to hypokalaemia
Imipramine and related antidepressants	(a) Monoamine oxidase inhibitors (b) Hypotensive agents	(a) Risk of hyperthermia, coma & convulsions (b) Antagonism of hypotensive effect
Monoamine oxidase inhibitors	(a) Amphetamines, sympathomimetic drugs, foods containing tyramine (b) Oral hypoglycaemic agents (c) Imipramine and related antidepressants (d) Hypotensive drugs	(a) Risk of hypertensive crisis (b) Enhanced hypoglycaemic effect (c) Risk of hyperthermia, coma & convulsions (d) Enhanced hypotensive effect
Phenothiazines	Alcohol, barbiturates, hypnotics, reserpine	Enhanced depressant effect on central nervous system
Probenecid	Salicylates	Antagonism of uricosuric action
Propranolol	(a) Oral hypoglycaemic drugs (b) Quinidine (c) Ether	(a) Enhanced hypoglycaemic effect (b) Depressant effect on myocardium (c) Increased risk of cardiac arrhythmia
Tetracycline	Oral iron	Reduced absorption & hence lower blood levels of antibiotic

IV

Immune Mechanisms and Disease

INTRODUCTION

The purpose of the immune mechanism is to defend the body against infection. The immune reaction is stimulated by contact of the lympho-reticular system with micro-organisms and also with certain other foreign materials which are antigenic. The immune system functions through the production of antibody and it may be described functionally as the antibody-forming system or morphologically as the lympho-reticular system. It consists of the collections of reticulum cells, macrophages, lymphocytes and plasma cells found in the spleen, lymph nodes, thymus and Peyer's patches of the gastro-intestinal tract. When an antigen meets a lymphocyte in a non-immune individual the lymphocyte reacts by enlarging and undergoing mitosis. The daughter cells may then either differentiate into plasma cells and synthesize specific immunoglobulin or divide further into a population or clone of sensitized lymphocytes which will react specifically with the antigen. The capacity of antibody to combine with antigen is attributed to the combining sites. An antigen is a macromolecule capable of reacting with antibody on account of a mosaic of molecular outlines which are potential antigen determinants. Many of these molecular configurations are inert because they are similar to self antigens.

The immune response is not confined to bacteria and viruses. Individuals respond immunologically to tissues of other species (hetero-immunity) or to tissues of another individual of the same species (iso-immunity), and may in auto-immune disorders react against their own tissues. The consequences of incompatible blood transfusion and rejection of tissue grafts are manifestations of the immune mechanism.

IMMUNE REACTIONS

Immune reactions are of two types: humoral and cellular. The humoral defences are circulating antibodies which attack bacteria and other foreign constituents and render them more susceptible to phagocytosis. Such antibodies are responsible for resistance to most of the bacterial infectious diseases and the aim of artificial immunization is either to stimulate the development of the patient's own antibodies to the infecting agent or, in the form of passive immunity, to protect the non-immune individual by transferring antibody (gamma globulin) from immunized persons. The primary antibody response which occurs following first contact with an antigen is a limited response of low intensity and short duration. During the

TABLE I

Name	*Function*	*Serum Level* (mg per 100 ml)
IgG :	Acquired antibacterial and antiviral antibodies	800–1600
IgM :	19s Macroglobulin; includes blood group antibodies	50–200
IgA :	7s gamma globulin which appears in secretions	150–420
IgD :	Immunological function unknown	
IgE :	Reagin antibody	

primary antibody response germinal centres develop in the lymph follicles at the same time as the plasma cells begin to proliferate. On a subsequent contact with antigen a secondary response occurs. This is a much more extensive and intense response as a result of which antibody may be produced for many months or years.

Antibody globulin is now called immunoglobulin. In man there are five different types of immunoglobulin and differences in structure between these groups coincide with variations in biological behaviour (Table 1). Most antibodies have a molecular weight of about 160,000 and when their rate of sedimentation is measured they have a sedimentation constant of about 7 Svedberg units (7s). There is, however, another group of antibodies which move faster on electrophoresis, have a greater molecular weight (900,000) and have a sedimentation constant of 19 Svedberg units (19s). Immunoglobulin G, or IgG, constitutes three-quarters of the protein within the electrophoretically defined gamma area of serum. It is a 7s antibody and constitutes the majority of the acquired antibacterial and antiviral antibodies. It is distributed equally between the blood and interstitial tissues and it is the only immunoglobulin which passes across the placenta to reach the foetal circulation. This transfer is not due to simple filtration but to an active cellular process. IgM or macroglobulin is so named because of its high molecular weight (900,000), and is predominantly intravascular. It is a 19s globulin and includes the blood group antibodies. IgG and IgM antibodies combine with antigen to form either soluble complexes or precipitates, depending on the relative proportion of antigen to antibody. They activate complement and this enables them to neutralize toxins, bacteria and viruses and to promote phagocytosis. If the reaction occurs across a vascular membrane the result will be an Arthus reaction consisting of oedema and haemorrhage (p. 84). Complement consists of nine different substances which act as a cascade analogous to the clotting mechanism. Some of the substances making up complement are only present in trace quantities; others can be measured in milligrams. Two of these substances (C 3 & 5) release histamine from mast cells, another (C5) is chemotactic to polymorphs, and others cause damage to cells by forming micelles in the surface layer of cells (C8 & C9). IgA is a 7s gamma globulin synthesized by plasma cells at mucosal surfaces and appearing in secretions in which its concentration is often much higher than that of IgG. IgA antibodies do not activate the complement system: they are mainly protective and are not involved in hypersensitivity reactions. They have been aptly described as an antiseptic paint. The immunological function of the IgD group of antibodies is unknown. IgE possesses reagin activity and may be the anaphylactic antibody in man (p. 83).

Each immunologulin consists of four polypeptide chains. Each has a basic molecular unit of two heavy chains (molecular weight 50,000) joined to light chains (molecular weight 25,000). The heavy chains are specific to the type of immunoglobulin but there are two light chains (k and λ) which are common to all classes of immunoglobulin. The specificity of different antibodies is due to differences in the sequence of aminoacids in those parts of the polypeptide chains which form the antibody combining sites. In normal antibody forming cells immunoglobulin synthesis is so well balanced that none of these peptide chains escape from the cell. In myelomatosis, however, the malignant proliferation of plasma cells results in an imbalanced production of the heavy and light chains of immunoglobulin molecules and the excess of free light chains escapes into the circulation and is filtered through the renal glomeruli as Bence-Jones protein. Such incoordinate production of immunoglobulin is a manifestation of the greater malignancy of the cell and hence augurs a worse prognosis for the disease. It must however be realized that rarely are humoral factors solely responsible for protection against infection, as the scavenger action of cells such as polymorphs and macrophages is also necessary.

Cellular immunity, on the other hand, is mediated by immunologically competent cells or lymphocytes and is not associated with humoral antibody production. Indeed the antibody in cell-mediated immunity remains fixed to the cell surface. The lymphocyte is a cell which, in the absence of antigenic stimulation, circulates through the blood and lymph node back into the circulation again over a period of more than ten years. It performs a policing role awaiting recognition of foreign material. When it encounters foreign material it is able to recognize it as such and responds by multiplication and transformation, which are the ingredients of this type of immune response. Resistance to tuberculosis, for example, depends on cellular and not humoral immunity and the Mantoux reaction is a cellular reaction to antigen injected into the skin. Mycobacteria, fungi and many protozoa have cell walls resistant to the effects of humoral antibody so that cellular immune mechanisms are largely responsible for immunity to these agents. In cellular immunity the antigen must first penetrate a cell and the latent interval between exposure to the antigen and development of the sensitized state varies from a couple of days to many weeks. Cellular immunity thus depends on the release of sensitized lymphoid cells into the circulation and it has no need of circulating antibody. Lymphoid cells house two distinct mechanisms—an afferent mechanism concerned with recognition of antigen, and an efferent mechanism that gives rise to the changed reactivity that follows recognition. A receptor group exists on the surface of a lymphocyte which has a molecular configuration similar to that of the receptor group of an antibody molecule. Such a recognition unit is probably part of the structure of the cell wall. Many lymphocytes can produce a small amount of immunoglobulin and the actual production of antibody can be demonstrated. It seems probable that the receptor group is indeed a minute amount of the antibody the cell is destined to produce. It is well known that delayed hypersensitivity reactions (see later) can be conveyed to normal animals by transfer of lymphocytes.

The humoral antibody response is quick but the cell-mediated response is delayed. The clinical characteristics of these two responses are summarized in Table 2. The lymphoreticular system is concerned with both types of immunity, and many immune reactions require the synergism of a humoral and cell-mediated response. Humoral antibody is conveyed by the mere transfer of serum, cellular antibody by the transfer of sensitized cells. Patients with hypogammaglobulinaemia lose their ability to form humoral antibody but retain their ability to form cellular antibody. The lymphoid cells include fixed reticulum cells, macrophages, lymphocytes and plasma cells. These cells are characterized by their proliferation in response to antigenic stimulation—the so-called reactive hyperplasia of histologists. Lymphocytes are the most numerous cells in lymphoid tissue and they may be large, medium or small. Their morphology, however, gives no indication of their origin, life span, function or fate.

TABLE 2

	Cell-mediated response	*Humoral response*
	(delayed hypersensitivity)	(Arthus reaction)
Time of maximal response	24–48 hours	4–8 hours
Appearance:		
(a) macroscopic	erythema and induration	oedema and haemorrhage
(b) microscopic	mononuclear cells	polymorphs
Production of passive immunity	cells	serum
Systemic manifestations	fever	deposition of immune complexes in organs

Cell mediated immunity is adapted to dealing with antigens that tend to be immobilized peripherally and do not reach the lymphoid tissues. Humoral antibody production is dependent upon antigens reaching the lymphoid tissues and being ingested by macrophages. The medulla of the lymph node is stimulated by the processed antigen and germinal centres are formed. Circulating small lymphocytes are sensitized on contact with a peripheral antigen and then proceed to a local lymph node where they enter the paracortical area and proliferate. They first differentiate into large cells which subsequently divide into a new population of lymphocytes or immunocytes. Recognition thus leads to proliferation and the resulting effector cells act on the antigen.

A small lymphocyte antigenically stimulated develops into a blast cell and may either multiply into a further generation of lymphocytes or in an appropriate environment initiate a clone of plasma cells. The way in which the activated cell develops will depend on its origin—if it is of bone marrow origin it will transform to a plasma cell, and if it is of thymic origin to a lymphocyte.

There are thus two distinct populations of lymphocytes, one dependent on the presence of the thymus ('T' lymphocytes) and the other being dependent on gut-associated lymphoid tissue and independent of the thymus ('B' lymphocytes). Both are concerned with immune responses. They differ in their distribution and in their life span. The former constitute the greater part of the recirculating pool of lymphocytes and have a long life, whilst the latter are more restricted to lymphoid tissue and have a short life. Thymus-dependent lymphocytes are responsible for delayed hypersensitivity and homograft immunity. They do not give rise to plasma cells and produce only minimal amounts of IgM. Gut-dependent lymphocytes give rise to plasma cells producing IgM, IgG, or IgA antibodies. For some types of antibody, production only results from the co-operation of both types of cell but a wide range of other antibodies do not require the co-operation of thymus-dependent cells. Both the thymus-dependent or 'T' lymphocytes and the bone marrow or bursa derived 'B' lymphocytes contain antigen sensitive cells with specific antibody on their surface. Morphologically 'T' lymphocytes and 'B' lymphocytes can not be distinguished but it has recently been shown that 'B' cells carry a heavier density of immunoglobulin on their surface than 'T' lymphocytes and thymocytes. By using radioactively labelled antiglobulin it is possible to identify 'B' lymphocytes. Using this method it has recently been shown that 34 per cent of the circulating blood lymphocytes are bone marrow derived or 'B' lymphocytes and 45 per cent of spleen and marrow lymphocytes have a similar origin.

It is, however, facile to think of the immune response as simply the switching on by antigen of a specialized population of cells which will eventually synthesize antibodies. At least three types of cell are necessary but the nature of their interactions is not fully understood. These are (1) macrophages (2) reactor cells (3) effector cells. Firstly the macrophage is required to process the antigen. The processing of antigen leads to the presentation of antigen-determinants at the cell surface and this is a prerequisite for the stimulation of thymic-dependent lymphocytes. The processing of antigen requires the coupling of an antigen fragment to a species of RNA and the transfer of this so-called immunogenic-RNA to the precursors of antibody-forming cells. Secondly reactor cells are required to identify the foreign nature of the antigen and to initiate the immune response. Thirdly effector cells must then actually synthesize the antibody. Both reactor and effector cells have similar histological appearances. In fact the round cells with the high nucleus to cytoplasm ratio which we describe as lymphocytes are a heterogenous collection of cells with different origins, functions, fates and life spans. The reactor cells are cells of thymic origin with a long life span and are components of the circulating lymphocyte pool. Effector cells on the other hand are short-lived and reside predominantly within the follicular zones of the lymph nodes. Animal experiments have demonstrated that thymus-derived cells identify foreign antigenic material and can initiate the production of antibody-producing cells. These antibody-forming cells do not, however, originate in the thymus but in the bone marrow. It seems that cells derived from the thymus react with the specific antigen and multiply before in some way directing another population of cells derived from the bone marrow cell to produce antibody.

HYPERSENSITIVITY

The term hypersensitivity is applied to the abnormal immunological reactions produced in certain individuals when re-exposed to antigens that are innocuous to normal individuals. A good deal of ambiguity has arisen over the use of the words allergic and hypersensitive. It is therefore important to define these terms precisely. Antigen or allergen stimulates an allergic response. This produces a state of altered reactivity or an allergic state. Such a state of altered reactivity may be beneficial to the host as in establishing a state of immunity, or it may be harmful to the host and produce a state of disease. When allergic reactions afford protection they are called immune reactions. Hypersensitivity can be regarded as an allergic reaction in an individual sensitized by previous exposure to the antigen and in whom the allergic process constitutes the disease. The distinguishing feature of immunity is the lack of clinical reaction on exposure to a dose of micro-organism that would have caused disease in susceptible subjects. Hypersensitivity can, like immunity, be mediated by circulating antibodies or be of the delayed type and mediated by sensitized lymphoid cells.

Hypersensitivity reactions are of four varieties and each of these may be responsible not only for hypersensitivity reactions to bacterial, viral and protozoal infections but also for certain drug-induced diseases and auto-immune disorders. They are:

Type 1 hypersensitivity (anaphylactic)
Type 2 hypersensitivity (cytotoxic)

Type 3 hypersensitivity (Arthus reaction with damage by antigen-antibody complexes)
Type 4 hypersensitivity (delayed hypersensitivity)

The first three of these reactions are induced by humoral antibodies and the fourth is mediated by sensitized lymphoid cells and is the so-called delayed hypersensitivity reaction. These types of reaction may occur together for the allergic response usually acts as a co-ordinated system.

Type 1 hypersensitivity (anaphylactic). In this type of reaction antibody is fixed on the surface of cells. When an antigen meets antibody in this situation an immunological reaction takes place on the cell surface and the cell membrane permeability is increased and histamine, serotonin and plasma kinins escape. The cells, however, are not damaged or killed and the hypersensitivity results from the pharmacological effects of the escaped substances. Most antibodies in man do not stick to cells but certain patients do produce an abnormal type of antibody called a reagin which readily becomes attached, especially to mast cells. IgE is the reagin antibody in man. IgE antibody does not precipitate with antigen and does not fix complement. The tendency to form this reagin and hence to become sensitized is inherited and is called atopy, and its manifestations are often accompanied by eosinophilia. Atopic subjects comprise approximately 10 per cent of the population. The reagin antibodies are produced on exposure to various antigens such as pollen and animal dusts. Urticaria, hay fever and asthma are typical examples of this type of hypersensitivity. Reagin antibodies may develop to inhaled, ingested or injected antigens. Desensitization is associated with the development of blocking antibodies and its effectiveness will depend on the amount of antigen to which the patient is subsequently exposed (as for example the pollen count). It is surprising that a different type of antibody (blocking) can be developed to the same antigen but the different route of administration utilized in desensitization may be relevant as demonstrated by the parenteral administration of an antigen normally inhaled.

Type 2 hypersensitivity (cytotoxic reactions). In this type of reaction the antigen is carried on the surface of the cell. The antigen may be a component of the tissue cell or a hapten which has become associated with the tissue cell. When antibody, in the presence of complement, meets the fixed antigen the cell is damaged and even destroyed. In haemolytic anaemia resulting from ABO blood group incompatibility, Rhesus disease of the new-born or auto-immune haemolytic anaemia the red cell is damaged by circulating antibody with consequent haemolysis. The thrombocytopenic purpura following apronal (Sedormid) or quinidine is an example of a drug hapten forming an antigenic complex with a tissue protein; antibody damages the complex, causing thrombocytopenia.

Type 3 hypersensitivity (Arthus reaction with damage by antigen-antibody complexes). In this type of reaction disease is caused by antigen-antibody-complement complexes. This is the mechanism of the Arthus reaction. The Arthus reaction occurs when there is a high concentration of conventional antibody (IgG) in the circulation and a high concentration of soluble antigen lying extravascularly in the tissue spaces. The wall of small blood vessels is one of the commonest sites of antigen-antibody reaction as antibody is present in the circulation and antigen often lies in the extravascular space. When antigen in the tissue reacts with IgG antibody across the walls of small blood vessels the various components of complement are fixed at the site and the kinins and other pharmacological mediators of inflammation are liberated. Vascular damage occurs leading to oedema, erythema and purpura.

In addition antigens form stable combinations with antibodies at varying concentrations and most of these do not cause harm. When there is an excess of antigen in the circulation unstable antigen-antibody complexes are formed and these are deposited in the walls of small arterioles, especially those of the kidney and heart, or in basement membranes, and cause local arteritis in a manner similar to that of the Arthus reaction, producing areas of localized tissue damage. An acute inflammatory process affecting the small blood vessels is thus produced. Later hyaline intimal thickening (fibrinoid) becomes prominent and this fibrinoid material contains antigen, immunoglobulin and components of complement. This type of reaction, unlike reagin antibody effects, damages tissues as a result of necrosis and haemorrhage. This is the mechanism of serum sickness hypersensitivity and some of the sensitivity reactions to penicillin and sulphonamides when lesions such as arthritis, glomerulonephritis and allergic arteritis predominate. It is also the way in which the tissue lesions of systemic lupus erythematosus and some other connective tissue disorders are caused. Serum sickness resolves when the supply of antigen is used up. If there is a continuous supply of antigen as in SLE the disease is self-perpetuating. Alternatively, these antigen-antibody complexes may be taken up by polymorphs and cause rupture of the cell lysosomes. Lysosomes are intracellular vesicles, which contain a number of hydrolytic enzymes whose function is to digest material taken into the cell by phagocytosis. If these enzymes are released into the circulation they may cause inflammation. Damage by antigen-antibody complexes is probably a part of many diseases believed to be due to a hypersensitivity mechanism.

Type 4 hypersensitivity (Delayed or cellular hypersensitivity). In this type of reaction tissue damage and disease are wrought by immunocytes which are sensitized mononuclear cells or lymphocytes that are altered in some way by contact with antigen to contain something in the nature of an antibody. Although the development of sensitized lymphocytes is an important defence mechanism in many parasitic, viral and bacterial infections, it may cause considerable destruction of tissues in the vicinity of the infective agent. The caseous necrosis of tuberculosis is an example. The damage in dealyed hypersensitivity is caused by infiltration by sensitized lymphocytes which replace tissue containing the antigen. Contact dermatitis, tuberculin sensitivity and certain bacterial and parasitic infections are examples of this delayed type of sensitivity. This is the mechanism of the tissue damage wrought in many auto-immune diseases which will be considered later.

Immunological tolerance

The immune reaction is essentially protective and the fact that it could be harmful has only recently been recognized. Thus anaphylaxis may be fatal and serum sickness may be a serious disease. The immune mechanisms cannot differentiate the harmful from the harmless antigen and the immune response occurs with equal enthusiasm against either. However, the body is able to recognize its own tissues, for the immune apparatus can differentiate between what is 'self' and what is 'not self'. The breakdown of this ability leads to auto-immune disease, in which the body produces humoral and cellular antibodies against its own tissue components.

The process by which a lymphocyte can recognize self components has been the subject of a good deal of debate. Originally it was believed that every body cell carried a means of identification. It was called a 'self marker' and it was supposed that lymphocytes could actually recognize these badges of the home team. When recognition failed an immune response resulted. More recently it has become accepted that it is the lymphocytes that carry the recognition units and that for a foreign protein to be recognized it must find a corresponding receptor on the lymphocyte. A preconceived recognition unit for every potential antigen must therefore exist and the lymphocyte must also carry a sample of the antibody it could make when stimulated. The varieties of recognition unit must be enormous for there are over 2,000 types of Salmonella alone, each of which produces its own specific immune response.

It appears that there are in the body a multitude of antigen-sensitive lymphocytes bearing individually one type of this vast array of recognition units. Such diversity of lymphocytes is not, however, quite so difficult to accept when one appreciates that the production of every protein is controlled by a specific gene, so that before any antibody protein can be synthesized the gene controlling its production must pre-exist (p. 24).

The specific lack of response of the lympho-reticular system to the body's own antigens is known as immunological tolerance and the breakdown of this tolerance leads to auto-immune disease. Auto-immune disease has been defined as a condition in which structural or functional damage is produced by the action of immunologically competent cells or antibodies against normal components of the body. The antibodies produced against the body's own antigens are called auto-antibodies. They must be distinguished from iso-antibodies which are produced against antigens of another member of the same species (for example blood group incompatibility and graft rejection) and from hetero-antibodies which are produced against antigens of a different species.

How this tolerance develops is uncertain but it is known that there is a period in early life when the lympho-reticular system responds to contact with an antigen, not by the development of antibody but by the development of tolerance.

There are three possible responses of an immunologically competent cell or immunocyte to contact with the appropriate antigenic determinant.

(1) Destruction: this is especially likely to occur if the immunocyte is physiologically immature.

(2) Proliferation without an essential change in character of the cell (i.e. memory cells).

(3) Proliferation and antibody production as a clone of plasma cells.

The acquisition of tolerance may be explained by postulating that in foetal life antigen inhibits cell activation instead of stimulating it. Even after foetal life the dose of antigen to which a cell is exposed or the way the antigen is presented to the cell may determine whether antibody production or tolerance results. It has recently been postulated that direct access of antigen to lymphocytes results in cell death. In this way those lymphocytes which bear corresponding receptors are eliminated and tolerance ensues. Immunization, on the other hand, is brought about by the presentation of antigen to lymphocytes by a second cell, the macrophage. If this is the explanation of tolerance failure to eliminate clones of lymphocytes reacting with self antigen would provide a basis for auto-immune reaction. If after the acquisition of tolerance the antigen is continuously present and in contact with the lympho-reticular system, this tolerance may persist indefinitely. It seems that immunologically competent cells which come into contact with an antigen before their maturation is complete become tolerant, whereas cells which encounter the antigen when they are fully mature respond by making antibody.

Experimentally, tolerance to a specific antigen can be induced by injecting the antigen into an animal foetus some time before antibody production begins. This time varies from species to species but is usually about the time of birth. The reactivity of the antibody forming tissue is thus largely determined by the antigens present when these tissues are reaching maturity. In the freemartin, in which non-identical twins of cattle share a common placental circulation, there is a mutual exchange of circulating cells and tolerance is established to cells of the second twin which would have otherwise been antigenic. Tolerance is thus a function of foetal life and the altered reaction of the lympho-reticular system is a feature of immaturity of the antibody-forming tissues. It must be realized, however, that immunological tolerance is not absolute. It can occasionally be broken down by a strong antigenic stimulus where it would have remained intact had the stimulus been weaker. Furthermore, exposure to antigen before birth does not induce unresponsiveness once and for all. For tolerance to last, restimulation with antigen is required. Experimentally tolerance can be prolonged indefinitely by the appropriate timing of injections of bovine serum albumin into rabbits. Just before the tolerance induced by the previous injection is lost another injection is given and in this way tolerance to this foreign protein may be prolonged indefinitely.

Red cell iso-antibodies appear in the circulation during the second half of the first year. It is probable that these antibodies develop as a result of an immune response to intestinal bacteria with antigens that cross-react with A or B blood group substances. If the individual carries A or B antigens on the surface of the red cells he will have become tolerant to these antigens during embryonic life and will therefore not develop those iso-antibodies which appear in the serum of those who do not carry these antigens.

MECHANISMS OF AUTO-IMMUNITY

Auto-immune haemolytic anaemia, thyroiditis, systemic lupus erythematosus, pernicious anaemia, myasthenia gravis, Sjogren's disease, rheumatic fever and rheumatoid arthritis are a few of many diseases now recognized to be associated with auto-immunity. How the disease actually arises in these situations is still largely a matter of speculation but there appear to be three processes which may give rise to auto-immunization. They are:

(1) Alteration in the antigen

(2) Defect of the immunocyte

(3) Breakdown of tolerance

An alteration in the antigen. Many tissues of the body to which tolerance has been established may be altered as a result of infection, irradiation or drugs so as to modify them antigenically and render them foreign to the lympho-reticular or antibody forming system. Certainly in the experimental animal pertussis vaccine has been used successfully in association with adrenal and testis extracts to induce adrenalitis and orchitis respectively. Alternatively, there may be a somatic mutation in the tissue so that a component of the tissue to which the body was previously tolerant now becomes antigenic. It has been suggested that escape into the circulation of a tissue antigen to which tolerance had not been acquired might provoke an auto-immune reaction. 'Segregated antigen diseases' were proposed as a group of auto-immune diseases in which the relevant tissue antigen was inaccessible to the lympho-reticular system and so failed to establish immunological tolerance in early life. When the lympho-reticular system encounters this substance after immunological maturity has developed, an immune response is stimulated without there being any inherent abnormality of the lympho-reticular system. The resulting disease was essentially a localized auto-immune process confined to one specific tissue and the antibodies are specific for that particular tissue; that is, they are organ-specific antibodies. There are certainly a number of auto-immune diseases with organ-specific antibodies and pathologically they are characterized by infiltration and replacement of the organ containing the antigen by sensitized lymphocytes, the disease being due to a deficiency of the secretion normally produced by the tissue involved. Infiltration and destruction of the parietal cells of the stomach leads to atrophic gastritis with impaired production of intrinsic factor. Local antibody to intrinsic factor occurs in the gastric juice of all patients with pernicious anaemia. A circulating auto-antibody to intrinsic factor may combine to ensure a deficiency of this carrier protein of vitamin B_{12} so that pernicious anaemia results. Infiltration and destruction of thyroid parenchyma leads to impaired thyroxine production and hypothyroidism. It may be that some antigens are inaccessible and so do not provoke tolerance. The lens protein is probably an example.

It was originally believed that thyroglobulin was segregated from lymphoid tissue because cell membranes had provided a barrier that prevented it reaching lymphoid tissue and so it had never had the opportunity to induce tolerance. However, this is probably not true as local thyroid damage does not produce subsequent antibodies to thyroglobulin and indeed, in monkeys at any rate, thyroglobulin is a normal constituent of the lymph leaving the thyroid.

Auto-immunization with antibody formation is readily achieved experimentally with brain, testis, thyroid, adrenal, uveal tract and lens antigens. These tissues contain organ-specific antigens and are antigenic in animals without admixture of Freund adjuvant. Inaccessible antigens do not provoke tolerance in the normal individual. When infection occurs with a micro-organism which happens to carry a major antigenic determinant equivalent to one of the inaccessible body antigens, the normal response takes place, giving rise to antibody and an increased population of immunocytes. This does not in itself give rise to an attack on the cells carrying the equivalent body antigen any more than simple immunization of a rabbit with a thyroid extract provokes damage to the thyroid. In both cases some additional aggressiveness of the immunocyte is needed and this may be either genetic in origin or invoked by the use of Freund's adjuvant in the experimental situation. When rabbits are immunized with rabbit thyroglobulin combined with a hapten, the antibodies which are formed react not only with the altered thyroglobulin but also with the unaltered thyroglobulin. It may therefore be possible for the auto-immune disease to be induced by an immune response to an altered body constituent and be maintained by the normal tissue.

The crystalline lens protein of the eye and constituents of the uveal tract are segregated and if they enter the circulation following injury they may stimulate antibody production with resulting damage to the lens or uveal tract. The condition of phaco-anaphylactic endophthalmitis is believed to be the result of a hypersensitivity to lens protein, which sometimes follows the removal of a cataract in man. The escape of lens protein during cataract operations may lead to an immune reaction and result in inflammatory changes around the lens of the opposite eye. This condition is likely to be the result of auto-immunization to a constituent of lenticular protein. Certainly lens protein is antigenic and patients with the disease show sensitivity to lens protein injected intradermally.

Sympathetic ophthalmia is an uveitis due to auto-immunity; in this condition an immune response to tissue antigens escaping from the ciliary body and iris, as a result of perforating injury, stimulates an inflammatory reaction in the contralateral eye about two to six weeks later. This is associated with circulating antibodies to uveal antigens and the disease responds to corticosteroid therapy. A similar disease can be induced in animals by injecting extracts of ciliary body together with Freund's adjuvant. Spermatozoa only appear after foetal life and they are sufficiently distinct antigenically to act as antigens even in the animal of their source. Indeed it has been shown that spermatozoa acquire during maturation an antigen that is absent from immature germinal cells. The penetration of spermatozoa into the interstitial tissues of a testis following obstruction to the vas deferens may lead to the development of sperm antibodies.

Modification of antigen leading to antibody production is the cause of a thrombocytopenic purpura due to apronal (Sedormid) and quinidine. Antibodies are formed to the complex of platelet and drug and the resulting agglutination leads to thrombocytopenia. In vitro, the antibody does not react with platelets unless the drug is added. The foreign non-antigenic substance is known as a hapten. It is not itself antigenic but when combined with a plasma or tissue protein it becomes antigenic. In quinine purpura the antibody is directed towards the platelet as modifed by the drug. Malarial infestation of red blood cells may render them antigenic and precipitate the haemolysis characteristic of black-water fever.

Mycoplasma pneumoniae infections are commonly associated with the presence of cold agglutinins in the serum which react with the patient's own red cells and may produce a mild haemolytic anaemia. These antibodies are macroglobulins (IgM) reacting against the I antigen on the red cells. There is no cross-reaction between these cold agglutinins and antibodies against the mycoplasma and it seems that the infecting organism in some way modifies the 'I' antigen of the red cells and stimulates an immune response.

Methyl dopa often results in the development of antibodies directed against Rhesus antigens normally present on the patient's own erythrocytes. The drug seems able to unmask these antigens which are normally present on the cell surface and to alter them in such a way that they produce an immunological reaction.

There are two distinct types of drug allergy depending on whether the antibody response is humoral or cell mediated. If the response is humoral antibody production it takes the form of a serum sickness type of disease or more rarely an anaphylactic response. If the drug induces a cell-mediated immune response the individual will develop a contact sensitivity whenever he takes the drug.

In certain situations the converse to apronal purpura may occur, in which the hapten is endogenous and the protein exogenous. This is believed to be the mechanism whereby streptococci precipitate such diseases as rheumatic fever and glomerulonephritis. Reiter's syndrome following bacillary dysentery, gonococcal urethritis or the non-gonococcal urethritis due to mycoplasma probably have a similar basis. In acute glomerulonephritis a streptococcal infection of the pharynx is followed by the development of circulating streptococcal antigen of which the nephritogenic streptococcal antigens become fixed to the renal glomeruli. As antibody production against the streptococcus occurs circulating antibody reacts with the antigen fixed to the kidney causing acute glomerulonephritis.

Alternatively antibodies produced against bacteria may cross-react with normal tissue components. It has been shown that antibodies arising as the result of Group A haemolytic streptococcal infections cross-react with the human heart owing to the existence of common antigens between the infecting organism and cardiac muscle. Such an immune reaction may be responsible for the production of the heart lesions of rheumatic fever. A similar cross-reaction between intestinal bacteria (Esch. coli) and colonic epithelium is believed to play a role in the pathogenesis of ulcerative colitis. It has been shown experimentally that rabbits tolerant of bovine serum albumin will produce antibodies that cross-react with this antigen if immunized with sheep serum albumin. Similary rabbits immunized with conjugated thyroglobulin produce antibodies that cross-react with normal thyroglobulin and they also develop lesions in the thyroid gland.

A defect of Immunologically Competent Cells. The antibody-forming cells or immunocytes may alter as a result of mutation and these altered cells may not recognize the normal tissue components as belonging to the body. This is believed to be the mechanism of the auto-immune haemolytic anaemia secondary to such frankly neoplastic diseases of lympho-follicular tissue such as Hodgkin's disease, chronic lymphatic leukaemia and lymphosarcoma, and a similar mechanism probably occurs in idiopathic auto-immune haemolytic anaemia as well. It is significant that autoimmune haemolytic anaemia seldom occurs in other types of malignant disease such as carcinoma. Experimentally, alteration in the immune mechanism may be achieved by grafting adult lymphoid tissue into recipient neonatal animals. The neonatal recipient is unable to reject the graft owing to the immaturity of its antibody-forming tissue, but the grafted lymphoid cells do not tolerate the tissues of the recipient and initiate a graft versus host reaction which precipitates 'runt disease'. Thus in this disease an abnormal clone of cells is injected from outside. The animal fails to thrive, appears stunted and dies in a few weeks, but before death it may show an auto-immune type of haemolytic anaemia as well as arthritis and arteritis. Not only is there circulating antibody to red cells, but 'cell-bound antibodies' to many of the host antigens are also produced. The most convincing parallel to auto-immune disease can be found amongst mice of a particular inbred strain called the New Zealand Blacks. They develop auto-immune haemolytic anaemia and nephritis due to a genetic predisposition to mutation of their immunologically competent cells, probably precipitated by virus infection (p. 207).

A breakdown of Tolerance. Immunological tolerance may, under certain circumstances, break down. Disorder of the cellular recognition system results. The maintenance of tolerance is dependent upon the persistence of antigen and tolerance could break down if for some reason the contact between antigen and the lymphoreticular system were broken and later renewed. Alternatively, the suppressing mechanism which must exist to destroy any abnormal immunocytes that arise (the 'forbidden clones') may break down. In such 'disturbed tolerance diseases' auto-antibodies to many tissue components arise and the pathological lesions are widespread. This mechanism possibly explains the manifestations of systemic lupus erythematosus where antibodies to red cell antigens, platelet antigens, constituents of cell nuclei, thyroid antigens and others may be formed. In this situation circulating auto-antibodies are formed and cellular immunity develops to antigens which are not foreign and which have been continuously present in the circulation and thus freely accessible to the antibody-forming system. These antigens are widely distributed in the body. In the case of deoxyribonucleic acid (DNA), to which the anti-nuclear factor is an antibody, it is even present in the antibody-forming cells themselves. Tolerance to DNA must exist in the normal state. Furthermore, antibodies are also formed against substances which are not good antigens, such as the constituents of cell nuclei, normal platelets and proteins of the clotting mechanism. These antigens fail to stimulate auto-antibody production when injected into experimental animals.

In diseases due to a disturbance of immunological tolerance the mechanism must be a disorder of the immunological system itself. Arteritis is a characteristic feature of these disorders and the pathological changes are due to the deposition of antigen-antibody complexes in the walls of the small blood vessels with the consequent activation of the complement cascade (p. 78). Systemic lupus erythematosus (SLE) is the most familiar example of this group of disorders. In the families of patients with SLE there are often abnormalities of gammaglobulin synthesis, such as hypergammaglobulinaemia and hypogammaglobulinaemia, suggesting a familial disturbance of the antibody-forming system.

To summarize, auto-immune disorders can be divided into two fundamentally different categories. They may be the result of a primary disturbance of the antigen, in which case antibody formation is specific for an antigen of the particular organ and the lesions of the disease are due to lymphocyte invasion and destruction of that organ. Thyroiditis and pernicious anaemia are examples. Alternatively, the disease process may be due to a primary disturbance of the antibody-forming system, namely a disorder of tolerance. Such a disorder is an abnormality of the cellular recognition system. Here the antibodies are various and are not restricted to any one organ, and the lesions are widespread resulting from the deposition of immune complexes in small blood vessels.

Although segregation into these two categories is useful in order to understand the factors causing auto-immune disease, it is not precise. Auto-immune disorders are a spectrum of diseases in which these two groups form the extremes. Even in disturbed antigen diseases there must be some enhanced reactivity of the lympho-reticular system. Half the relatives of patients with auto-immune thyroiditis have circulating antibodies to thyroid antigens without clinical evidence of disease, although focal lesions in the thyroid are often present. Patients with one disease not infrequently have auto-antibodies characteristic of other disorders in the group. Indeed, patients sometimes have more than one auto-immune disease and the association of thyroiditis with pernicious anaemia is a good example. Furthermore, there is a group of auto-immune diseases in which the tissue infiltration by sensitized lymphocytes is confined to a single organ but antibody production is more general and not specific for any one organ. Myasthenia gravis and Sjogren's disease are examples. In these disorders the tissue infiltration and damage is limited to a single organ, the muscle and salivary glands respectively, but circulating antibodies are formed to a wide variety of antigens and circulating anti-nuclear factor is commonly found in both these conditions.

Diseases in which auto-immunity is recognized as playing an important part may thus be considered as:

1. A predominant disturbance of the antigen.

2. A predominant disturbance of immune tolerance.

3. An intermediate group in which tissue infiltration is limited to a single organ but circulating antibody formation is widespread.

4. A group in which bacterial or viral infection initiates auto-immune disease, the disease usually going into remission when the infection is eradicated.

Group 1. Disturbed antigen diseases.

(a) Hashimoto's disease.
(b) Primary sporadic myxoedema.
(c) Atrophic gastritis (pernicious anaemia).
(d) Idiopathic Addison's disease.
(e) Granulomatous orchitis.
(f) Sympathetic ophthalmia.
(g) Phaco-anaphylactic endophthalmitis.
(h) Some cases of acute polyneuritis.
(i) Some cases of acute encephalopathy (e.g. following rabies vaccination).

Group 2. Disturbed tolerance disease.

(a) Systemic lupus erythematosus.
(b) Rheumatoid arthritis.
(c) Dermatomyositis.
(d) Auto-immune haemolytic anaemia.

Group 3. Intermediate group.

(a) Sjogren's disease.
(b) Myasthenia gravis.
(c) Discoid lupus erythematosus.
(d) Ulcerative colitis.
(e) Diffuse interstitial fibrosis of the lungs.

Group 4. Diseases initiated by steptococcal, mycoplasma or viral viral infections.

(a) Rheumatic fever.
(b) Acute glomerulo-nephritis.
(c) Auto-immune haemolytic anaemia secondary to mycoplasma or viral infections.

ANTIBODIES AND DISEASE

Both circulating antibodies and lymphocytes have the capacity to produce tissue damage and disease. Humoral auto-antibody in the circulation can only cause damage where the antigens are easily accessible, such as the formed elements of blood and vascular endothelium. In auto-immune haemolytic anaemia red cell damage is caused by circulating antibody. However, circulating antibody is unable to produce lesions in solid tissues, where a barrier prevents penetration of the antibody to the surface of the antigen-bearing cell. In solid vascularized tissue auto-immune damage is wrought to parenchyma and blood vessels by direct invasion of lymphocytes and other immunologically competent cells coming from the circulation, and it is these lymphocytes that are the important factor in the pathogenesis of most auto-immune diseases. Hence there is often little correlation between the titre of circulating antibodies and the pathological changes in the tissues. It is, however, possible that the circulating antibodies participate in the production of disease by entering the tissue through the lesions induced by the lymphocytes. Certainly serum from patients with Hashimoto's disease will kill thyroid cells in tissue culture. In the rejection of homografts, whether of skin or kidneys, there is direct destruction of tissue and blood vessels and it is the sensitized lymphoid cells coming from the recipient's circulation that are responsible, the antigen being present in the cells of the graft. The passive transfer of living lymphoid cells from sensitized donors to normal animals has produced encephalitis, auto-immune haemolytic anaemia, thyroiditis and glomerulonephritis when the passive transfer of serum had failed.

The circulating humoral antibodies may often be a by-product of the disease rather than the cause (as occurs with antibodies to heart muscle arising after myocardial infarction), and the mere demonstration of circulating auto-antibodies does not establish with certainty the immune nature of the disease.

It is difficult to prove that a disease is caused by an auto-immune disturbance. The mere demonstration of auto-antibodies is not enough and the injection of such antibodies into a normal human being, to see if they cause disease, is obviously not justified. Much of the evidence of an auto-immune aetiology must therefore depend on animal experiments and the demonstration of certain points is necessary before an auto-immune aetiology can be seriously considered. These include:

1. The presence of specific antibodies against some tissue constituent in patients with the disease.

2. The antigen should be capable of inducing lesions similar to the disease when injected into an experimental animal.

3. The disease of the experimental animal should be transferable to a normal animal by means of serum or suspensions of lymphocytes.

AUTO-IMMUNE DISEASES

It will be profitable to consider certain diseases in which an auto-immune aetiology is beyond reasonable doubt. It is often difficult to be certain that a disease is caused by auto-immune mechanisms. There are, however, five clinical criteria upon which a diagnosis of auto-immunity is judged. They are:

1. Hypergammaglobulinaemia: a gammaglobulin concentration of more than 2 g. per 100 ml.
2. Circulating antibodies to the relevant antigen.
3. Lymphoid invasion of the relevant tissue.
4. Response to corticosteroid therapy.
5. Association with other auto-immune diseases.

Auto-immune Haemolytic Anaemia

Auto-immune haemolytic anaemia is one of the disturbed tolerance diseases and it was one of the earliest disorders shown to be due to auto-immunity. In this disease fixed immunoglobulin is found on the red cells of the patient with haemolytic anaemia. This immunoglobulin can be eluted from the cell and shown to behave as a specific antibody to known red cell antigens, which are present on the red cells of most normal people. The red cells of patients with auto-immune haemolytic anaemia are not antigenic when transfused into subjects of compatible blood group. Thus there does not appear to be any abnormality in the antigen, but for some reason the lympho-reticular system has produced immunocytes reacting against an apparently normal red cell antigen. This antibody is demonstrated by the Coombs', or anti-globulin, test. In this test anti-human globulin is prepared by the injection of human serum into rabbits. The rabbit serum then contains an anti-human gammaglobulin factor which, when mixed with red cells coated with human gamma-globulin, causes the cells to agglutinate.

It is not surprising that in neoplastic disease of lympho-reticular tissues such as chronic lymphatic leukaemia, lymphosarcoma and Hodgkin's disease, abnormal lymphocytes should be produced. Some of them synthesize antibodies reacting against normal red cell antigens and when this happens a secondary auto-immune haemolytic anaemia results. In most cases of auto-immune haemolytic anaemia there is no apparent disease of the lympho-reticular tissue and the abnormal antibody-producing cells are assumed to have arisen by somatic mutation. The presence of antibody on the red cells leads to the sequestration of the cells in the red pulp of the spleen, probably because these coated cells adhere to one another in the slowed circulation of the spleen pulp and they then cannot fit through the small exits into the spleen sinuses. Immune mechanisms may cause thrombocytopenia and leucopenia in a similar way.

Connective Tissue Disorders

Systemic lupus erythematosus, polyarteritis, dermatomyositis, progressive systemic sclerosis and rheumatoid arthritis are diseases of connective tissue which are believed to be auto-immune in nature, although this is not proven. The histological feature of this group of diseases is fibrinoid degeneration of collagen and intercellular connective tissue, and this gave the name 'collagen diseases' to these disorders. In addition diffuse vasculitis of terminal vessels with infiltration of tissues by lymphocytes and plasma cells is characteristic. The term 'fibrinoid' was introduced to describe material which had the histological appearance of fibrin. Fibrinoid is of diverse origin but the main sources are nucleoprotein, gammaglobulin and fibrin. Firbrinoid degeneration of connective tissue probably represents degraded antibody complexes in collagen fibres.

In systemic lupus erythematosus circulating antibodies occur to a wide variety of tissue constituents including erythrocytes, leucocytes, platelets and even to nucleic acid constituents, which are present in the antibody-forming cells themselves. The false positive serological tests for syphilis are also reflections of abnormal antibody production. The LE cell which is characteristic of SLE arises from a reaction between the nucleus of a damaged polymorphonuclear leucocyte and antibody in the circulating plasma. As a result the nucleus swells, loses its structure and is phagocytosed by a normal leucocyte. This phagocytosed nuclear material within a living leucocyte provides the characteristic picture of the LE cell. The antinuclear factor is a gammaglobulin in the serum of patients with SLE which reacts with antibody-like specificity with somatic cell nuclei. Although anti-nuclear factor is characteristic of SLE and occurs in all cases, it is also seen in many patients with uncomplicated rheumatoid arthritis, Sjogren's disease and other connective tissue disorders. High titres of anti-nuclear antibodies may be present without overt disease and may occur in patients with chronic discoid lupus, in whom the lesions are localized to the face. Many of the antigens to which antibodies develop in systemic lupus do not stimulate antibody production when injected into experimental animals.

The disease is believed to be due to the proliferation of immunologically competent cells which react against normal body constituents. The body tissues involved are vascular endothelium, with consequent diffuse vasculitis which may be followed by thrombosis and secondary ischaemic lesions, red cells, white cells, platelets and constituents of collagen. This results in auto-immune haemolytic anaemia, leucopenia and thrombocytopenia, and fibrinoid degeneration of connective tissue. It is believed that arteritis is related to the deposition of antigen-antibody complexes (p. 84).

Renal disease in SLE and in chronic serum sickness shows many similar features as in both it results from the glomerular localization of soluble immune complexes. The production of relatively small soluble complexes results in glomerulitis as these are less easily cleared from the plasma by the reticulo-endothelial system. It is these antigen-antibody-complement complexes in the circulation that do the damage. They initiate an acute inflammatory process when they are deposited in the small blood vessels. Later hyaline intimal thickening (fibrinoid) becomes prominant and this material contains gammaglobulin, antigen and components of complement. Animal experiments have shown that immune complexes do damage small blood vessels in the kidney, and in patients with systemic lupus erythematosus there is evidence of deposited complexes in the glomerular lesions and in the skin lesions. The presence of auto-immune haemolytic anaemia in 25 per cent of patients with systemic lupus erythematosus suggests common aetiological factors.

There is less evidence that polyarteritis, dermatomyositis and progressive systemic sclerosis are auto-immune disorders, but the considerable overlapping of these diseases with SLE suggests common aetiological factors. The overlap of connective tissue disease is also seen in Sjogren's disease, which is frequently associated with a rheumatoid type of arthritis and less frequently with vasculitis. There is also a high incidence of circulating rheumatoid factor even when rheumatoid arthritis is not present, and antibodies to thyroglobulin are frequent.

There is evidence that auto-immunity has a contributory part to play in the pathogenesis of rheumatoid arthritis. The disease is characterized by the presence of circulating antibodies such as rheumatoid factor, which is an antibody to altered human gammaglobulin. One of the ways gammaglobulin is altered is by combination as antibody with antigen. Hypergammaglobulinaemia is a feature of the active phase of rheumatoid arthritis and both systemic lupus erythematosus and Sjogren's disease are often associated with rheumatoid arthritis. Rheumatoid factor is a macroglobulin with a molecular weight of about one million and such macroglobulins are often antibodies, as for instance the ABO blood group iso-agglutinins. As with most other auto-immune disorders the circulating antibody does not cause the disease and the transfusion of serum containing rheumatoid factor to normal volunteers is without effect. Furthermore, patients with hypogammaglobulinaemia frequently develop a rheumatoid type of arthritis. The damage in auto-immune disease is usually wrought by sensitized lymphocytes infiltrating the tissue containing the antigen. The inflammatory tissue which infiltrates the synovium of affected joints in rheumatoid arthritis is characterized by the presence of plasma cells, lymph follicles and germinal centres, and is similar to the infiltrating tissue in auto-immune thyroiditis and other disturbed antigen disorders. This suggests that antibody production is going on in the joints themselves and it is highly probable that it is connected with the arthritis. The plasma cells in the joint synovium and in rheumatoid nodules are actively producing the rheumatoid factor.

The patient's own gammaglobulin is probably damaged in the joint by some unknown mechanism and this precipitates, in predisposed subjects, the local production of antibody with its accompanying cellular proliferation. The proliferating tissue is then damaged by the use of the joint and a vicious circle ensues. The importance of a predisposition is suggested by the familial incidence of the disease. Although the nature of the process that damages the patient's own gammaglobulin in the joints is unknown, the recent isolation of mycoplasma from the synovial membrane of patients with rheumatoid arthritis, systemic lupus erythematosus and Reiter's syndrome is possibly relevant. Although this organism is sometimes just a saprophytic invader of damaged cells, certain strains do produce a polyarthritis when injected into animals. The animal disease shows some similarity to rheumatoid arthritis and responds, like the human disease, to treatment with gold salts.

AUTO-IMMUNITY AND THE THYROID

Chronic Thyroiditis

The best example of a disease due to a 'disturbed antigen' is lymphadenoid goitre which is also called chronic thyroiditis or Hashimoto's disease of the thyroid gland. This condition occurs almost exclusively in women and is characterized by infiltration of the thyroid gland with lymphocytes, which may form germinal centres in the gland. It occurs in all degrees of severity from infiltration by a few microscopic foci of lymphocytes to complete destruction of the gland. The gland may be enlarged and firm, as in typical Hashimoto's disease, or there may be no detectable goitre and the patient presents with primary hypothyroidism as a result of destruction of thyroid tissue. Primary sporadic myxoedema is indeed usually the end result of a silent auto-immunizing thyroiditis. The serum of patients with lymphadenoid goitre contains antibodies which react with human thyroglobulin and extracts of thyroid tissue. The raised serum gammaglobulin and positive flocculation tests characteristic of the disease are manifestations of the immune response to antigens released from the thyroid.

It has been shown experimentally that when partially thyroidectomized animals are injected with extracts of their own thyroid they not only produce circulating antibodies to constituents of their own gland, but the remaining portion of the gland develops histological changes resembling the appearance of Hashimoto's thyroiditis. The transfer of suspensions of lymphocytes from animals in whom this experimental thyroiditis has been induced will provoke the disease in a normal animal.

The high incidence of various thyroid disorders in the relatives of patients with lymphadenoid goitre suggests that there may be some constitutional abnormality of the thyroid. The severity and course of the disease in auto-immune thyroid disorders will obviously be related to the capacity of the immune system to react with the thyroid antigen and to the strength of the antigenic stimulus provided by the thyroid. The hyperplastic thyroid of thyrotoxicosis will produce a greater stimulus than a normal thyroid and there is a high incidence of auto-antibodies in this condition. The lympho-reticular system is probably hyper-reactive in patients with lymphadenoid goitre and this is supported by the fact that in a small proportion of cases other auto-immune diseases co-exist, notably pernicious anaemia and Addison's disease.

The diagnosis of this condition depends on the detection of antibodies to thyroglobulin in high titre, either by a simple precipitation test using extracts of thyroid as antigen, or by more refined tests using red cells treated with tannic acid as carriers of the antigen. These red cells agglutinate when contact is made with sera containing antibody (tanned red cell haemaglutination test). The treatment of auto-immune thyroiditis with thyroxine suppresses pituitary thyrotophic hormone production with consequent atrophy of the thyroid gland and hence reduction of the antigenic stimulus.

Autoantibodies and the Thyroid

There is an undoubted clinical association between thyrotoxicosis, Hashimoto's thyroiditis, and primary myxoedema. Even before effective methods of treatment were available a percentage of patients with hyperthyroidism who survived their illness eventually developed myxoedema. Indeed, hypothyroidism was considered to occur ultimately in a large proportion of these patients. We now know that the tendency for thyrotoxic patients treated surgically to become myxoedematous can be correlated with the degree of lymphocytic infiltration of the gland and with the presence of circulating throid antibodies. Progressive exophthalmos with pretibial myxoedema may occur in patients who have never been hyperthyroid, and in many of these instances there is histological evidence of lymphocytic thyroiditis. Patients with euthyroid Hashimoto's disease may subsequently develop thyrotoxicosis. Primary myxoedema and chronic thyroiditis are basically the same disease. It is not known why in some instances of chronic thyroiditis the thyroid tissue unobtrusively disappears whilst in others there is goitre formation or true Hashimoto's disease. The goitre in these cases is due partly to the inflammatory reaction and partly to the effect of increased secretion of TSH provoked in order to maintain the thyroxine output of the damaged gland. It would seem that thyrotoxicosis, Hashimoto's thyroiditis and primary hypothyroidism are different manifestations of what is fundamentally the same disease process.

There is evidence of a familial tendency to develop these thyroid disorders, and this predisposition is genetically determined rather than a result of environmental factors. In a retrospective study of unselected twins in Denmark there were 41 probands with adult thyrotoxicosis who were identical twins; 12 of their co-twins were similarly affected and a further 6 co-twins had nontoxic goitres. In contrast, of 59 thyrotoxic probands from unidentical twins of the same sex, 2 co-twins had thyrotoxicosis and 3 had a nontoxic goitre. A recent report describing thyrotoxicosis in each member of 4 pairs of identical twins is also of interest, and a similar association of Hashimoto's thyroiditis in identical twins has been reported. Family studies provide further evidence of this genetic factor, for near relatives of patients with thyrotoxicosis quite commonly suffer from myxoedema.

Circulating thyroid antibodies are also common to the three thyroid disorders of thyrotoxicosis, Hashimoto's thyroiditis and primary myxoedema. Although most frequent in Hashimoto's disease, varying degrees of focal thyroiditis associated with circulating thyroid antibodies are found in most patients with thyrotoxicosis. These circulating antibodies reflect the presence of an auto-immune process within the thyroid gland even if they are not directly responsible for the damage wrought to the parenchyma. There is statistical correlation between the serological reaction and the degree of lymphocytic infiltration of the gland in Hashimoto's thyroiditis, myxoedema and thyrotoxicosis.

Four different thyroid antibodies have been recognized:

1. *Antibody to thyroglobulin.* This antibody was first detected by the agar diffusion method, but a more sensitive and semiquantitative method for detecting it is provided by the tanned red cell agglutination test. Sheep red cells are treated with tannic acid to make the cell surface more suitable for coating with human thyroglobulin. When such coated cells come into contact with antibody to thyroglobulin they agglutinate. Another method for detecting antibody to thyroglobulin is the immunofluorescence technique. Sections of normal human thyroid tissue are incubated with the test serum; if antibodies to thyroglobulin are present in the test serum they will become attached to the thyroglobulin of the thyroid tissue. The thyroid tissue is then washed and incubated with anti-human globulin conjugated with fluorescent dye. The fluorescent anti-human antibody will become attached to any human serum, so that any site of reaction between antibody in the test serum and antigen in the thyroid tissue will be shown by bright green fluorescent staining.

2. *Antibody to second component of colloid.* Antibodies are also formed to a colloid antigen which does not contain iodine and is therefore not thyroglobulin. They are demonstrated by the fluorescent technique but they do not appear to have clinical or pathological significance.

3. *Antibody to thyroid microsomes.* Many patients with thyroid disease have, in their serum, complement-fixing antibodies which react with the microsomal fraction of the thyroid cell. This antibody is directed against a particular component of the thyroid secretory cell. It can be detected by complement fixation or by the immunofluorescent technique, in which the cytoplasm of the secretory cells will be stained but not the content of the vesicles. Titres of the thyroid complement-fixing antibodies correlate closely with the titres of thyroid cytoplasmic antibodies as determined by the fluorescent conjugation method. This suggests that both techniques are measuring the same antibody. Antibodies which fix complement are known to be able to cause lysis of cells and are therefore more likely to play an aetiological role in tissue destruction.

4. *Long acting thyroid stimulater (LATS).* This thyroid-stimulating globulin will be considered separately.

Antibodies to thyroglobulin and to thyroid microsomes are a common occurrence in Hashimoto's thyroiditis (80–87 per cent), primary myxoedema (70 per cent), and to a less extent in thyrotoxicosis (42 per cent). Their incidence in simple goitre and carcinoma of the thyroid is only slightly higher than in normal individuals.

LATS, on the other hand, is found almost exclusively in thyrotoxicosis and can be demonstrated in 85 per cent of patients with the disease. Although there is no correlation between the presence of LATS and other thyroid antibodies, these findings suggest that an immunological disturbance plays an important role in all three thyroid diseases. The tendency to develop thyroid antibodies is familial and genetically determined. The presence of circulating antibodies in the relatives of patients with thyrotoxicosis, Hashimoto's thyroiditis and myxoedema is more common than overt clinical disease; indeed, 50 per cent of near relatives of patients with Hashimoto's thyroiditis have circulating thyroid auto-antibodies. In thyrotoxicosis there is also an increased incidence of thyroid antibodies in parents and siblings of adult patients. Circulating antibodies were present in 11 of 12 children with thyrotoxicosis and in one or other parent of 10 out of the 12 children. The occurrence of a dominant inheritance of antibodies in both thyrotoxicosis and lymphadenoid goitre is evidence that these disorders may have a common underlying genetic basis. Low levels of thyroid antibodies are, however, not uncommon in perfectly healthy people. It is not known how long these antibodies persist in such persons, nor whether the presence of antibodies precedes the evolution of thyrotoxicosis, but the frequency of thyroid antibodies in females is 50 times that of the estimated incidence of thyrotoxicosis in the female population. Other important influences are therefore involved. The presence of thyroid antibodies indicates a genetically determined predisposition to overt thyroid disease, which may manifest itself either as thyrotoxicosis, Hashimoto's thyroiditis or primary myxoedema. These three thyroid disorders may all be manifestations of an inherited instability of the immunological system. It is, however, not known what initiates the disease process in such a predisposed individual, nor why it should take the form of thyrotoxicosis in one individual and lymphadenoid goitre in another.

Thyrotoxicosis

Patients with hyperthyroidism have traditionally been divided into two groups. The younger patients tend to have diffuse thyroid enlargement with eye involvement, whilst in the older groups the thyroid enlargement is usually nodular and severe eye involvement is rare. Although many endocrinologists have tried to segregate these two groups of patients into those with classic Graves' disease and those with toxic nodular goitre, no convincing clinical, biochemical or immunological distinction has been established. Rare forms of thyrotoxicosis exist which are caused by an autonomous solitary toxic adenoma. In these cases the function of the rest of the thyroid gland is suppressed by the humoral feedback mechanism whereby raised concentrations of circulating thyroxine suppress pituitary production of thyrotrophic hormone (TSH). Even more rare is congenital thyrotoxicosis, in which hyperthyroidism is present at birth due to the placental transfer from the mother of a circulating humoral agent which stimulates thyroid activity.

In health thyroid function is regulated by a feedback mechanism between the pituitary and the thyroid, whereby rising levels of circulating thyroxine suppress the release of TSH from the pituitary gland. It is the level of free hormone in the plasma to which the pituitary responds and this is not synonymous with the level of protein-bound hormone. In addition, external stimuli such as cold, acting through the central nervous system, stimulate the hypothalamus to liberate TSH-releasing factor.

In thyrotoxicosis rising levels of circulating thyroxine fail to restrain the activity of the thyroid and indeed the tri-iodothyronine suppression test, in which the administration of tri-iodothyronine by mouth does not suppress the uptake of radioactive iodine, is one of the most useful confirmatory tests of thyrotoxicosis.

Recent advances in our knowledge of the aetiology of thyrotoxicosis stem from the observation that the thyroid-stimulating activity of the blood of a thyrotoxic patient is not due to TSH. It was noted that when the serum of a patient with thyrotoxicosis was injected into a guinea pig previously given radioactive iodine, the discharge of radio-iodine from the thyroid was unusually prolonged, with a maximum rise in blood radioactivity at 16–24 hours. This is quite unlike the short-lived response to TSH, which reaches its maximum at 2–3 hours (Fig. 8). This newly discovered thyroid stimulator was called long acting thyroid stimulator (LATS). The mouse is now used in preference to the guinea pig; in the mouse the peak response to TSH occurs after 2–3 hours and to LATS after 10–12 hours. When sera known to contain TSH and LATS are mixed the effect is additive.

Differences between TSH and LATS

Considerable further study has been made on the nature of LATS, and there is now little doubt that LATS is a true stimulator of thyroid function. It differs from TSH in a number of ways.

1. The more prolonged activity of LATS is due to its slower disappearance from the serum; it has in fact a half life 30 times that of TSH.

2. TSH resides in the pituitary gland but LATS does not. This correlates with the clinical evidence that hyperthyroidism may occur

after hypophysectomy. Furthermore, histological examination of the pituitary from patients with untreated hyperthyroidism suggests that their TSH secretion is suppressed. Indeed, recent determinations of human TSH by immunoassay failed to reveal detectable levels in thyrotoxic sera.

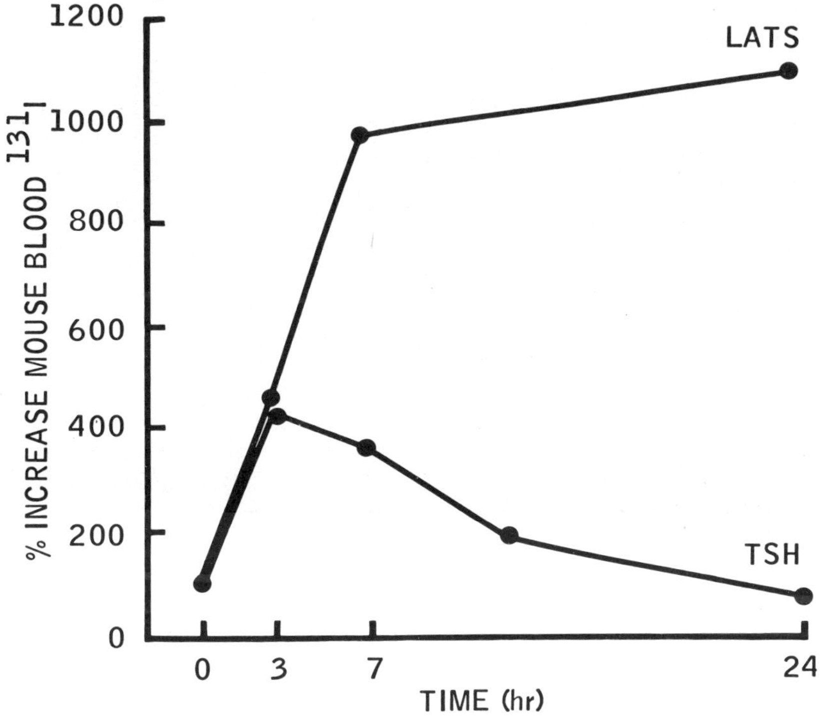

FIG. 8 TSH and LATS responses

3. TSH can be suppressed by thyroxine but LATS cannot. When thyrotoxicosis is overtreated, with the consequent development of hypothyroidism, TSH can be detected in the serum, demonstrating that the normal feedback mechanism is functional in these patients. The preservation of the negative feedback mechanism explains why thyroidectomy is so effective in achieving an exactly euthyroid state: thyroidectomy lowers the serum concentration of LATS, and after operation the LATS stimulus may be insufficient to produce enough thyroid hormone; however, TSH secretion will increase and stimulate thyroid activity until the patient is euthyroid. Experiments showing that LATS is fully effective in hypophysectomized mice have excluded the possibility that it is a factor derived from the

hypothalamus and acting by stimulating the release of TSH from the pituitary.

4. Chemical and immunological differences between LATS and TSH have been demonstrated. In particular, antisera to human TSH do not inactivate LATS.

Characterization of LATS

LATS has been shown to be a gamma globulin. It belongs to the IgG group of immunoglobulins, and antibodies to IgG destroy LATS activity but do not affect TSH. As LATS is an immunoglobulin it would be expected to arise from an antigenic stimulus. Intensive search has been made for the source of the antigen. It resides in the microsomes of thyroid epithelial cells, as LATS activity can be consistently removed from serum by incubation with thyroid microsomal fractions. This is not proof of an antigen-antibody reaction since humoral agents of any nature may be expected to bind to their target tissues.

Relationship of LATS to Hyperthyroidism

There is little doubt that LATS is the direct cause of most cases of thyrotoxicosis. Although LATS cannot be demonstrated in the unconcentrated serum of a large proportion of patients with undoubted thyrotoxicosis, this is due to the insensitivity of the bioassay method; when the serum is concentrated LATS can be detected in 85 per cent of all patients with hyperthyroidism. It is present just as frequently in patients with nodular goitres as in those with smooth goitres. When remission of the disease occurs following antithyroid drugs LATS activity disappears from the serum. Furthermore, there is a correlation between LATS activity and the radioactive iodine turnover per unit weight of gland. The evidence that LATS is the direct cause of hyperthyroidism is thus overwhelming. Furthermore, in neonatal thyrotoxicosis there is a high level of LATS which falls as the degree of hyperthyroidism in this self-limiting disease resolves.

There is little qualitative difference between the effects of TSH and those of LATS on the thyroid gland. It has been suggested that TSH acts physiologically by removing a tonic inhibition of an essential enzymatic process. Antibody to the hypothetical inhibitor could release the same enzyme system.

Thyrotoxicosis as an Auto-immune Disease

There is increasing evidence to suggest that thyrotoxicosis is an auto-immune disease. The following criteria are evidence of auto-immunity in clinical disease.

1. The direct demonstration of free circulating antibodies that are active at body temperature, or the demonstration of cell-bound antibodies by indirect means. LATS is a circulating immunoglobulin which satisfies this criterion. In addition, varying degrees of focal thyroiditis associated with circulating antibodies to thyroglobulin and to thyroid microsomes are found in most patients with thyrotoxicosis; indeed, thyroid antibodies are present in 85 per cent of patients with Graves' disease. Significant titres to the complement fixation type of antibody occur in 65 per cent of patients and to the tanned red cell agglutination type in 46 per cent.

2. The recognition of a specific antigen to which the antibody is directed. The specific antigen to which LATS is antibody has not been identified. It has, however, been shown to reside in the microsomal fraction of the thyroid epithelial cells.

3. The production of antibodies against the same antigen in experimental animals. LATS production has been provoked by the injection of thyroid homogenates.

4. The appearance of pathological changes in the corresponding tissues of an actively sensitized experimental animal that are basically similar to those of human disease. This criterion has not yet been satisfied. It has, however, been shown that hyperfunction of the thyroid gland can be induced in animals by injecting serum which has been produced as a result of the injection of thyroid homogenates.

5. The successful transfer of the disease by an antibody-containing serum or by immunologically stimulated lymphoid cells. Neonatal thyrotoxicosis provides the evidence for successful transfer of the disease by LATS produced in the mother and carried across the placenta to the foetus.

Other criteria which have been suggested as evidence of auto-immunity are the response of the disease to corticosteroids and the association of the disorder with other auto-immune disease. Thyrotoxicosis responds to corticosteroid therapy and the LATS levels fall. There is also clinical association of thyrotoxicosis with other auto-immune diseases. The most impressive connection is that of thyroid disease with pernicious anaemia. Histamine-fast achlorhydria occurs in 46 per cent of patients with primary hypothyroidism, and pernicious anaemia in over 12 per cent. Extensive deficiency of vitamin B_{12} without pernicious anaemia is more common than overt clinical disease. Achlorhydria is also seen in patients with thyrotoxicosis and the gastric mucosa often shows atrophy and lymphocytic infiltration with the formation of germinal centres. Over 19 per cent of mothers of patients with thyrotoxicosis show antibodies to gastric parietal cells, although there is no significantly increased incidence in other relatives. There is also a clinical association between thyroid disease and nontuberculous adrenal insufficiency, and conversely patients with idiopathic Addison's disease have a high incidence of thyroid and parietal cell antibodies. A similar association has been reported with idiopathic hypoparathyroidism.

The suggestive evidence that thyrotoxicosis is an auto-immune disease is thus impressive. The close association between thyrotoxicosis and other auto-immune thyroid disorders, and the dominant inheritance of thyroid antibodies in diseases known to have a familial incidence, add further support for this hypothesis. This does not, however, explain how the disease arises and here speculation is inevitable.

Selected Bibliography

ANDERSON, J. R. (1963) Auto-antibodies in Diseases of Man. Brit. Med. Bull. 19, 251.

GELL, P. G. H. and COOMBS, R. R. A. (1968) *Clinical Aspects of Immunology*. 2nd Ed. Blackwell, Oxford.

GLYNN, L. E. and HOLBORROW, E. J. (1971) *Auto-Immunity and Disease*. 2nd Ed. Blackwell, Oxford.

Leading Article (1965) Thymus and Auto-immunity. *The Lancet* 1, 1007.

Leading Article (1968) The Immunological Orchestra. *The Lancet* 1, 185.

MACKAY, I. R. and BURNETT, SIR MACFARLANE (1962) *Auto-immune Diseases*. Thomas, Springfield.

TURK, J. (1972) *Immunology in Clinical Medicine*. 2nd Ed. Heinemann.

V

Respiratory Failure

THE FUNCTION OF THE LUNG

The function of the lung is to provide a surface through which the blood can receive oxygen and excess carbon dioxide be removed. The pulmonary alveoli are the site of this exchange of gases. The mechanical requirements for respiration are the thoracic cage, the chest and abdominal muscles and the diaphragm. These provide the means of introducing air to the pulmonary circulation so that this gaseous exchange can take place.

Normal respiratory function keeps the partial pressure of oxygen and carbon dioxide in the blood within certain narrow limits and when these limits are exceeded lung failure may be said to have occurred. Respiratory or lung failure is thus present when, because of impaired respiratory function, the arterial partial pressure of oxygen (p O_2) is below 60 mm.Hg or the arterial partial pressure of carbon dioxide exceeds 50 mm.Hg. It must be realized that the p O_2 may also fall below this level if there is a right to left cardiac shunt and the p CO_2 may exceed the normal range in metabolic alkalosis but in neither of these conditions is there respiratory failure.

For the process of respiration to take place efficiently certain conditions are necessary.

1. *Ventilation:* the pulmonary alveoli must be adequately ventilated with air.

2. *Intrapulmonary distribution:* the air should be evenly distributed to the millions of alveoli throughout the entire lung.

3. *Perfusion:* the alveolar capillaries must be adequately and evenly perfused with blood.

4. *Diffusion:* this is the process by which oxygen and carbon

dioxide are exchanged between the alveolar air and the pulmonary capillary blood. The alveolar-capillary membrane must be adequate in extent and permeability to allow the diffusion of gases across its surface.

A number of different processes are thus necessary for normal respiration and defective function may involve any of them, and precipitate respiratory failure. Different pulmonary diseases may give rise to a single physiological disturbance and one disease may, in different situations, cause a variety of functional disturbances. For example, sarcoidosis may restrict ventilation, produce an alveolar-capillary block or cause no functional change.

The partial pressure of oxygen in the alveolar air is 100 mm.Hg. It is often called the oxygen tension. If plasma is exposed to this oxygen tension, only 0·3 ml. of oxygen would be taken up by 100 ml. of plasma. Whole blood will take up 20 ml. of oxygen at the same oxygen tension. The extra oxygen uptake is due to the presence of haemoglobin in red cells. Haemolglobin combines with oxygen reversibly becoming saturated at higher partial pressures of oxygen and unsaturated at lower ones. The haemoglobin is 98 per cent saturated at the normal oxygen tension. Over-ventilation of parts of the lung cannot therefore compensate for under-ventilation of other parts because oxygen tensions above normal cannot cause any significant increase in the arterial saturation of oxygen. At the lower ranges of oxygen tension encountered in the tissues small changes in tension are associated with large falls of saturation because the haemoglobin gives up more oxygen at the lower oxygen tensions. In the upper ranges of oxygen tension, however, a considerable reduction in the partial pressure of oxygen below the normal alveolar tension of 100 mm.Hg does not reduce the oxygenation of arterial blood significantly. This can be seen from the oxygen dissociation curve which relates the saturation of haemoglobin to the oxygen tension (p O_2) in the blood. (Fig. 9.) A fall of p O_2 to 60 mm.Hg occurs when alveolar ventilation is reduced by approximately one-half but it is not associated with a fall in arterial saturation below 90 per cent. At lower oxygen tensions the blood gives up relatively more of its oxygen with only a slight fall in the p O_2. Hypoxaemia begins when the oxygen tension falls to 60 mm.Hg but cyanosis cannot be detected with certainty until the saturation of haemoglobin falls to 75 per cent, which corresponds with an oxygen tension of 50 mm.Hg.

Hypoxia of even slight degree may stimulate an increase in cardiac output and erythropoiesis but does not cause serious damage until the tension of oxygen falls to 40 mm. of mercury and this is associated in the normal blood with an arterial saturation of about 50 per cent. An arterial oxygen tension of 20 mm.Hg causes death. The margin between the oxygen tension causing cyanosis and that which causes severe damage is narrow.

If ventilation is reduced by half, hypercapnia is likely to be present without hypoxaemia. In other varieties of lung failure

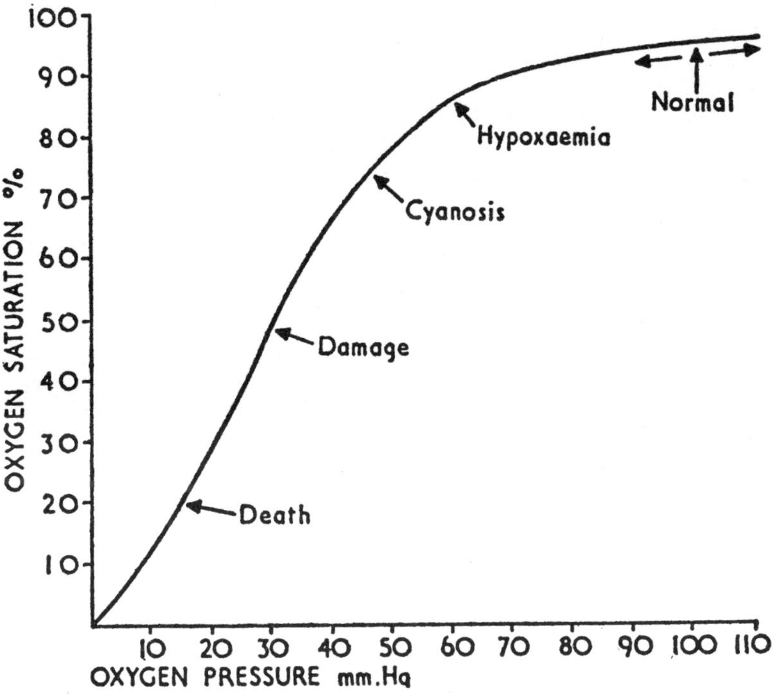

FIG. 9 Oxygen dissociation curve

hypoxaemia may be present without hypercapnia. These types of lung failure will be considered later.

Dyspnoea, which is a consciousness of the necessity for increased respiratory effort, is not the same as respiratory failure. It is usually a symptom of some defect in the action of the lungs as a pair of bellows. It may occur in the presence of normal blood gases as in physical exercise or asthma and conversely respiratory failure may on occasions occur without dyspnoea. If the patient complains of dyspnoea or difficult breathing there is likely to be some obstruction to ventilation. If the patient complains of excessive breathing rather than a true difficulty the cause is more likely to be alveolar in origin.

Stimuli for Respiration

The stimuli for respiration are, (I) Chemical: (a) through the respiratory centre in the medulla: this is the chief stimulus to respiration and is partly regulated by the p CO_2 and to a lesser extent by the pH of the blood, (b) through the aortic and carotid bodies: these chemoreceptors respond to anoxia. (II) Proprioceptive: these stimuli come from the lungs themselves, and are responsible for the increased ventilation associated with physical exercise, during which the p CO_2 usually remains normal. Pulmonary congestion sensitizes stretch receptors in the lung so that the rate of ventilation is increased though the depth of inspiration curtailed. (III) Voluntary Control: this is initiated from the cerebral cortex.

The two major contributions to normal respiratory function are thus:

1. Ventilation

Ventilation is the mass movement of air up and down the respiratory passages. Normally the alveoli, of which there are approximately 750 million, are ventilated by 5–6 litres of air per minute and this is achieved by the bellows-like action of the thoracic cage. The volume of this air is comparable to the cardiac output and hence the volume of blood perfusing the alveoli. The contraction of the muscles of inspiration causes expansion of the chest and this provides the negative intra-thoracic pressure which enables air to be inspired through the air passages. To ensure adequate ventilation of the lungs the respiratory muscles must overcome the elastic resistance of the lung tissue and the resistance of the airways to the flow of air through them. About one-quarter of the inspired air ventilates the conducting airway (dead space) and the remaining three-quarters constitutes alveolar ventilation. In medical practice the rate of respiration receives close attention and is usually recorded at frequent intervals in the patient's notes together with the temperature and pulse frequency. However the depth (tidal volume) is just as important as the rate of breathing for the ventilation of the alveoli.

Ventilation may be impaired on account of

(a) obstruction of the air passages,

or (b) reduction or restriction of the bellows-like action of the thoracic cage

or (c) diminished distensibility of the lungs.

The ciliary action of the bronchial mucous membrane normally keeps the bronchi free from foreign material, which sticks to the lining mucus and is swept towards the pharynx. This maintains the patency of the airway. When a larger quantity accumulates the cough reflex is initiated and it is expectorated. Infection may impair ciliary action with the result that mucus and foreign material accumulate, thereby narrowing the air passages and impeding ventilation. The removal of carbon dioxide from the alveoli depends on adequate alveolar ventilation. As the partial pressure of carbon dioxide in the arterial blood is in equilibrium with that in the alveoli, its concentration will rise in the arterial blood if air cannot be removed from the alveolus, and this is precisely what happens in ventilatory failure.

If alveolar ventilation is to be adequate each alveolus must get its share of the inspired air. When an alveolus is not ventilated but has a normal blood flow the result is a by-pass of active lung or what is in effect a right to left cardiac shunt. This may cause hypoxaemia. Conversely if an alveolus is ventilated, but has no blood flow, the air undergoes little or no exchange of oxygen or carbon dioxide and the result is an increase in the 'dead space' and wasted respiratory effort.

2. Diffusion

Diffusion is the process by which the interchange between the air and blood in the lungs takes place. After adequate alveolar ventilation has been achieved, diffusion of oxygen and carbon-dioxide across the alveolar membrane, interstitial tissue and capillary endothelium must occur. This raises the plasma p O_2 to rather less than 100 mm. of mercury and oxygen is then taken up by the haemoglobin of the red cells and the blood becomes 98 per cent saturated. When the blood reaches the tissues, where the oxygen tension is lower, oxygen is given up. The diffusing capacity of the lungs is determined by the surface area available for diffusion and the thickness of the alveolar-capillary membrane, as well as the tension of gas in the alveolus and the blood flow perfusing it. Normal diffusion presupposes an adequate alveolar ventilation and an adequate pulmonary circulation. Furthermore, the volume of the pulmonary capillary bed must be adequate to permit enough red cells to make contact with the alveolar gases. Normally total alveolar ventilation parallels the cardiac output so that blood and gas are distributed to different parts of the lung in equal proportions. (Fig. 10a.) In more technical terms the ratio of ventilation to perfusion in different parts of the lung should be uniform, and near to unity.

Lung Failure

Normal respiratory function keeps the arterial blood fully oxygenated and the carbon dioxide pressure within a narrow range. The diagnosis of respiratory failure depends on the demonstration of serious abnormality of these blood gases as a result of pulmonary disease. When breathing air a rise in alveolar p CO_2 is invariably associated with a fall in alveolar p O_2 and hence the oxygen tension

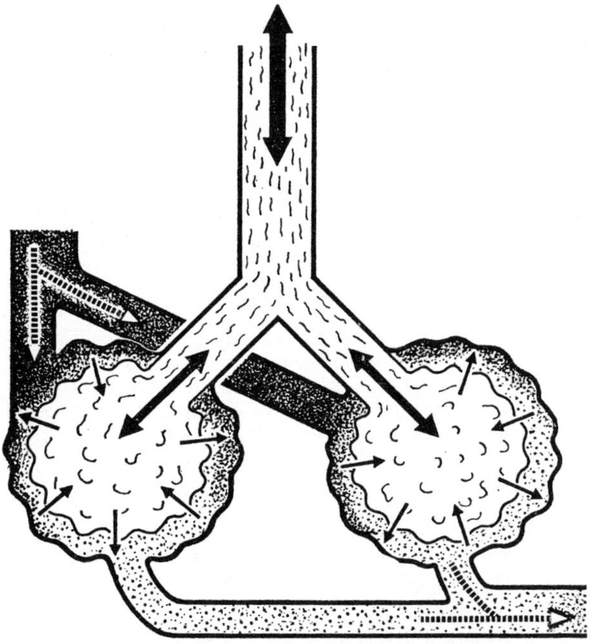

FIG. 10 (*a*) Normal distribution of air and blood to alveolus

in the blood as well. However the fall in the partial pressure of oxygen is not necessarily associated with arterial oxygen desaturation because of the shape of the oxygen dissociation curve. Hypoxaemia and hypercapnia thus do not run in parallel.

Respiratory failure may be:

(1) ventilatory, in which condition the alveoli are under-ventilated.

(2) alveolar, in which situation there is impaired transport of gases across the alveolar-capillary membrane.

(3) due to maldistribution of air and blood within the lung. This may be the result of the perfusion of unventilated areas of lung or the ventilation of unperfused areas. (Fig. 10b.) Such a maldistribution of air and blood may be associated with disorders of ventilation such as chronic bronchitis or may be associated with primary defects of diffusion such as pulmonary collapse or pulmonary infiltrations.

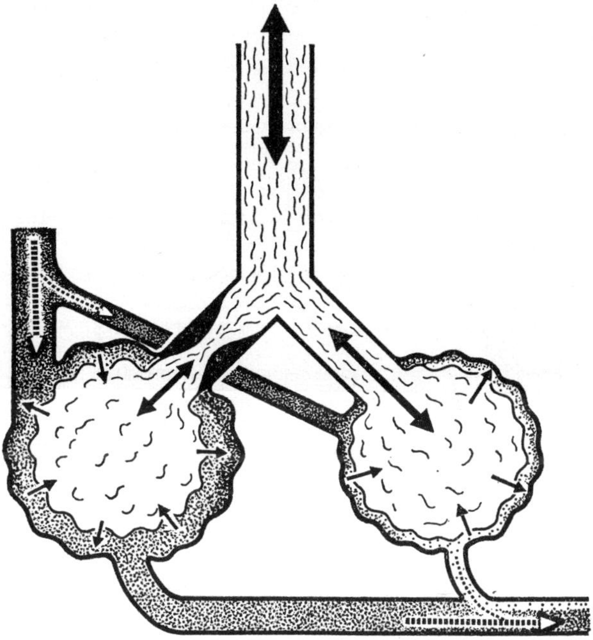

FIG. 10 (*b*) Maldistribution of air and blood to alveolus

When respiratory failure is due to a failure of ventilation the partial pressure of carbon dioxide in the blood is increased but the oxygen saturation falls little until ventilatory failure is severe. When respiratory failure, however, is the result of impaired diffusion or the result of a maldistribution of gas and blood within the lung, the arterial oxygen saturation becomes decreased whilst the partial pressure of carbon dioxide in the blood tends to remain normal. Thus the two types of respiratory failure may be distinguished by the presence or absence of hypercapnia.

Ventilatory failure

Ventilatory failure may be due to:

(i) obstruction of the air passages.

(ii) restriction of the thoracic muscles or diminished distensibility of the lung.

(iii) depression of respiratory centre.

Obstruction of air passages

The factors likely to produce obstruction of the air passages are (a) oedema of the lining mucous membrane or the presence of excessive mucus, as in bronchitis; or spasm of the constrictor muscles of

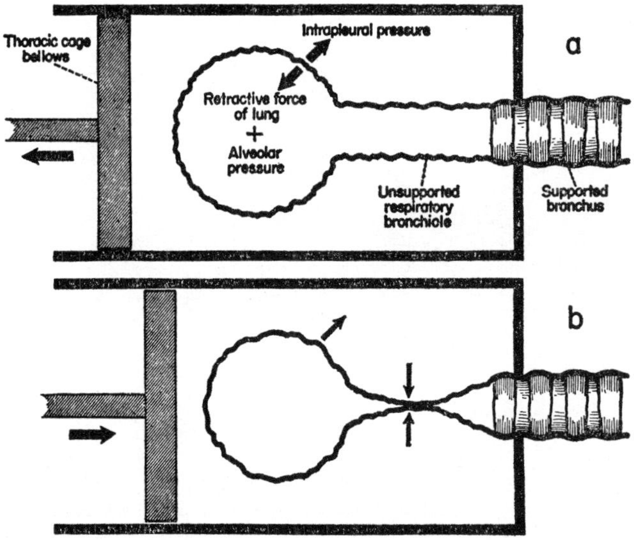

FIG. 11 Mechanism of air trapping

the bronchioles as in asthma. An important factor maintaining the patency of the airways is the elastic pull of the lung surrounding the smaller bronchioles. If this elasticity is impaired there will be a narrowing of the airway during expiration and the smaller bronchioles will tend to collapse towards the end of expiration. This is because during expiration, when the retractive force of the lung is reduced, the intra-pleural pressure may become positive relative to atmospheric pressure and cause collapse of the unsupported bronchioles. The air in the alveolus is then trapped. (Fig. 11.) The limiting factor in the performance of a maximum expiration in a normal person is the collapse of the intrathoracic airways due to the reduced elastic force of the shrinking lung being overcome by the rising intrathoracic pressure. In emphysema, when the elastic forces of the lung are compromised, this critical point of airway collapse is reached before expiration is complete. If the bronchioles collapse air is trapped distally and cannot get out. This leads to over-distension of the lungs and prevents fresh air entering the alveoli at the next inspiration. The loss of elasticity in the walls of the alveoli and smaller bronchioles is the most important mechanism of irreversible obstruction to the airways.

In this country airway obstruction is the commonest disorder of lung function and it is usually the result of asthma or chronic bronchitis. In asthma the airway obstruction is reversible. In chronic bronchitis because of constant increased production of mucus and intermittent inflammatory oedema, the airway obstruc- is more chronic and progressive. Once the elasticity of the walls of the alveoli and smaller bronchioles is lost the obstruction to the airways becomes irreversible and air-trapping, due to collapse of distal bronchioles, predisposes to emphysema.

Restriction of thoracic muscles

Ventilation may fail because of conditions which restrict the movement of the thorax and increase the work of breathing. For example, the function of the respiratory muscles may be impaired as a result of poliomyelitis, polyneuritis or myasthenia gravis, or from loss of mobility of the bony case due to kyphoscoliosis or gross obesity. Ventilation may also be impaired because the lungs have diminished distensibility such as might occur secondary to pulmonary fibrosis or pulmonary congestion or because of a pleural effusion or pneumothorax.

Kyphoscoliosis provides a problem of ventilation. Not only is there the mechanical disadvantage of the deformed chest, which may result in a great increase in the work of breathing but owing to impaired chest movement half of these patients have chronic bronchitis in addition. Similarly in obesity the work of breathing is greatly increased and the impaired respiratory excursion predisposes towards infection. Such a failure of ventilation results in hypercapnia and, if severe, hypoxia as well.

Depression of respiratory centre

Ventilatory failure may also result from a lack of respiratory drive due to brain damage. Here there is a failure to increase ventilation in response to hypercapnia or hypoxia. Such damage to the respiratory drive may result from drugs such as sedatives or may be due to intracranial lesions. It is sometimes associated with gross obesity and terminal diseases. Sometimes it is idiopathic and these patients have a normal ventilatory capacity but simply do not breathe enough. Measurement of the arterial carbon dioxide tension is the only clinical way of knowing whether a patient's alveolar ventilation is adequate or not.

The causes of ventilatory failure may be summarized as:

(a) Obstruction to the air passages.
1. Bronchitis.
2. Asthma.

(b) Restriction of the chest movements.
1. Kyphoscoliosis.
2. Obesity.
3. Muscular paralysis.
4. Pleural thickening or calcification.

(c) Depression of respiratory centre.
1. As a result of drugs, especially sedatives.
2. As a result of intracranial lesions.
3. In association with obesity.
4. In association with shock.
5. In terminal diseases.
6. Idiopathic.

Alveolar Respiratory Failure

This is due to impaired alveolar-capillary gas exchange, or what is in effect a loss of functioning alveolar surface. This loss may be an absolute reduction of total alveolar surface or a relative reduction due to under-ventilation of portions of lung which are adequately perfused with blood.

Normally the spaces between the alveoli and pulmonary capillaries are thin and gaseous exchange occurs freely. If the membrane or the interstitial spaces are thickened as a result of pulmonary oedema or destroyed by pulmonary disease, surgical removal of portions of lung, interstitial pulmonary fibrosis, or granulomatous and neoplastic infiltrations, diffusion may be impaired. The surface area for diffusion may also be decreased by diseases which disrupt area for diffusion may also be decreased by diseases which disrupt the normal alveolar structure such as pulmonary emphysema or cysts or by diseases which decrease the functioning capillary surface. In these conditions there is in effect a loss of the alveolar surface available for gas exchange. This causes a reduction of the oxygen saturation of the blood but as carbon dioxide is much more soluble and diffusible than oxygen its diffusion is less seriously affected. Clinically the reduction in the total number of alveoli available for gas exchange is more common than thickening of the alveolar membrane. More important still as a cause of diffusion defect is the relative loss of alveolar surface due to the perfusion with blood of alveoli which are not being adequately ventilated, because of air-trapping or pulmonary collapse. In these situations there is in effect a loss of alveolar surface available for gas exchange.

Alveolar respiratory failure may thus be due to:

(a) Maldistribution of gas and blood within the lung.

(b) Primary or idiopathic emphysema.

(c) Pulmonary oedema.

(d) Pulmonary fibrosis.

(e) Pulmonary granulomatosis, e.g. sarcoidosis, histiocytosis X.

(f) Loss of functioning lung tissue, as a result of pulmonary collapse, pleural effusion or surgical removal.

(g) Pulmonary vascular disease (causing reduction of pulmonary capillary circulation).

   1. Pulmonary hypertension.
   2. Thrombo-embolic disease.

Maldistribution of air and blood within the lung

The maldistribution of air and blood within the lung may be the result of (i) perfusion of unventilated areas of lung or (ii) the ventilation of unperfused areas of lung. (Fig. 10b.)

Perfusion of unventilated areas of lung (lowered ventilation–perfusion ratio)

When the perfusion of the alveoli by the pulmonary capillaries is normal but some of the alveoli are under-ventilated because of air trapping or collapse, there will be an increase in the partial pressure of carbon dioxide in the under-ventilated alveoli and a corresponding decrease in tension of oxygen in these alveoli. The blood leaving the under-ventilated area will contain an excess of carbon dioxide and will be inadequately saturated with oxygen. The excess carbon dioxide in the blood, because of its greater diffusibility, can be transferred in adequately ventilated parts of the lung but hyperventilation cannot increase the arterial oxygen saturation of the blood leaving the ventilated parts of the lung to more than 100 per cent. Thus, when the fully oxygenated blood is mixed with the shunted blood from the areas of lung perfused but not ventilated, the mixture is unsaturated. Such a disturbance may occur in many types of lung disease such as pulmonary collapse and ventilatory diseases. It also occurs in injuries to the chest involving lung contusion. In patients with pneumonia the cyanosis is usually due to shunting of unsaturated blood through the non-ventilated areas of consolidated lung. The distribution of air and blood are thus not in balance and the ratio of ventilation to perfusion has been lowered. Such maldistribution is the commonest cause of cyanosis of pulmonary origin. The volume of blood passing through the lung without being oxygenated must be 30 per cent of the total pulmonary flow before arterial saturation falls below 90 per cent.

Ventilation of unperfused areas of lung (raised ventilation–perfusion ratio)

The pulmonary circulation is an important factor in the maintenance of normal diffusion of gases and the volume of the pulmonary capillary bed must obviously be adequate to permit enough red cells to make contact with the alveolar gases. The blood only spends three-quarters of a second in passing through alveoli. Pulmonary hypertension therefore with occlusion of pulmonary arterioles will result in impaired perfusion of scattered alveoli which are normally ventilated. Thrombo-embolic disease will have a similar effect. Similarly, after haemorrhage or myocardial infarction there is a marked reduction in cardiac output and hence pulmonary blood flow. The pulmonary hypotension, which results, produces a pressure head inadequate to overcome the effects of gravity in different parts of the lung. The consequent ventilation of unperfused alveoli is wasted ventilation because gaseous exchange does not occur. In a severe case of emphysema, as a result of over-inflation of the lungs and ventilation of avascular bullae the 'dead space' may be so increased that 70 per cent of each breath is wasted.

In chronic bronchitis and emphysema areas of lung where avascular bullae are ventilated will have a high ventilation–perfusion ratio, and other areas of lung which are not ventilated because of air-trapping or collapse but which are perfused with blood will have a lowered ventilation–perfusion ratio.

Respiratory failure may thus be due to a failure of the bellows, a failure of the alveoli or a failure of the pulmonary capillaries and the symptom resulting from each will be shortness of breath.

Although respiratory function can be divided into ventilation, diffusion and the pulmonary circulation, the tests of respiratory function measure the overall function of the lungs rather than that of separate portions and many causes of ventilatory failure are associated with some defect in diffusion or in the pulmonary circulation. Patients with chronic bronchitis and emphysema suffer largely because of a failure of ventilation but as a result of chronic air-trapping and distension of the alveoli much of the alveolar surface is lost in the development of secondary emphysema and this causes a diffusion defect. Conversely, when the pressure in the pulmonary circulation rises, as in cardiac failure or mitral stenosis there is a diffusion defect but as the lungs become less distensible the work of ventilation will be increased and this may precipitate a secondary ventilatory failure.

Under-ventilation of alveoli results in an increase in alveolar carbon dioxide concentration, which in turn results in increased arterial carbon dioxide partial pressure. A rise in alveolar partial pressure of carbon dioxide must be associated with an equivalent fall in the partial pressure of oxygen. A fall in the partial pressure of alveolar oxygen need not, however, produce a significant change in the arterial saturation because of the shape of the oxygen dissociation curve. Alveolar under-ventilation can thus be quite severe without any appreciable change in the arterial oxygen saturation. Ventilatory failure is hence characterized by constant hypercapnia but hypoxaemia may, or may not, be present depending upon the severity of the ventilatory failure or any associated ventilatory–perfusion imbalance.

However, when the defect is due to impaired alveolar-capillary diffusion, oxygen transport suffers more severely than that of carbon dioxide because the latter is twenty times more diffusible. Thus respiratory failure due to a diffusion defect will result in a fall in arterial oxygen saturation often without an appreciable change in the carbon dioxide partial pressure.

COMPLICATIONS OF LUNG FAILURE

(i) *Cor pulmonale*

The combination of hypoxia and hypercapnia leads to pulmonary vasoconstriction and hence pulmonary hypertension. This causes right ventricular hypertrophy and often failure or cor pulmonale. It is the alteration in the blood gases that is responsible for pulmonary hypertension and not the destruction of pulmonary blood vessels by emphysema.

(ii) *Secondary polycythaemia*

In some patients persistent hypoxia results in secondary polycythaemia. The reason why this response to hypoxia is limited to certain patients is unknown.

(iii) *Raised intracranial pressure*

Hypercapnia causes cerebral vasodilatation and an increase in the filtration pressure for the cerebro-spinal fluid. This may give rise to a raised intracranial pressure and even papilloedema.

CLINICAL DIAGNOSIS OF RESPIRATORY FAILURE

The clinical diagnosis of respiratory failure resolves itself into the diagnosis of hypoxia and hypercapnia. The clinical diagnosis of hypoxia is difficult and usually depends on the presence of certain central nervous system symptoms, such as mental confusion or symptoms similar to alcoholic intoxication, in the presence of central cyanosis. Hypoxia is a more accurate term than anoxia though they tend to be used as synonyms. Although cyanosis requires a certain threshold level of reduced circulating haemoglobin to be exceeded, there is very considerable variation in its detection by different observers. The visual impressions of cyanosis are unreliable and most observers cannot detect it unless the arterial oxygen saturation is below 75 per cent. Furthermore, cyanosis may be present with a normal oxygen saturation in patients with polycythaemia and may be absent with severe reduction in oxygen saturation if the patient is anaemic. Oxygen deficiency may therefore be severe under certain circumstances in the absence of cyanosis and may be absent in the presence of cyanosis in other situations. In many patients a pigmentation of mucous membranes occurs which is indistinguishable from cyanosis and this may also give rise to difficulty in assessing oxygen saturation. The direct measurement of arterial oxygen tension by arterial puncture is a necessary investigation for the precise diagnosis and management of respiratory failure.

Carbon dioxide retention is a characteristic feature of ventilatory failure. The clinical diagnosis depends on a number of physical signs, which are not specific but are nevertheless helpful. There is tachycardia, a bounding pulse with signs of peripheral vasodilatation, such as a raised pulse pressure and warm extremities. Muscle twitching, mental confusion and a flapping tremor of the hands are later signs. The important factor in the development of the symptoms and signs of hypercapnia is not the absolute blood level but the rise

in the blood level precipitated by an acute episode. Direct measurle
ment of the arterial carbon dioxide tension is the most usefu-
investigation in ventilatory failure.

Treatment of Respiratory Failure

The treatment of respiratory failure resulting from impaired alveolar-capillary gas exchange is by the administration of oxygen. In this situation there is no elevation of the arterial p CO_2 and there is no danger of depressing the respiratory centre by the administration of oxygen. The other aspects of treatment concern the management of the cause of the alveolar-capillary diffusion defect.

The problem of respiratory failure with chronic elevation of the p CO_2 is much more complex because here the unlimited administration of oxygen will remove the anoxic stimulus for respiration and so depress respiration and cause carbon dioxide narcosis. Nevertheless, the patient is hypoxic and this state requires urgent correction. The admixture of hypoxia and chronic elevation of p CO_2 is the combination of ventilatory failure and alveolar failure characteristic of chronic bronchitis and emphysema. Treatment should comprise:

(1) *Rest and warmth.*

(2) *The treatment of the infection.*

The common organisms are the pneumococcus and haemophilus influenzae. Pneumococcal infections are characterized by green purulent sputum and haemophilus infection by yellow purulent sputum. This is a useful guide for the choice of antibiotic as there is no time to await bacterial culture and sensitivity results. As only 50 per cent of haemophilus organisms are sensitive to penicillin, the antibiotic of choice is a tetracycline or ampicillin. Pneumococcal infections respond to penicillin.

(3) *Relief of hypoxia.*

In respiratory failure hypoxia is of enhanced importance as a stimulus to respiration, and carbon dioxide narcosis will follow unlimited oxygen therapy. Nevertheless the relief of severe hypoxia is of urgent importance as untreated it will cause metabolic acidosis due to the accumulation of lactic acid and lead to cardiac, cerebral and renal damage. Whilst a patient is breathing air hypoxia is the complication likely to kill him and not hypercapnia. This is because when the p CO_2 rises in the alveolus the p O_2 falls and the hypoxaemia will cause serious damage before the hypercapnia reaches dangerous levels. Oxygen therapy should therefore be given but by using a combination of oxygen and air the concentration of oxygen administered can be adjusted so as not to exceed 30 per cent. This will permit the relief of severe hypoxia but the relief will be inadequate to remove the stimulus of hypoxia to respiration. If greater concentrations of oxygen are used, depression of ventilation occurs with alarming rapidity and can cause death from carbon dioxide narcosis within an hour. Thus, though hypercapnia is of no real danger to the patient breathing air, when he is breathing oxygen especially in concentrations exceeding 30 per cent it becomes potentially lethal. Carbon dioxide narcosis is unlikely to occur at oxygen concentrations below 35 per cent but if it does it should be treated with analeptic drugs. The oxygen should always be humidified and this requires an efficient nebulizer as bubbling through water is not adequate. The method of administering oxygen should be comfortable for the patient as it will be necessary to continue treatment for many hours. Many of the disposable masks allow a substantial degree of re-breathing and are therefore potentially harmful. The disposable venti-mask (Oxygenaire) and Edinburgh mask (British Oxygen Co.) are satisfactory and do not require humidification artificially as when the Venturi principle is used the gas breathed is naturally humidified by the room air. In the Venturi principle a fine jet of oxygen at a flow of 2 litres per minute induces a flow of air of about 50 litres per minute giving an inspired oxygen concentration of approximately 24 per cent. By increasing the amount of added oxygen to a side tube, controlled concentrations of up to 30 per cent oxygen can be given.

Oxygen therapy must be continuous as intermittent therapy is dangerous. Its administration should therefore not be left to the whims of the patient or nursing staff. Serial measurements of the p CO_2 are desirable so that the inspired oxygen concentration can be adjusted accordingly. The aim of oxygen therapy is to raise the oxygen saturation of the blood to about 80 per cent. This will prevent severe hypoxia and yet avoid removing the stimulus for respiration.

In acute pulmonary conditions such as lobar pneumonia, pulmonary embolus or pneumothorax there is little danger of carbon dioxide retention and 100 per cent oxygen therapy is safe.

4. *Clearing the airway.*

The production of coughing is of the utmost importance. It clears the airway and also prevents the pulmonary collapse, which so often accompanies shallow breathing. Frequent physiotherapy, even if no more than tipping and turning the patient, is of the greatest benefit. Amateur attention at frequent intervals is far better than expert attention only twice daily. Bronchoscopy may occasionally be indicated to clear the airway. When consciousness is impaired the tongue may fall back and obstruct the airway and the cough reflex will be suppressed. Correct posture of the patient is therefore important.

5. *Respiratory stimulants.*

When as a result of CO_2 narcosis the patient is drowsy and failing to expectorate the purulent sputum which is lining the bronchi and causing obstruction of the airway, the intravenous administration of nikethamide will stimulate the respiratory centre and rouse the patient to clear his airway: 2–10 ml. should be given slowly intravenously. Not only does this stimulate the patient to clear his airway but it also causes him to take deep breaths which is an important part of treatment as shallow respiration diminishes alveolar ventilation, predisposes towards pulmonary collapse and further deterioration of lung function. Other respiratory stimulants, such as amiphenazole, prethcamide or aminophylline have been advocated but are only really effective intravenously, although some benefit may be achieved by intramuscular injection. The therapeutic dose is near to the dose that causes convulsion so caution is necessary in administering these stimulants.

6. *Intermittent positive pressure respiration.*

Some patients require artificial ventilation to lower their p CO_2 and they are usually the individuals whose bronchial secretions are sticky and difficult to expectorate. Intermittent positive pressure respiration is indicated when controlled oxygen therapy is not producing improvement. For positive pressure respiration to be used effectively it is necessary that an endotracheal tube be passed or a tracheostomy performed. Endotracheal tubes cannot be left *in situ* for long periods and tracheostomy is therefore advisable if positive pressure respiration is to be instituted. The appropriate rate and volume of respiration must be determined for the individual patient and the p CO_2 should be estimated to ensure that ventilation is adequate.

7. *Tracheostomy.*

Tracheostomy is required when the patient is unable to cough and bronchial secretions obstruct the airway despite suction, physiotherapy and bronchoscopy. Once tracheostomy is performed it enables more effective aspiration of mucus in patients, who will not, or cannot, cough effectively. It also enables intermittent positive pressure respiration with a cuffed tracheostomy tube to be performed and it reduces the 'dead space' air. For many patients in whom respiratory failure is not due to primary disease of the lung but the result of neuromuscular paralysis from poliomyelitis or polyneuritis, the need for positive pressure assisted ventilation is the main indication for tracheostomy.

8. *Broncho-dilators.*

Broncho-dilators, in the form of aerosols, are helpful if given with an efficient nebulizer and will improve reversible airway obstruction (see Chronic Respiratory Failure). Injection of intravenous aminophylline is indicated if obstruction is severe.

9. *Treatment of Cor pulmonale.*

Cor pulmonale is a complication of the altered blood gases and is reversible if the lung failure can be corrected. Treatment of the respiratory disorder is thus the most important factor. Diuretics and digoxin may however be indicated as a temporary measure or, if the lung failure cannot be corrected, on a more continuous basis. There is however a risk of precipitating cardiac arrhythmias if digitalis is used in respiratory failure.

Chronic Respiratory Failure

There is no satisfactory treatment for this condition. The avoidance of exacerbating factors, such as smoking and fog, will improve ventilation. Broncho-dilators may decrease the airway obstruction. Oxygen from a lightweight portable oxygen cylinder may improve the exercise tolerance of the respiratory cripple and make an enormous difference to his way of life. Aerosols containing adrenaline, isoprenaline or orciprenaline are useful and pressurized inhalers or medihalers are convenient though expensive. It is essential to teach the patient the correct use of an inhaler to gain the maximum therapeutic effect. As there is now no doubt that cigarette smoking is a major factor causing airway obstruction one of the most important aspects of treatment is to persuade the patient who smokes to stop. In an occasional patient surgical removal of emphysematous bullae or segments of emphysematous lung may be of real benefit. Although there is some evidence that patients with chronic ventilatory failure frequently have a defective drive to breathe, the results of treatment with respiratory stimulants have been disappointing.

The oral broncho-dilator agents are sympathomimetic drugs or aminophylline compounds. These include:

1. Ephedrine or ephedrine resinate (Asmapax) for prolonged action.

2. Isoprenaline. Sublingual administration is necessary for maximum absorption. A disadvantage of this drug is that it may cause palpitations.
3. Orciprenaline. This is preferable to isoprenaline as cardiac side effects are not prominent.
4. Choline theophyllinate (Theophylline).

Selected Bibliography

CAMPBELL, E. J. M. (1965) Respiratory Failure. *Brit. Med. J.* 1, 1451.
CAMPBELL, E. J. M., DICKINSON, C. J. and SLATER, J. D. H. (1968) *Clinical Physiology*. 3rd Ed. Blackwell, Oxford.
COMROE, J. H. and others (1962) The Lung. 2nd Ed. *Year Book*.

VI

Radioactive Isotopes in Clinical Medicine

A rational understanding of the use of radioactive isotopes must be based on an elementary knowledge of the structure of the atom and of the fundamental particles. We shall first deal with the radioactive particles, and then consider the types of radiation and the measurement of radioactivity.

FUNDAMENTAL PARTICLES

There are four fundamental atomic particles—the proton, the neutron, the electron, and the positron. The *proton* has mass and a unit positive electrical charge. The *neutron* has mass and no charge. The *electron* has very small mass compared with the proton and neutron, and has unit negative electrical charge. The *positron* is the positively charged counterpart of the electron, having equal mass and unit positive charge.

The atom is composed of a positively charged central nucleus surrounded by a number of electrons. The nucleus is made up of protons and neutrons. The number of protons determines the positive charge and is known as the *atomic number*. The number of protons plus neutrons is the *atomic mass number* and determines the *atomic weight*. The number of orbital electrons surrounding the nucleus of an atom is equal to the number of protons in the nucleus. Hence the atom is electrically neutral. Since chemical reactions concern only interactions between the outer electrons, the chemical properties of an atom are determined by the number of orbital electrons—that is, they are characterized by the atomic number.

An *element* is matter consisting of atoms having the same atomic number. The number of neutrons in the atom of an element may vary and therefore its atomic mass number may vary. A *nuclide* is a species of atom characterized by its atomic number, atomic mass number, and nuclear energy state. *Isotopes* are nuclides having the same atomic number but different mass number. For example, hydrogen with atomic number one occurs in nature as a mixture of the nuclides hydrogen–1 with mass number one (that is, one proton in its nucleus), and hydrogen–2 (deuterium or heavy hydrogen) with mass number two—that is, one proton and one neutron in its nucelus. Hydrogen–1 and hydrogen–2 are both isotopes of hydrogen and are chemically indistinguishable. The terms isotope and radioactive isotope are frequently used when nuclide and radioactive

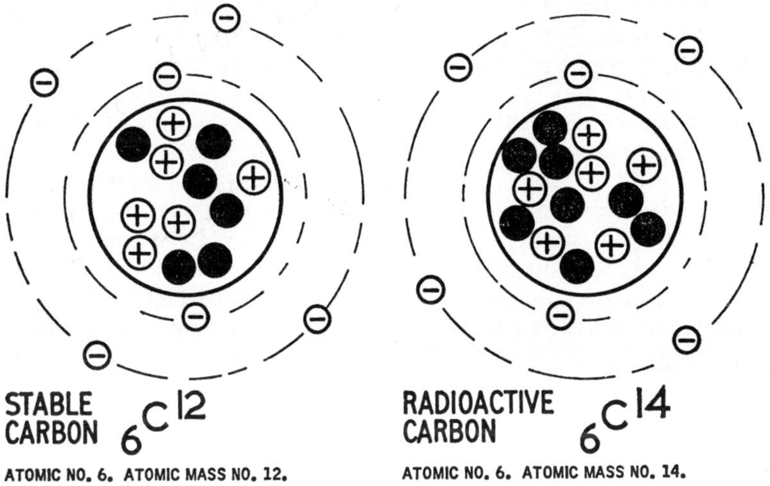

FIG. 12 Atomic structure of stable carbon and radioactive carbon

nuclide would be more accurate. Atomic weight is not quite synonymous with atomic mass number. The atomic weight for a given specimen of an element is the mean weight of its atoms expressed in atomic mass units, for many elements consist of a mixture of different nuclides of that element.

Isotopes may be stable or radioactive. In *stable isotopes* the relative number of protons and neutrons are found to lie within quite close limits. In *radioactive isotopes* this balance is upset owing to an excess or deficiency of neutrons, with the result that the nuclei become unstable. They tend to change into stable configurations by processes known collectively as radioactive decay. This involves spontaneous disintegration with emission of radiation. The atomic structure of radioactive carbon, which has six protons and eight neutrons, and that of stable carbon, which has six protons and six neutrons, is illustrated in Fig. 12.

The artificially produced radioactive isotopes may be grouped roughly into two categories, those produced in a nuclear reactor and those produced in a cyclotron. In nuclear reactors the target elements are bombarded with neutrons. The nuclides produced, therefore, are usually isotopic with the stable target elements, and have more neutrons in their nuclei. The radioactive isotope of hydrogen, tritium, has a mass number of three and the ratio of neutrons to protons is 2:1. Isotopes with excess neutrons in the nuclei tend to decay by the emission of beta rays. In the process of producing isotopes in a cyclotron the target material is bombarded with protons, deuterons, or alpha particles. The radioactive products are thus isotopes of a different element from the target. They are deficient in neutrons, and therefore tend to decay by emission of positrons.

Each radioactive substance, whether naturally occurring, produced in a nuclear reactor, or in a cyclotron, is characterized not only by the type and energy of radiation given off but also by the rate of disintegration. The *half-life* is the time taken for one-half of the original number of unstable atoms to disintegrate. Half-lives of different isotopes vary enormously. For example, carbon-14 has a half-life of over 5,000 years, while silver-109 has a half-life of only 39 seconds. The unit of radioactivity is the *curie*, which may be defined as that activity in which the number of disintegrations per second is $3{\cdot}7 \times 10^{10}$.

Within the nucleus the particles are in constant motion, and therefore they collide frequently. In these collisions energy transfers take place, so that all particles do not have the same kinetic energy. In a stable nucleus no particle ever acquires sufficient energy to overcome the potential barrier and to escape from the nucleus. In an unstable nucleus, owing to the presence of an excess number of neutrons, there is an excess of energy among the particles, so that there is a probability that one particle will acquire sufficient kinetic energy to overcome the barrier and to escape from the nucleus.

TYPES OF RADIATION

The type and energy of radiation given off by radioactive substances is the same for any one nuclide. The primary radioactive decay process is always either the emission of a charged particle (alpha particle, beta particle, or positron) or the capture by the nucleus of an orbital electron. These processes alter the charge on the nucleus, giving rise to a chemically different element. Any one of these may be accompanied by gamma rays or *x* rays. In medical diagnosis the beta particles and gamma rays are the most commonly encountered forms of radioactivity.

Beta particles are electrons and have limited tissue penetration dependent on their energy. Even energetic beta particles are only able to penetrate about one centimetre of tissue, so they are not suitable for the study of deep organs. Gamma rays are not particulate, but are electromagnetic radiations of the same nature as light, though of much shorter wavelength, and therefore of much higher energy. They may be considered as being made up of discrete amounts of energy or photons. They have a much greater power of

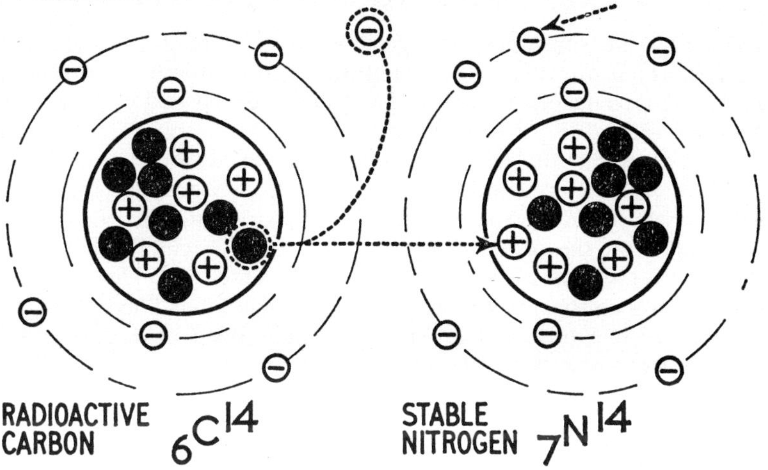

FIG. 13 Diagrammatic representation of the decay of radioactive carbon

penetration than beta particles, and this power is dependent upon their energy.

Isotopes having an excess of neutrons usually decay by emission of negative beta particles. Decay of an isotope by emission of a beta particle may be thought of as the conversion of a neutron into a proton and electron, with the immediate ejection of the electron from the nucleus (Fig. 13.) The loss of a unit of negative charge means that the nucleus has effectively gained a proton in place of a neutron, and the resulting nucleus is that of the next highest element in the periodic system. To maintain electrical neutrality the atom must acquire an extra orbital electron. The decay of radioactive isotopes has thus fulfilled the dream of the alchemist. Radioactive carbon decays by emission of a beta particle and becomes stable nitrogen (Fig. 13.) Similarly phosphorus-32 disintegrates with the emission of a beta particle, and thereupon becomes stable sulphur. This may be represented by the equation:

$$^{32}P_{15} \rightarrow {}^{32}S_{16} + \beta-$$

The beta particles from a particular isotope have varying energies up to a maximum characteristic of that isotope. Phosphorus-32, sulphur-35, carbon-14, and hydrogen-3 are beta emitters. In some isotopes the available energy in the radioactive nucleus is not accounted for completely by beta decay, and excess energy is then emitted as a gamma ray. This occurs with such isotopes as iodine-131, iodine-132, sodium-24, and potassium-42.

MEASUREMENT OF RADIOACTIVITY

Radioactive substances are detected by virtue of the radiation they emit. Ionization and excitation of the atoms is produced in the absorbing medium through which they pass. The beta rays produce ionization directly by their electrical charge. The gamma rays, by interaction with the atoms in the absorbing medium, produce so-called secondary electrons which behave in the same way as beta particles. Some radiation detectors—namely, the ionization chamber, the proportional counter, and the Geiger counter—depend on the ionization produced in a gas. Essentially each of these instruments consists of two electrodes in a chamber filled with gas, across which a potential difference is maintained. The passage of ions between the electrodes gives rise to an electric current or a series of pulses, both of which may be measured.

The scintillation detector consists of a 'phosphor,' such as a sodium iodide crystal, a photo-multiplier tube, and associated electronic equipment. When radiation energy is absorbed in the phosphor each quantum absorbed gives rise to a number of light quanta (photons). These cause emission of electrons from the photocathode of the photo-multiplier tube, which in turn give rise to a pulse at its output. The size of these pulses is proportional to the energy of the absorbed radiation and the number of pulses to the intensity of the absorbed radiation. The pulses are measured and counted by the associated electronic equipment.

Ionization chambers are the least sensitive of detectors. The Geiger counter and the scintillation counter are equally sensitive to beta radiations, but the scintillation counter has much greater sensitivity to gamma radiation than the Geiger counter.

APPLICATIONS OF RADIOACTIVE ISOTOPES TO DIAGNOSIS

The use of radioactive isotopes in diagnosis is based on the fact that it is possible to tag many of the substances normally present in the body with a radioactive label. Because it is possible to detect minute quantities of radioactive material, only very small doses need be given. The body pool of the material is therefore not appreciably altered, and metabolism is not disturbed. Thus in studies of iodine metabolism the ratio of radioactive atoms administered to stable atoms in the body pool is of the order of 1 to 1,000 million. By measuring radioactivity in the body, in blood samples, or in the excreta it is possible to gain information about the fate of the labelled substance, and hence of the chemically identical inactive material. Hence it is theoretically possible to trace the absorption, distribution, and excretion of any substance normally present in the body, provided that it can be tagged with a suitable radioactive label.

If the investigation necessitates tracing the path of the material through the body by means of external counting over the body surface it is obviously essential to use an isotope that emits gamma radiation or positrons. If, however, only measurements on blood samples or excreta are required it is possible to use pure beta emitters. Recently whole-body counters have been introduced which measure the total radioactivity in the body, and these are of great value in absorption studies. Another development has been that of more sensitive scanning devices, which are used in studying the distribution of radioactive isotopes in various organs and tissues. Furthermore, the recent production of isotopes with shorter lives has made it possible to give higher radioactive doses without increasing the radiation hazard. This is of particular advantage to the scanning techniques, which now enable most organs of the body to be visualized.

Five main groups of diagnostic uses may be defined.

1. Metabolic Studies

The use of radioactive materials in metabolic studies is based on the fundamental property that all isotopes of an element are chemically identical. The radioactive isotope is used as a true isotope tracer—that is, when introduced into the body (in whatever form) it behaves in the same way as the inactive element. Thus isotopes of iodine are used to measure thyroid function, and isotopes of calcium enable kinetic studies of bone formation and destruction to be performed. The distribution of iron-59 from the serum to the bone marrow, liver, and spleen may be followed and its incorporation into the haemoglobin of the red cell used as a measure of bone-marrow function. Orthoiodohippurate (Hippuran) labelled with iodine-131 may be used to assess renal vascularity and to detect differences in renal blood supply due to such conditions as renal artery stenosis.

2. **Absorption and Distribution Studies**

The fate of labelled substances given by mouth can be followed to assess their absorption, utilization, and excretion. In most of these studies the isotope is a true isotope tracer. For example, iron absorption can be measured with radioactive iron; vitamin-B_{12} absorption may be investigated with vitamin B_{12} tagged with radioactive cobalt. In studies of fat absorption, on the other hand, triolein labelled with iodine-131 may be used, but this is not a true isotopic tracer.

3. **Body Composition by Dilution Studies**

By introducing an isotope into a compartment, such as the blood or extracellular space, it is possible to measure the volume of that compartment by determining the dilution of radioactivity when equilibrium has been reached. In this way iodine-131-labelled human serum albumin is used to estimate the plasma volume; chromium-51-labelled red cells to measure the red-cell volume; and bromine-82 to determine the extra-cellular water. The total body exchangeable potassium can be measured with potassium-42, and total exchangeable sodium with sodium-24 or sodium-22.

4. **Physical Tracing Studies**

In this type of study the isotope is not necessarily used as a true isotopic tracer. In other words, it does not trace the path of the corresponding inactive isotope. For example, xenon-133 is used in measurements of blood flow in muscles, and in lung-function studies; krypton-85 is used to detect intracardiac shunts. Neither of these elements is normally present in the body. The survival of red cells may be followed and the organ of sequestration revealed by labelling red cells with radioactive chromium. Though chromium is normally present in the body, it does not take part in the metabolic process of the red cell, and the labelling of cells with chromium-51 is simply used as a convenient tag to trace their fate.

5. **Scanning of Organs and Tissues**

Scanning is a technique which is used to determine the distribution of radioactive isotopes within the body or within one particular organ. In the conventional scanner the radiation detector, which is a scintillation counter, 'sees' only a small cross-sectional area of the body at a time. The activity 'seen' at each point is registered, and a 'map' of the activity seen over the scanned area is recorded. Various methods of presentation have been used, and the recently improved display systems present the information gathered by the scanner more effectively. Mechanical printing of black marks, which are closer together for higher count rates (PLATE VI), has been followed by photoscanning and by 'colour print-outs,' where the colour of the mark is selected by the count rate. A pictorial representation of the degree of radioactivity is thus achieved. This is advantageous, as the eye can detect quite small variations in colour pattern from point to point much more easily than in monochrome. More recent developments are stationary detectors such as the gamma camera, autofluoroscope, and other devices which can view the whole of the area simultaneously. Thus when selective concentration of an isotope in a tissue occurs it is possible to examine the distribution of that isotope by means of scanning. A toxic nodule in the thyroid may be identified by its selective concentration of iodine-131 (PLATE VI). Areas of absent function on the radioactive scan ('cold' areas) suggest the presence of tumours, abscesses, and similar lesions (PLATE VII). Iodine-131 may be used to localize tumours of the thyroid, and chlormerodrin labelled with mercury-197 to delineate tumours of the kidneys. Of even greater practical application is the localizing of brain tumours with chlormerodrin labelled with mercury-197, with human serum albumin labelled with iodine-131 or with radioactive technetium.

We now propose to deal with some of these applications in detail.

METABOLIC STUDIES

Iodine Isotopes

Isotopes of iodine are the most commonly used isotopes in clinical medicine, and, as they have also thrown considerable light on the physiology of the thyroid gland, they will be considered at some length. Iodine is present in the diet as iodide and is readily absorbed from the gut into the blood stream, being trapped by the thyroid and excreted by the kidneys. In the plasma, iodine exists partly as inorganic iodide (less than 1 mcg. of iodide per 100 ml.) and partly as protein-bound or hormonal iodide (4 to 6 mcg. per 100 ml.). The average daily diet contains 100 to 200 mcg. of iodide and about 55 mcg. are taken up by the normal thyroid each day.

Owing to the presence of specific enzymes the thyroid gland is able to trap these small amounts of circulating iodide into its substance. The iodide is then converted to iodine and bound to organic compounds of tyrosine to form the thyroid hormones thyroxine and tri-iodothyronine, which are then either secreted into the circulation or stored in the gland as thyroglobulin. The initial trapping of iodide is blocked by substances such as perchlorate and the subsequent organic binding of iodine is inhibited by drugs such as the thiouracils and carbimazole.

The most commonly used isotope of iodine is iodine-131, which has a half-life of 8 days and emits both beta particles and gamma rays. The beta particles are completely absorbed within the thyroid gland and cannot be measured externally. It is therefore the gamma emission that is important for diagnostic purposes. In certain situations another isotope of iodine, iodine-132, is advantageous. This has a half-life of only 2·3 hours, so that the radiation dose to the thyroid is only 1 per cent of that with iodine-131. This may be of importance when repeated studies are necessary or when radiation must be kept to an absolute minimum, as in pregnancy or in children. Furthermore, if the isotope studies are to be repeated a few days later the short half-life is a great advantage, as no appreciable remaining radioactivity will be present after a day or two (only 0·05 per cent remains after 24 hours).

Tests of Thyroid Function

Tests of thyroid function depend, firstly, on the rate of uptake of the iodine isotope by the gland, and, secondly, on the proportion that reappears in the circulation as labelled hormone bound to the plasma proteins. The functional activity of solitary thyroid nodules can also be assessed by special scanning procedures. Nevertheless, it must be remembered that the clinical state of the patient depends on the amount of *stable* iodide taken up by the thyroid which is converted into thyroid hormone and secreted into the circulation.

A commonly used diagnostic test of hyperthyroidism is the uptake of iodine-131 by the thyroid gland after an administered dose of the isotope by mouth. The value of this depends on the fact that the rate of trapping of iodide by the thyroid gland in general parallels the rate of secretion of thyroid hormone into the circulation. A few exceptions exist. If the thyroid store of iodine is low the uptake of iodine-131 will be high. When stores are low most of the iodide derived from the peripheral degradation of thyroxine is reutilized, and little is allowed to escape in the urine. The thyroid hypertrophies to maintain a normal output of thyroid hormone by trapping a greater proportion of the circulating iodide from the blood. This gives rise to the hyperplastic, non-toxic goitre of iodine deficiency, puberty, and pregnancy, in which the increased uptake of iodine-131 is not associated with an increased secretion of thyroxine.

The normal range of uptake varies from 20 to 55 per cent of the administered dose of isotope at 24 hours. Values exceeding 55 per cent are suggestive of hyperthyroidism, and values less than 20 per cent of hypothyroidism. The test is more reliable in overactivity than underactivity of the thyroid, and the chemical estimation of the protein-bound iodine concentration in the serum is a better test of hypothyroidism. Though in euthyroid patients the uptake by the thyroid gland is maximal at 24 hours, in many cases of hyperthyroidism the maximum uptake is reached earlier, and by the time the 24-hour reading is taken the level has fallen, because some of the isotope has been secreted into the blood as labelled thyroxine. This accounts for the fact that one in ten patients with hyperthyroidism shows a normal 24-hour uptake. Readings should therefore be taken at four and six hours after administration of the isotope as well.

It is also advisable that the 24-hour uptake should be combined with some other test of thyroid function, and this usually takes the form of a measure of the iodine-131, which has reappeared in the circulation as labelled hormone bound to plasma proteins. In hyperthyroidism a high concentration of protein-bound iodine-131 is present in the serum after the dose of isotope, and this reaches a peak at about 48 hours. The normal value does not exceed 0·3 per cent of the administered dose per litre of plasma. An alternative measure is the proportion of total plasma radioactivity that is bound to protein at 24 hours. The unbound portion represents the administered dose that has not been taken up by the thyroid. The protein-bound fraction represents that which has been taken up by the thyroid and which has reappeared as circulating thyroxine bound to protein. Normally the proportion of the protein-bound fraction is less than 35 per cent, while in hyperthyroidism it is usually greater than 50 per cent.

It is important to remember that the protein-bound iodine-131 is not a true measure of the plasma-thyroxine concentration. The former depends not only on the rate of secretion of thyroid hormones but on the size of the iodine pool within the thyroid and the proportion of the isotope dose that has accumulated within the thyroid. In hyperthyroidism the iodine pool within the thyroid is usually normal, and a raised protein-bound iodine-131 concentration reflects an increased hormonal secretion rate. If, however, the thyroid iodine pool is reduced, which will happen if the patient has had a previous thyroidectomy or previous iodine-131 therapy, and also if the patient has lymphocytic destruction of the gland (chronic thyroiditis), a raised radioactive protein-bound iodine level may mean no more than a reduced iodine pool. Moreover, if the amount of stored thyroxine (thyroglobulin within the acini of the gland) is reduced radioactive thyroxine will be present in greater concentration, and the same hormone output will contain more radioactive protein-bound iodine.

Nevertheless, a combination of the 24-hour uptake by the gland and some measure of the rate of reappearance of labelled thyroxine enable most cases of hyperthyroidism to be diagnosed accurately.

If doubt remains in differentiating a simple goitre from a toxic gland a suppression test with tri-iodothyronine may be performed. This depends on the fact that normally 120 mcg. of tri-iodothyronine daily for one week will suppress pituitary thyrotrophic hormone and considerably reduce the amount of isotope taken up by the gland (usually to less than 35 per cent of the uptake at 24 hours). In hyperthyroidism, on the other hand, the activity of the thyroid gland is usually unaffected by administered tri-iodothyronine. Hence a measure of iodine-131 uptake before and after treatment with tri-iodothyronine is often helpful in difficult cases.

In pregnancy the administration of iodine-131 is contra-indicated. The most satisfactory test for hyperthyroidism in pregnancy is measuring the iodine-132 uptake and the effect of tri-iodothyronine suppression. The protein-bound iodine and basal metabolic rate are raised in normal pregnancy, and are therefore of little help.

IN VITRO TRI-IODOTHYRONINE UPTAKE TESTS

A number of procedures have been introduced to measure indirectly the amount of free thyroid hormone in the plasma. The uptake of tri-iodothyronine by a resin-sponge has proved the most useful. Circulating thyroxine is bound to a plasma protein called the thyroxine-binding globulin. Tri-iodothyronine is similarly but less firmly bound. In hyperthyroidism the thyroxine-binding sites are largely saturated. Any added tri-iodothyronine will therefore tend to be taken up by alternative binding sites such as red blood cells, or by exogenous material such as a resin-sponge. In hypothyroidism on the other hand thyroxine-binding globulin is poorly saturated and will therefore take up more avidly any added tri-iodothyronine.

The principle of the test is based on the competition for added radioactive tri-iodothyronine between the thyroxine-binding protein of the patient's plasma on the one hand and an ion-exchange resin on the other. Iodine-131 labelled tri-iodothyronine is added to the patient's serum and without delay a resin-sponge added to the mixture. After incubation for one hour the radioactivity in the tube is counted. The serum is then discarded and the radioactivity in the resin-sponge counted, after it has been washed. The percentage uptake of the sponge can then be calculated. In hypothyroid patients it is between 16 and 26 per cent, in euthyroid patients between 25 and 36 per cent and in hyperthyroid patients between 34 and 55 per cent. There is however some degree of overlap. The test has the advantage that is not invalidated by the previous administration of iodine-containing compounds. The disadvantage of the test is that quantitative changes in the total thyroxine binding globulin capacity will affect the results. Thus in pregnancy, as in patients on oral contraceptives, where there is an increase in thyroxine binding globulin the resin uptake will be reduced. Drugs which interfere with thyroid hormone binding will similarly upset the test. Salicylates for example are partly bound to thyroxine binding globulin and this reduces the binding capacity for thyroid hormone. In liver diseases there is an alteration in the plasma protein, which affects the test.

Thyroid Scanning

The distribution of iodine-131 in the gland may be investigated by scanning techniques (PLATE VI). If a solitary nodule takes up iodine more freely than the rest of the gland it is likely to be benign, whereas if it does not take up any isotope the nodule is likely to be a cyst or possibly neoplastic. Substernal extension of the gland and ectopic thyroid tissue may also be identified by scanning, while this technique is also of use in detecting metastases from those carcinomas of the thyroid which are metabolically active.

All these isotope investigations, as well as the chemical estimations of plasma-iodine concentrations, will be affected by alterations in the inorganic iodide pool of the body, such as may occur in states of iodine deficiency or as a result of increased dietary intake of iodine. It is the total amount of iodide trapped by the gland, converted to thyroid hormone, and secreted into the circulation that determines the clinical state of the patient. It is therefore important that the inorganic iodide pool should be normal if the isotope measurements are to be significant. An increase in the size of the pool will decrease the uptake of isotope, and a decrease in the size of the pool will increase the uptake of isotope. It has been shown that a single dose of 1 mg. of stable iodide by mouth will reduce the isotope uptake of a hyperthyroid patient to normal, and that 10 mg. will reduce it to inappreciable levels. One millilitre of Lugol's solution contains 130 mg. iodine, which is equivalent to a normal iodine requirement for 1,000 days. The iodine pool would thus be increased tremendously if such doses were taken. Many cough mixtures contain a large amount of iodine, and organic iodide is contained in compounds used as radiographic contrast media. These will suppress the radioactive-iodine uptake and invalidate the test. Though the kidney rapidly excretes the dyes used for pyelography, the contrast media used for cholecystography, bronchography, and myelography may continue to release iodide for many months or even years. Hence it is of the utmost importance that patients referred to hospital for investigation of thyroid function should not receive iodine therapy before coming. The taking of antithyroid drugs will also suppress the isotopic iodine turnover.

Though iodine-131 tests are less reliable for the diagnosis of hypothyroidism, they provide a useful distinction between primary and secondary hypothyroidism when undertaken before and after the administration of thyroid-stimulating hormone.

Bone-marrow Function

The utilization by the red blood cells of iron-59 given intravenously can be used as a measure of bone-marrow function. Daily measurements of radioactivity in the red cells will demonstrate the rate of incorporation of iron into the haemoglobin molecule, and this provides a measure of effective erythropoiesis—that is, erythropoiesis which results in the production of viable red cells that survive an appreciable time in the circulation. The amount of iron leaving the plasma can be calculated from a knowledge of the rate of disappearance of iron-59 from the plasma and the concentration of the serum iron. This is called the plasma-iron turnover, and it measures the total erythroid activity, which includes both effective and ineffective erythropoiesis. Ineffective erythropoiesis includes erythropoiesis which does not result in viable red cells because the red-cell precursors are destroyed within the bone-marrow or because the red cells produced are so defective that they survive only a few minutes or hours in the blood. Plasma-iron turnovers are of little value as a measure of bone-marrow activity, and they are largely used for research studies of iron metabolism. Scanning over the body surface will reveal the distribution of radioactive iron in the bone-marrow, liver, and spleen, and may be of help in determining whether extra-medullary haemopoiesis is taking place in such organs as the spleen. The presence of extramedullary haemopoiesis can be assumed when iron-59 curves resembling those seen by scanning the bone-marrow are found also to occur over the liver or the spleen. When the bone-marrow is aplastic most of the iron goes to the liver. These patterns of iron metabolism may be of help in diagnosing disorders of the bone-marrow.

A disadvantage of the iron-isotope test is that it cannot measure any *increase* in bone-marrow function. Thus the bone-marrow may increase its output sixfold in chronic haemolytic states, but the red cell uptake of radioactive iron will be reduced because the rapid destruction of labelled red cells leads to a loss of iron-59 from the blood. In both haemolytic anaemia and iron deficiency, for example, the marrow curve of iron-59 uptake will fall more rapidly than normal, as the iron leaves the bone-marrow in the red cells at an enhanced rate.

Kidney Function

Iodine-131-labelled orthoiodohippurate (Hippuran) may be used to study renal function. An initial rapid rise in isotope concentration over the kidneys following intravenous administration represents the filling of the renal blood vessels. This is called the vascular phase. Differences in the rate and degree of this initial uptake between the two kidneys may permit the detection of renal artery stenosis in the assessment of patients with hypertension. A subsequent slower rise in isotope concentration represents active tubular transport. This is the secretory phase. The final stage of rapidly decreasing concentration coincides with the excretion of the dye into the bladder and is called the excretory phase. Non-functioning kidneys show a slight initial uptake, followed by a flattening of the curve. Ureteric obstruction will be characterized by a normal uptake with a delayed excretory phase.

In addition to these studies the glomerular filtration rate may be measured with iodine-131 labelled inulin.

STUDIES OF ABSORPTION AND DISTRIBUTION

Iron Absorption

Ferrous iron is absorbed from the duodenum and upper part of the small intestine in quantities that depend on the body needs. Thus as the iron stores fall more iron is absorbed. Ferric iron must be reduced to the ferrous state before it can be absorbed, and ascorbic acid, among other reducing agents, will achieve this. Iron transfer across the mucosal cell is part of an active metabolic process during which a proportion of the iron absorbed is delivered to the transferrin of the plasma and the remainder deposited as ferritin within the mucosal cell. The deposition of iron as ferritin prevents excessive absorption from the gut as the iron is lost to the body when the mucosal cells exfoliate. After absorption iron becomes attached to a beta-globulin called transferrin, and is cleared quickly from the plasma by the bone-marrow, where it is incorporated into the haemoglobin molecule of the developing erythrocyte. The total serum-iron level remains at about 120 mcg. per 100 ml., and transferrin is normally only one-third saturated. Iron excreted in the faeces represents the amount unabsorbed, and a measure of the fraction absorbed may therefore be obtained from the difference between the amount in the faeces and the dose given by mouth. Normally the amount of iron absorbed is not more than 30 per cent, but in iron deficiency this figure may increase to 80 per cent. Seventy to one hundred per cent of the absorbed iron will reappear in the circulating erythrocytes within a period of ten days. The remainder is deposited as iron stores in the form of ferritin or haemosiderin in the liver, spleen, bone-marrow, and reticuloendothelial system.

Studies of the absorption of radioactive inorganic iron salts in a fasting subject give information of only limited value, for ferrous salts are absorbed more readily than food iron in both normal people and patients with iron deficiency. Indeed, in patients who have undergone partial gastrectomy food iron may be absorbed poorly but ferrous chloride readily. The difference is due in part to the necessity of reducing the food iron to the ferrous form before absorption takes place, and in part to the solid content of the test meal and the formation of insoluble iron compounds, such as phytates and phosphates, when the iron is taken in food. In order to study iron absorption under natural conditions, the absorption of iron incorporated biosynthetically into foods, such as eggs and vegetables, may be studied, but the labelling process is tedious. Tests of iron absorption have therefore been developed in which the labelled iron is added to a meal of standard iron content. Though this is not an exact reproduction of the conditions by which food iron is absorbed, it has been shown to provide a reliable measure of absorption of dietary iron.

Double Isotope Technique

A double isotope technique for measuring iron absorption has recently been introduced, and this obviates the necessity of stool collection. One isotope of iron (iron-59) is injected intravenously, and another isotope (iron-55) is given by mouth at the same time. The intravenous isotope is used to determine the percentage of plasma iron that is used for haemoglobin synthesis: this is the amount which appears within the circulating red cells after a period of ten days. From the relative amount of the orally administered isotope in the red cells at the same time it is possible to calculate the amount of oral isotope that has been absorbed. Both the isotopes of iron can be counted separately. Liquid scintillation counting is required for the iron-55, and this necessitates separating the iron from the blood by a process of digestion and precipitation. The accuracy of these methods is reduced if iron is not absorbed adequately, or, if as a result of iron overloading, the radioactive iron does not appear in the circulating haemoglobin in an appreciable concentration.

A happy solution to many of the problems of absorption in haematological studies, and indeed to the studies of absorption in general, is the development of a reliable whole body counter. The measurement of total body radioactivity immediately after a dose of a radioactive isotope, and then again a week or more later, provides the information necessary to determine the amount absorbed. A suitable body counter would obviate the need for stool collections, and, as it would mean counting body radioactivity on only two occasions, it would be ideal for out-patient use. It is obviously important that the count recorded should always be proportional to the radioactivity in the body and independent of any localization of this radioactivity. The crystal must therefore be placed at a distance from the patient. The use of two detectors, one above and one below the patient, has improved the accuracy of such a total body counter. Rapid developments are taking place in the field of counting whole body radioactivity, and there is little doubt that this method will provide the most acceptable and accurate measure of absorption of radioactive compounds before long.

Vitamin-B_{12} Absorption

Certain species of streptomyces synthesize vitamin B_{12}, a vitamin containing one atom of cobalt per molecule. If radioactive cobalt is added to the culture medium of the organism the synthesized vitamin is radioactive. Pernicious anaemia is characterized by a deficiency of intrinsic factor, and vitamin B_{12} cannot be absorbed from the ileum unless intrinsic factor is present. The radioactive cobalt bound to the vitamin may be traced after its oral administration, and if the labelled vitamin is absorbed then intrinsic factor must be present. The reverse, however, is not necessarily true, because vitamin B_{12} may not be absorbed on account of intestinal disease, such as regional ileitis, malabsorption syndrome, or tropical sprue. The principle of the test is to give labelled vitamin B_{12} by mouth and to calculate the amount absorbed. This may be done by counting the amount excreted in the faeces, a normal person losing 20–50 per cent of the administered dose, while a patient with pernicious anaemia loses 85–100 per cent of the dose. An alternative method is to measure the concentration in the blood after the administration of an oral dose, though this requires a large dose of isotope. The favoured test is, however, the Schilling test, which measures the urinary excretion of isotope. This test depends on detecting in the urine the amount of isotope that has been absorbed into the blood and excreted by the kidney. To prevent accumulation and storage of the radioactive vitamin in the body a large dose of non-radioactive vitamin B_{12} (1,000 mcg.) is given parenterally about an hour or two after the oral administration of the labelled vitamin. Urine is collected for 48 hours and the radioactivity measured. A normal person will excrete 15–50 per cent of the administered dose, but a patient with pernicious anaemia less than 7 per cent. The Schilling test is not reliable if there is renal failure. Repetition of the test after the administration of intrinsic factor will restore absorption to normal in the patient with pernicious anaemia, but will not improve the malabsorption of vitamin B_{12}, secondary to states of intestinal malabsorption. An alternative method of measuring vitamin-B_{12} absorption is to determine the liver uptake by external counting after an oral dose of labelled vitamin B_{12}.

The cobalt isotope originally used was cobalt-60, which has a half-life of five years. Other isotopes of cobalt have a shorter half-life and permit larger doses to be given and hence enable plasma levels to be determined. Cobalt-58 with a half-life of 71 days has been used for this purpose. Peak plasma concentrations occur 8 to 12 hours after an oral dose in a normal person.

Intestinal Fat Absorption

Fats labelled with iodine-131 have been used to determine the digestive and absorptive capacities of the intestinal tract. By giving triolein labelled with iodine-131 by mouth it is theoretically possible to estimate the unabsorbed fraction of fat in the faeces over a period of 48 hours. There is, however, little correlation between the degree of malabsorption as estimated by labelled triolein and that obtained by the chemical determination of fat excretion in patients with steatorrhoea. This is hardly surprising, as dietary fat consists of a mixture of long- and short-chain saturated and unsaturated fats and triolein may not be representative of these. Furthermore, the iodine label may become detached from the triolein and absorbed separately. Hence some patients with steatorrhoea appear to 'absorb' labelled triolein normally. Thus the clinical application of the isotope method is limited, and the chemical estimation of fat excretion remains the most reliable test of steatorrhoea. Nevertheless, it is true that most patients whose excretion of labelled triolein exceeds 5 per cent of the administered dose have malabsorption. Carbon-14-labelled fats have been used in research studies on animals: the half-life of the isotope is, however, over 5,000 years, so that the hazard of radiation precludes its general use in man.

ISOTOPES IN DILUTION STUDIES

The body content and distribution of water and electrolytes may be measured with the appropriate isotope, using the dilution principle. The estimation of plasma volume, red-cell volume, and exchangeable body sodium and potassium is largely restricted to research purposes. Nevertheless, the measurement of the plasma volume may be of value in states of dehydration following burns, in chronic protein deficiency, and in congestive cardiac failure. In states of dehydration the serum electrolyte concentrations are no reflection of the body content of the electrolytes. In polycythaemia rubra vera the red-cell volume is always increased and may often be twice normal. Occasionally there is a concomitant increase in plasma volume, so that the concentration of the haemoglobin and the packed cell volume may be near normal, though the total red-cell mass is greatly increased. In these situations the estimation of the red-cell volume may be of great value. A known quantity of red cells labelled with chromium-51 is injected, and a sample is taken 10 minutes later, when mixing has occurred. The red-cell mass may then be estimated from the degree of dilution that has occurred. The increased red-cell mass is an important diagnostic criterion to differentiate true polycythaemia from relative polycythaemia, in which the haemoglobin is raised but the red-cell mass is normal.

Similarly the concentration of electrolytes in the blood is not a true guide to the body's content of these elements if the plasma volume is altered. Plasma-volume determinations may then be helpful. This is done by injecting a known quantity of iodine-131-labelled human serum albumen into the circulation and withdrawing blood at a suitable interval after injection to measure its dilution and so estimate the plasma volume. Since human serum albumen will ultimately diffuse into the extracellular space, the specimens of blood for estimation of the isotope dilution must be withdrawn as soon as possible after mixing in the blood, and this is usually done at about ten minutes. If longer intervals are allowed to elapse there may be diffusion of the albumen into the extracellular space.

Isotope studies are useful for the measurement of exchangeable body potassium. As 90 per cent of the body potassium is intracellular, the serum concentration is a poor indicator of the total body potassium, especially if an associated loss of sodium has led to reduction of the extracellular volume. The isotope potassium-42 equilibrates with intracellular exchangeable potassium in about 24 to 48 hours. From the dilution of the isotope injected, therefore, the total exchangeable body potassium can be calculated.

PHYSICAL TRACING STUDIES

Red Cell Survival

Chromium, as sodium chromate, readily penetrates red blood cells and becomes firmly bound to the globin portion of the haemoglobin molecule. Labelling of red blood cells with chromium-51 permits evaluation of red-cell survival, and this method has replaced the Ashby differential agglutination technique, which could not be used to study the survival of a patient's own cells in his own circulation. The procedure involves withdrawal of a 20-ml. sample of blood and adding the isotope. An interval of 30 to 60 minutes allows the chromium to become attached to the haemoglobin of the red cells. The cells are then washed with normal saline, and a known amount of the labelled blood is reinjected. Samples are taken at intervals on subsequent days over the next two weeks. When the logarithm of the radioactivity (counts per minute) is plotted against time the points lie on a straight line and the time taken for half the radioactivity to disappear is apparent. The results of cell survival are usually expressed in terms of the half-time disappearance of the chromium isotope; the normal is about 28 days. Though this apparent survival curve differs appreciably from the survival curve obtained by the differential agglutination method, the results with chromium-51 are consistent and more accurate. The difference is largely due to the fact that chromium elutes from the red cells at a constant rate. Because this rate is constant it can be allowed for. Formulae are available for calculating the mean cell survival from these data. These calculations are accurate if cell survival is short but are less reliable when the cell life approaches normal.

In patients with a haemolytic process the site of red-cell destruction can be recognized by in-vivo surface counting, and this is an invaluable procedure before submitting a patient with haemolytic anaemia to splenectomy. Moreover, by measuring the survival of normal group O cells in the patient's circulation and the survival of the patient's cells in a normal compatible recipient, the nature of the haemolytic disease can be assessed. If, on the one hand, the patient's cells survive normally in a recipient then the haemolysis must be due to a lytic factor in the patient's serum. If, on the other hand, the patient's cells do not survive normally in a recipient the cells must be abnormal. The red cells from normal donors will survive their usual span in patients with diseases such as congential spherocytosis, sickle-cell disease, or paroxysmal nocturnal haemoglobinuria, where the haemolysis is due to intrinsic defects in the red cells. Conversely, spherocytic or sickle cells will be rapidly destroyed when transfused into normal people.

Leucocytes may also be labelled with chromium-51 and their survival measured. Various isotopes have been used for the measurement of platelet survival, but the in-vitro labelling of isologous platelets with chromium-51 has been the most extensively employed. A normal platelet survival of 8–10 days is obtained, and in idiopathic thrombocytopenic purpura the survival is found to be constantly reduced, being 1–3 days in the chronic varieties and shorter in more acute forms. The number of platelets in the peripheral blood has been shown to depend exclusively on the rate of platelet destruction. A compensatory increase in bone-marrow production does not seem to occur, as it does with the red-cell series in haemolytic disease. This suggests that the autoantibodies which influence the destruction of platelets also affect megakaryocyte function.

The labelling of red cells with chromium-51 also provides a sensitive measure of gastrointestinal bleeding. Normally only negligible amounts of radioactivity can be detected in the faeces in patients whose cells have been labelled with radioactive chromium. A comparison of the amount of chromium-51 in the stool with that in the circulating blood yields a quantitative figure of the volume of blood being lost.

Renogram

The clearance of hippuran by the kidney is a measure of renal plasma flow. By labelling the hippuran with iodine-131 it is possible to record the clearance pattern by external counting. A difference in pattern between the two kidneys represents a difference in renal circulation. This provides a useful screening test for hypertensive patients to permit the segregation of hypertensive patients with unilateral renal disease. This is only a screening test and further investigation is necessary if the isotope studies suggest a unilateral lesion. The interest in renograms has waned a little since it has become realized that hypertension in a patient with a narrowed renal artery is often not the result of the stenosis and that even when it is it may not be relieved when the stenosis is corrected.

Left to Right Cardiac Shunts

The radioactive gas krypton-85 may be used to detect intracardiac shunts. The gas is administered to the patient by inhalation and is carried through the pulmonary capillaries and veins to the left atrium. The instant at which the gas is inhaled is recorded by a Geiger counter placed in the inflow to the face mask. Blood from the right side of the heart is withdrawn through a cardiac catheter and directed through a scintillation counter, so that the moment of the appearance of radioactivity in the right side of the heart is also recorded. If there is no shunt the time interval is equal to the complete circulation time—that is, 15–25 seconds—whereas if there is a left to right shunt present the time interval is shorter—namely, about 5 seconds.

Determination of Blood Flow

The clearance of a freely diffusible indicator from extracellular tissue is determined only by the blood supply, and hence is a measure of local blood flow. This principle has been used to measure the blood flow in skeletal muscle, employing the radioactive gas xenon-133. The xenon is dissolved in saline and injected directly into muscle tissue; subsequently its clearance rate is measured by placing a scintillation counter directly over the injection site. This technique permits a clear-cut differentiation between limbs with a normal circulation and limbs with occlusive vascular disease.

Lung-function Studies

It is sometimes desirable to measure the function of small regions of lung as, for example, in assessing the pulmonary disability being caused by localized bullae. This may be done using the radioactive gas xenon-133. The radioactive xenon is dissolved in saline and injected through a catheter either into the femoral vein or the superior vena cava. When the xenon reaches the pulmonary capillaries it becomes transferred into alveolar gas because of its low solubility. The radioactivity is detected by scintillation counters placed at different areas over the chest, and the regional perfusion may be evaluated from the maximum counting rate. The regional ventilation may also be assessed from the rate of disappearance of the radioactivity from the region.

SCANNING OF ORGANS AND TISSUES

Brain Tumour Localization

Attempts have been made recently to discover compounds which will localize in tumour tissue. By labelling these compounds with a radioactive element it would then be possible to identify and locate such tumours. Useful preparations are now available for the detection of brain and liver tumours. For brain tumours chlormerodrin labelled with mercury-197 has been used with good effect. The localized concentration of this substance in tumours probably results from a breakdown of the vital barriers that prevent the entrance of certain substances into normal tissue.

Iodine-131-labelled human serum albumen has also been used to detect brain neoplasms, but in this instance the selective concentration in the tumour is not due to a breakdown of normal cell barriers but reflects the greater proportion of extracellular fluid that is characteristic of tumour tissue in the brain. Radioactive technetium is also distributed in extracellular fluid, and, with its suitable energy and shorter half-life, it promises to be a useful isotope for the detection of brain tumours. Most tumours (80 per cent confirmed positives) can be detected and localized by this method, but, as the radioactive compound must reach the tumour through the blood, vascular and inflammatory masses will also show a high uptake of radioactivity, so that it may be impossible to distinguish them from tumours. A technique such as this, which causes little distress to the patient, is likely to replace air-studies and cerebral angiography as screening procedures. Brain scanners are now available in which the distribution of radioactivity is displayed by the mechanical printing of coloured marks. The colour of the mark at any point is determined by the counting rate detected by the scintillation scanner at that point. Six colours may be selected from a multi-coloured ribbon. The highest counting rates are recorded by blue marks and lesser degrees of radioactivity are represented by purple, red, yellow, and green marks, and the lowest rates by black. Quite small variations in the colour pattern are visible to the human eye and the tumour may thus be visually portrayed.

Hepatic Tumours

Tumour masses may be identified in the liver by using an isotope which is taken up by normal liver cells and which will thus reveal tumours as 'cold areas.' As the Kupffer cells extract colloid particles from the blood, colloidal gold, labelled with gold-198, is taken up by the Kupffer cells and fixed there, so that a subsequent scan will show a reduced uptake if there is a tumour, abscess, or cyst. Rose-bengal is a dye rapidly taken up by liver cells and excreted into the bile. Tumours and masses, which do not contain functioning liver tissue, will not take up the dye. When the dye is labelled with iodine-131 tumours appear as 'cold areas' on the radioactive scan. (PLATE VII). Hepatic scans may provide information about the size, shape, position, and internal detail of the liver. Their major application is in the diagnosis of localized disease or space-occupying lesions within the liver. Nevertheless, equivocal results from such scans are unfortunately frequent.

Other Tumours

Chlormerodrin labelled with mercury-197, being concentrated in the renal tubules, has been used for the detection of renal tumours. These, being 'non-functioning' renal tissue, will appear as 'cold areas' on the radioactive scan. Renal abscesses and cysts cannot, however, be differentiated from tumours on a radioactive scan. Furthermore, renal scanning does not give the anatomical detail of arteriography, and hence its application is limited.

Selenomethionine labelled with selenium-75 behaves like the amino-acid methionine, and localizes in pancreatic tissue. The normal pancreas takes up the isotope uniformly, but tumours may appear as 'cold areas' on the radioactive scan, and in chronic pancreatitis there is often diffuse inhibition of isotope uptake. Unfortunately the liver also takes up the isotope, and it is necessary to precede this investigation with a liver scan, using colloidal gold labelled with gold-198, to determine the position of the liver edge. It is premature to assess the value of this method of detecting pancreatic tumours, but the diagnosis of tumours in this region is notoriously difficult, and, as the pancreas remains one of the few organs defying radiological demonstration, the value of an isotope method would be great.

Methionine is a constituent aminoacid of the polypeptide hormone parathormone. It is therefore taken up by the parathyroid glands. Selenomethionine labelled with selenium-75 has been used to detect parathyroid tumours for a localized increase in uptake on the radioactive scan due to the adenoma can sometimes be identified.

Scanning of the Lungs

Scintillation scanning of the lungs with iodine-131 macro-aggregated human serum albumen is a safe and effective way of demonstrating pulmonary perfusion. Ordinary albumen would pass through the lung capillaries without obstruction, but techniques are available for preparing aggregates of human serum albumen with a particle size of 10 to 100 microns. Following intravenous infusion these particles are trapped in the pulmonary capillaries during their passage through the lung field. Thus the distribution of these particles in any segment of lung is proportional to the pulmonary blood flow. The albumen may be labelled with iodine-131 or technetium-99 and the distribution of the radioactive aggregates measured by a scintillation counter. The albumen aggregates do not cause any permanent obstruction to pulmonary capillaries as they are readily metabolized, and indeed disappear from the lungs with a half life of five to ten hours.

The radioactive scan is likely to become of increasing importance in the diagnosis of pulmonary embolism. Small pulmonary emboli may be missed by the scan but major emboli will not escape detection and it is the major emboli that often provide the greatest diagnostic difficulty. Greater certainty in the diagnosis of this disorder is needed as so much more can now be done for these patients with embolectomy and anti-coagulant therapy. The scan is however not specific for pulmonary emboli. The appearance on a scan of a pulmonary embolus in a large lobar artery is indistinguishable from that of a lobar pneumonia. Indeed similar lung scan patterns occur in pulmonary neoplasms and pulmonary fibrosis also. Pulmonary angiography remains a superior technique for the diagnosis of pulmonary emboli and is required before surgical embolectomy.

The lung scan however causes little disturbance to the patient and may provide the diagnosis.

Other Applications

Red blood cells damaged by heat are rapidly destroyed in the spleen. If such cells are labelled with chromium-51 and reinjected subsequent in-vivo counting over the spleen area will enable the position of the spleen to be delineated.

RADIOACTIVE ISOTOPES IN TREATMENT

Thyrotoxicosis

There is no doubt that iodine-131 therapy is the most convenient form of treatment for the patient with thyrotoxicosis, as it entails merely drinking some tasteless fluid. The chief consideration which limits its use in thyrotoxicosis is the fear of inducing malignant changes in the thyroid gland subsequently. There are, however, no reports of cases of carcinoma which can be attributed to iodine-131 therapy for thyrotoxicosis despite the treatment of many thousands of patients during the last 28 years. Nor does the incidence of leukaemia exceed that which would be expected on the basis of chance association. Nevertheless, the possibility of radiation-induced mutations occurring after 28 years cannot be excluded, and it has been the practice in Britain to limit this form of treatment to patients over the age of 40 years, those with a life expectancy of less than 20 years, or those in whom there is some good reason to avoid surgery. Radioactive iodine therapy should not be used in thyrotoxic children nor in a patient who is lactating or who might be pregnant.

The substance most frequently used in Britain is sodium iodide-131. This contains the radioactive isotope of iodine having an atomic weight of 131, or Iodine-131. This isotope decays to half its initial activity in a period of 8 days. In the process of decay it emits two types of radiation. The first is known as beta radiation and consists of fast electrons. These can penetrate tissue to a distance of about 2 mm. and thereby produce the major part of the therapeutic effect. The second type is known as gamma radiation which is more important for diagnostic purposes.

The treatment involves oral administration of between 5 and 10 millicuries (mCi) of sodium iodide (I-131) solution. It is a colourless, tasteless fluid.

Treatment may be carried out on outpatients, although it should be remembered that the urine is radioactive for a few days and should not be allowed to contaminate any surface. Where possible, the patient's domestic arrangements should be regulated so that he or she does not come into close contact with children or pregnant women for a week or so after receiving the dose. This applies to any patient who has received radioisotope treatment.

One of the disadvantages of this form of treatment is the increased incidence of myxoedema that develops subsequently. Within the two-year period following treatment the overall incidence of hypothyroidism is 9 per cent, which differs little from that following surgery. With the passage of time, however, it increases steadily, and after eight years the incidence of hypothyroidism is 30 per cent and ultimately it may reach 40–50 per cent of the patients treated.

Radioactive iodine therapy has also been used for euthyroid patients with incapacitating angina of effort or refractory congestive cardiac failure. By inducing hypothyroidism, and thus lowering the rate of metabolism, the demand on the heart are reduced. This may benefit patients with refractory cardiac failure. The advent of propranolol has reduced the application of this form of treatment for patients with angina of effort.

Carcinoma of the Thyroid

The most effective treatment of carcinoma of the thyroid is complete surgical excision. If this is not possible or practicable, iodine-131 therapy may be used for the well-differentiated tumours, and external irradiation if the tumour is undifferentiated. When iodine-131 therapy is used all normal thyroid tissue must first be destroyed with a large dose of iodine-131 (75 to 100 mCi), so that with a subsequent dose the tumour cells will be encouraged to concentrate sufficient iodine-131 to effect their self-destruction.

Polycythaemia rubra vera

After administration phosphorus-32 passes to tissues that have a high phosphate content and which metabolize phosphate rapidly. It is therefore largely deposited in bone as calcium phosphate, for this comprises the major phosphate pool in the body, and it is also incorporated into the nucleoproteins of nuclei of rapidly dividing cells. This includes bone-marrow cells, particularly when the mitotic rate is increased as in polycythaemia rubra vera and leukaemia. Irradiation of the bone-marrow will result, and since phosphorus-32 has a half-life of 14·5 days this irradiation will last for several weeks. Phosphorus-32 disintegrates with the emission of a beta particle, and thereupon becomes stable sulphur. This beta particle can penetrate tissue to 7 mm., and this is how phosphorus-32 exerts its radiation effect. In leukaemia radioactive phosphorus is of value only in the chronic myeloid variety, and even in this condition it is not as effective as busulphan (Myleran). Its greatest therapeutic application is in polycythaemia rubra vera, in which remissions of the disease can be achieved in most cases. Radioactive phosphorus does not begin to have effect for 30–60 days after administration, and thus the packed cell volume should first be reduced by venesection. Remissions of several years after a single dose are common. Four to five millicuries of phosphorus-32 should be given intravenously, and the position reviewed after a month or two, though no further dose should be allowed for a period of three months.

One disadvantage of this form of therapy is that the incidence of leukaemia in patients with polycythaemia rubra vera treated with phosphorus-32 is higher than in patients treated by other means. If polycythaemia rubra vera is untreated patients survive for about five years and death is usually the result of thrombosis or haemorrhage, particularly in the cerebral and coronary vessels. A few patients will develop myelosclerosis or acute myeloblastic leukaemia as a natural outcome of the disease. With phosphorus-32, on the other hand, the mean survival has been increased from 5 to 14 years and it is possible that part of the increased incidence of acute leukaemia in the treated patients is related to the reduction of thrombotic and haemorrhagic causes of death. On the other hand, the incidence of leukaemia after the treatment of polycythaemia rubra vera with busulphan (Myleran) or pyrimethamine (Daraprim) is not increased, though the mean survival of such patients is precisely the same as after radioactive phosphorus. Cytoxic drugs have their own hazards and phosphorus-32, because of its ease of administration and absence of other serious side-effects, remains preferable except perhaps in the younger patient. Venesection is the quickest way of reducing the red-cell mass and should always be tried first.

Teletherapy

In cobalt teletherapy the isotope cobalt-60 is used to deliver 1·2–1·3-million-volt radiation, which is equivalent to *x* rays generated at a peak voltage of 3 to 4 million volts. Cobalt 'bombs' have replaced radium units, since cobalt-60 may be prepared by activation of stable cobalt in a nuclear reactor, which is more economical than the use of naturally occuring radioactive radium—which is scarce and expensive and does not have the same intensity of radiation. The only disadvantage of cobalt compared with radium is that its half-life is a good deal shorter. Radium has a half-life of more than 1,500 years, but the half-life of cobalt is 5·3 years, so that the isotope has to be replaced in cobalt units from time to time.

Implant Techniques

Several isotopes can be made up into needles for implantation, and the emission of their gamma rays provides local irradiation; cobalt is a good substitute for radium for this purpose and both are used in the treatment of carcinoma of the uterine cervix. Tantalum is more malleable than cobalt, and is preferable for use in wires to implant tumours of curved surfaces such as the bladder. It can be bent into any shape or form.

Radioactive gold (Au-198), as gold wire, may be cut into short pieces and has replaced radon seeds. The short half-life has an advantage of enabling the implant to be left in place permanently and not removed at a subsequent operation.

Yttrium-90 has been used as an implant for the pituitary to irradiate the gland, particularly in patients with carcinomatosis from primary growths in the breast and prostate. It has the advantage of avoiding operation, as the implant can be passed through a needle into the sella turcica through the nose and the sphenoidal sinus under radiological control. This is not without hazard and hypophysectomy probably carries no greater risk.

Radioactive Solutions Injected into a Cavity

In certain types of bladder tumour where there is diffuse disease and where total cystectomy is not desirable the bladder may be irradiated from within by injecting colloidal gold labelled with gold-198. There is no systemic absorption of the colloidal solution and it may, diluted with urine, be removed after three hours, when adequate irradiation will have been achieved.

Gold-198 has been used as a colloidal solution to prevent the reaccumulation of malignant effusions of the pleura and peritoneum. Most of the fluid is first drained off and the radioactive gold colloid (50–140 mCi) then instilled into the cavity. The patient is tipped into various positions to ensure that all the endothelial surface comes into contact with the radioactive fluid. The rationale of the treatment is that the endothelial surfaces are subjected to intense local irradiation. This usually results in a reduction in the rate of production of the protein-rich fluid. The treatment is palliative only, but by reducing the rate at which fluid re-accumulates the patient's comfort is substantially increased. The indications for intrapleural and intraperitoneal administration of radioactive isotopes have been reduced since the introduction of more recent cytotoxic drugs such as cyclophosphamide.

Selected Bibliography

BELCHER, E. H. and VETTER, H. (1971) *Radio-Isotopes in Medical Diagnosis*. Butterworths.

SILVER, S. (1968) *Radioactive Nuclides in Medicine and Biology*. 3rd Ed. Lea and Febiger.

Various Authors (1969) *Diagnostic Uses of Radioisotopes in Medicine*. Hospital Medicine Publications Ltd.

VII

Shock

Shock is a state of acute circulatory failure in which the cardiac outputs is inadequate to provide normal perfusion of the major organs. It represents a failure of blood flow rather than a failure of blood pressure. Whilst shock is accompanied by a fall in arterial blood pressure, a fall in blood pressure is not necessarily indicative of shock. Shock can arise from a variety of causes and produce variable clinical signs according to the state of deterioration and the underlying disease. Direct bedside measurements of blood flow are not available so that physicians must usually rely on indirect evidence of inadequate perfusion. Shock is therefore a clinical syndrome and is characterized by systemic arterial hypotension (brachial blood pressure less than 80 mm. of mercury), sweating and signs of vaso-constriction. These signs include pallor, cyanosis, a cold clammy skin, and a low volume pulse. They may be associated with clinical evidence of poor tissue perfusion such as mental apathy, confusion or restlessness and oliguria. In haemodynamic terms, shock is a state of circulatory failure associated with a low cardiac output and high peripheral resistance.

Shock results from many situations which give rise to inadequate perfusion of tissues and organs. It may occur because of increased resistance to blood flow, pooling or loss of blood, or because of cardiac insufficiency, but the end result of impaired tissue perfusion is the same. As perfusion depends on blood flow and not blood pressure, the sphygmomanometer reading is a poor indicator of circulatory failure. Nor is the cardiac output an entirely dependable measure of tissue perfusion. In conditions such as hepatic cirrhosis the cardiac output is raised because blood is shunted through arterio-venous communications and this reduces vascular resistance. If this raised cardiac output is reduced to normal levels effective blood flow to vital organs may be inadequate. Recent studies suggest that a rise in rectal temperature associated with a fall of skin temperature is a more useful measure of circulatory failure. This divergence of temperature reflects the inability of the core of the body to lóse heat as a result of generalized vasoconstriction. Failing precise identification of the haemodynamic abnormality in shock there is an inevitable temptation to reverse the most easily recognized sign, namely that of the lowered arterial blood pressure. However the use of vasopressor drugs may aggravate an already inadequate tissue blood flow. The treatment of shock must be based on a knowledge of the haemodynamic disturbance.

The constant defect in shock is a reduction in the perfusion of tissues. This is usually precipitated by a fall in cardiac output and stroke volume. A compensatory increase in systemic vascular resistance is inadequate to maintain arterial blood pressure. Impaired perfusion of tissues results, leading to hypoxaemia, metabolic acidiosis, lactic acidaemia and hyperkalaemia. In many situations cardiac function may be enhanced more by reducing peripheral resistance and ensuring more effective tissue perfusion than by raising peripheral resistance artificially in an attempt to increase arterial blood pressure and enhance coronary perfusion.

Three main factors affect cardiac output.

1. *The filling pressure of the right heart.* This is the central venous pressure, which is due in part to the volume of blood distending the veins and partly to the venous tone. The tone of the veins controls the degree to which the veins constrict the blood within.

2. *The functional efficiency of the heart and the resistance of the pulmonary circuit.*

3. *The peripheral resistance.* This depends mainly on the degree of arteriolar constriction and to a lesser extent on the viscosity of the blood. The degree of arteriolar (and venous) constriction is controlled by autonomic nervous activity, although the precapillary sphincters are under local metabolic control and not adrenergic control.

In shock what matters is the circulating blood volume not the volume of blood. Sequestration of blood in various areas of the vascular bed because of severe constriction of venules reduces the circulating blood volume and hence the venous return to the heart. The heart is just as dependant on the peripheral circulation for proper function as on its own coronary circulation. A disturbance of this balance between arteriolar and venous resistance to blood flow is responsible for the fatal outcome of shock due to various causes. Furthermore there is evidence that left ventricular contractility may be impaired in shock even after the circulating blood volume and venous return have been restored to normal.

The Peripheral Circulation

The blood volume is approximately 5 litres. The heart puts out this volume each minute, a stroke volume of 70 ml. being ejected 70 times per minute in the resting subject. Only 15 per cent of the

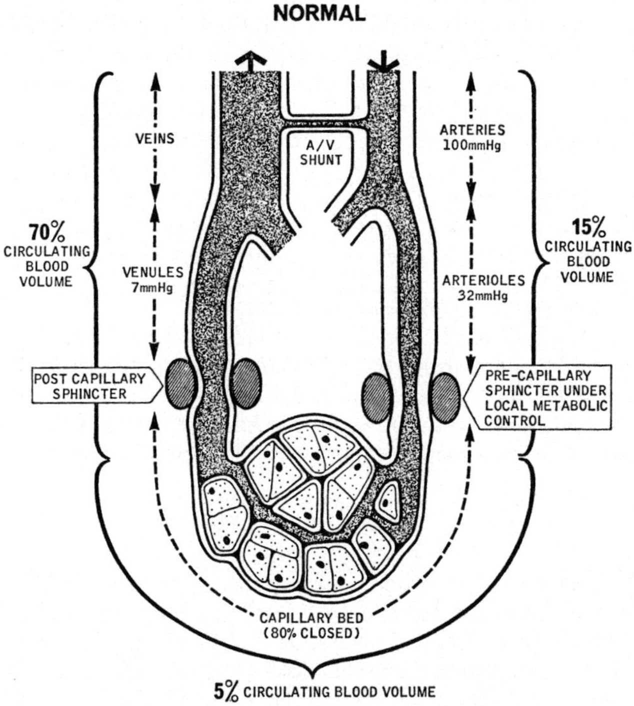

FIG. 14 Diagrammatic representation of the normal peripheral circulation

blood volume lies in the arterial bed so that variations in arteriolar calibre have little affect on the vascular capacity. (Fig. 14.) The arterioles are extremely muscular vessels and the tone of the arteriolar muscle varies the blood flow enormously. Because the greatest decline in pressure occurs at this level the arterioles are called resistance vessels. Arterioles are normally fairly widely open to permit free perfusion of the tissues. As the main resistance to blood flow lies in the arterioles, it follows that the greatest pressure drop occurs in traversing them. The degree of fall in pressure is dependant upon the degree of arteriolar constriction. The mean arterial pressure falls from 100 to 32 mm. of mercury in the arterioles. In the erect subject pressure is affected by gravity, so that in dependent parts such as the dorsalis pedis arteries, it may be 170 mm. of mercury (mean arterial pressure of 100 mm. of mercury plus hydrostatic pressure of 70 mm. of mercury) whilst in cerebral arteries it may be only 70 mm. of mercury at a time when the aortic pressure is 100 mm. of mercury. When the arterioles constrict the pressure gradient increases so that the hydrostatic pressure of blood entering the capillaries decreases. This alters the equilibrium between the formation and reabsorption of tissue fluid by the capillaries, and permits the assimilation of tissue fluids by these vessels. The capillary beds only contain 5 per cent of the circulating volume so that unless capillary dilatation is widespread this in itself will not influence vascular capacity greatly. Eighty per cent of all capillaries are normally closed at any one time. These capillaries open in rotation on demand of the cells adjacent to them. The pre-capillary sphincter relaxes as oxygen tension in the tissues falls and as the concentration of metabolic products rises. Mast-cells secrete histamine when anoxic to cause capillary sphincters to open. The histamine is immediately inactivated in the blood. Also the accumulation of metabolites such as lactate, pyruvate, ketones, and the products of tissue protein breakdown will cause relaxation of pre-capillary sphincters. Tissues themselves can thus call on arterioles for more blood flow.

Over two thirds of the circulating blood volume lies on the venous side of the circulation, particularly in the venules. Hence the venous system is called the capacitance system. The veins are less muscular than arterioles but are also under autonomic nervous control. The pressure in veins is only about 7 mm. of mercury. They have a relatively large diameter and correspondingly low resistance. The tension of venous musculature although not great has a critical influence on venous return and on venous pressure. The calibre of the veins may vary considerably and these changes will affect the capacity of the circulation enormously. Passive assumption of the erect posture will reduce the cardiac output by 25 per cent. Nervous adjustment through the sympathetic nervous system is intended to prevent pooling in the capacitance system. Failure of venous tone with pooling of blood in venules and capillaries is associated with a large fall in cardiac output and failure of the peripheral circulation. Failure of arteriolar tone on the other hand with consequent arteriolar dilatation is associated with hypotension but blood flow remains normal and there is only a transient decrease in the venous return to the heart.

Blood expelled by the left ventricle flows round the systemic circulation to the right atrium because of the continuous pressure gradient that exists along its route. The blood pressure is the lateral pressure exerted on the walls of the vessels by the contained blood. The systolic pressure is the maximum pressure during systole, and the diastolic pressure the lowest pressure during diastole. The systolic pressure may fluctuate during exertion and anxiety with variations in cardiac output, but the diastolic pressure is a measure of peripheral resistance and depends mainly on the tone of the arterioles. The pulse is the rise in pressure produced by ventricular systole.

When estimating blood pressure with a sphygmomanometer, the arm cuff is inflated to a pressure at which blood flow is completely impeded. The obstruction is gradually reduced to a point at which spurts of blood give rise to pulsations which are audible through a stethoscope placed over the artery distal to the cuff. This sound is normally well correlated with the systolic blood pressure. The diastolic blood pressure correlates with the disappearance of the sounds. The loudness of the sounds depends on the force with which blood spurts through the occluded artery. In shock the blood flow is reduced and the sounds are often not loud enough to give true or clear-cut systolic and diastolic pressures. The sphygmomanometer readings thus do not reflect the true intra-arterial blood pressure in states of shock. Cuff pressures and peripheral pulses may disappear when the intra-arterial pressure is 110/70. It is generally true that when the real arterial pressure is below 90 mm. of mercury the indirect measurements of blood pressure underestimate by approximately 15 mm. of mercury.

The arterial blood pressure is produced by three factors. Firstly the amount of blood expelled by the heart into the aorta. Secondly the elasticity of the arterial system. Thirdly the arteriolar resistance which controls the escape of blood from the arterial system. Identical pressures can be achieved by high cardiac output and low arteriolar resistance as by low cardiac output and high arteriolar resistance. Tissue perfusion is however very different in these two situations. Hence during exercise the cardiac output may increase five-fold but there is little change in the mean arterial blood pressure as vasodilation of arterioles in muscle reduces peripheral resistance.

The left ventricle forces blood into the aorta. The energy thus developed is used to accelerate the blood, to distend the walls of the aorta, to increase the pressure in the arterial system, and to overcome resistance to flow. As in all hydraulic systems the pressure within the circuit is determined primarily by the pump (heart) and the characteristics of the pipeline (arterial system). The aorta is distensible so that a localized bulge occurs in the tube when the volume is increased. This bulge passes down the walls of the tube, the lateral pressure of the tube rising in each area where the volume is increased and falling as the pressure wave passes on. The rise in pressure during systole is limited by the elasticity of the aorta. During diastole, when the pressure tends to fall, the artery walls recoil and energy stored during systole is reconverted into kinetic energy. The arterial system is made up of a series of flexible tubes whose elasticity varies in different areas. The ascending and thoracic aorta are freely distensible and increase in volume with change in pressure from diastolic to systolic levels, whilst the carotid, femoral and more peripheral arteries hardly change their volume at all. The pressure wave thus travels more slowly in the aorta than in the peripheral arteries. The rise in pressure along the arteries causes an escape of blood from the arterial system through the arterioles and capillaries. The resistance offered by the arterioles and capillaries determines the diastolic blood pressure. The precise pressure in the peripheral arteries is predominantly dependent on the degree of incontinence of the system. Thus it is more dependant on the degree of arteriolar dilatation than it is on the elastic qualities of peripheral arteries.

The Maintenance of the Circulation

The normal regulatory mechanisms for the circulation, that is the baroreceptors, and the autonomic innervation of the arterioles and venules, are geared to cope with the adjustments necessary in postural alterations, physical exercize and acute trauma. The adrenergic system regulates blood pressure, the distribution of blood, the capacity of the venous system and the force and rate of cardiac contraction. The autonomic nervous system can adequately compensate for ten per cent alterations in blood volume, moderate systemic infections and a good deal of myocardial damage, by shunting blood away from visceral organs into cerebral, coronary and skeletal muscle beds. Furthermore an increase in venous constriction adds additional blood to the effective circulation. Supplementing the sympathetic nervous response is the release of adrenaline and noradrenaline from the adrenal medulla. The price that has to be paid for the adrenergic maintenance of blood pressure is inadequate and potentially lethal under-perfusion of viscera, lungs and kidney. This vasoconstriction is the mainstay of the body's response to hypovolaemia and yet if prolonged becomes a destructive force responsible for its ultimate dissolution. The hazards of vasoconstriction are apparent from the effects of prolonged administration of noradrenaline to the experimental animal. Haemoconcentration and hypovolaemia are followed by a fall in cardiac output and hypotension.

Inadequate perfusion of tissues results with consequent acidosis and relaxation of pre-capillary sphincters with the production of irreversible shock.

The haemodynamic response to shock inevitably produces inadequate perfusion of viscera in order to preserve the circulation to the brain and coronary vessels. (Fig. 15.) If this is prolonged, the

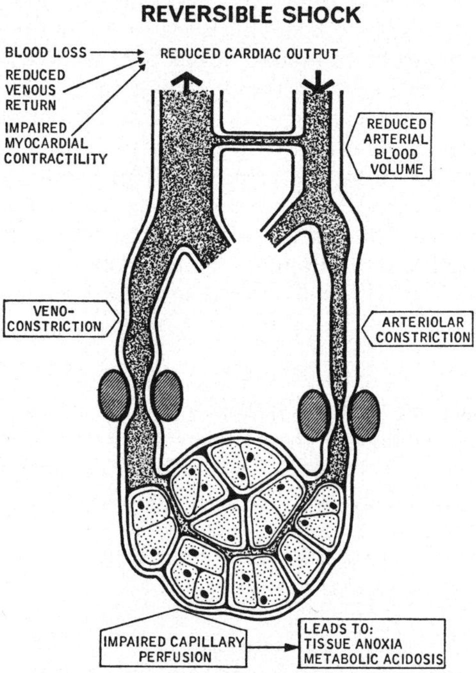

FIG. 15 Diagrammatic representation of the peripheral circulation in reversible shock

effects are diastrous. (Fig. 16.) The ischaemic intestine permits the transfer of toxic bacterial products and proteins across its wall into the blood. Renal ischaemia leads to production of angiotension with its intense vasoconstrictor effects. Furthermore the ischaemic kidney can no longer maintain a normal electrolyte and acid-base balance. Anoxic tissues release proteolytic enzymes and vasoactive substances such as bradykinin, serotonin and histamine.

Teleologically vasoconstriction due to sympathetic over-activity occurred in states of oligaemia. This resulted in selective vasoconstriction of skin and visceral vessels in order to maintain cerebral and coronary blood flow in the face of a reduced cardiac output, because the arterioles of the cerebral and coronary circulations are insensitive to adrenergic activity. Such a response can however only persist for a limited period because the peripheral vessels themselves also become ischaemic. Relaxation of the precapillary sphincters and an increased pressure within the capillary then occurs. Plasma

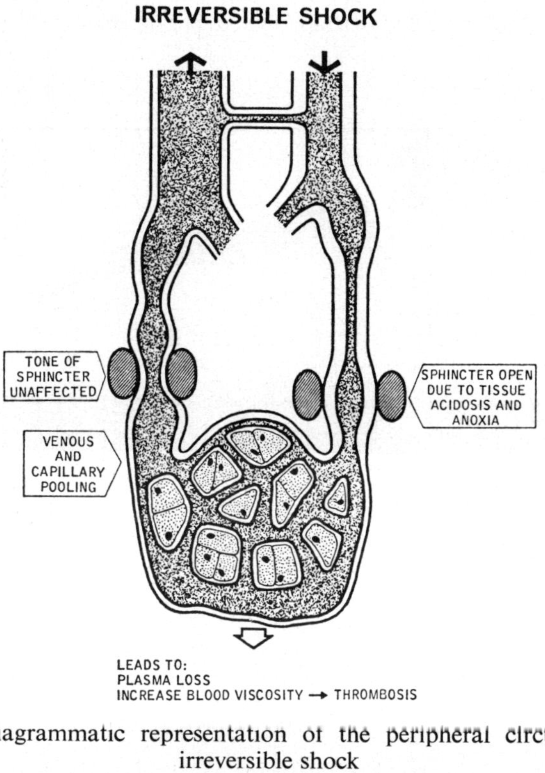

FIG. 16 Diagrammatic representation of the peripheral circulation in irreversible shock

is lost through exudation from the circulating volume. The shock is then uncompensated and anoxia leads to local haemorrhage especially in the gut. For this reason the dog with prolonged oligaemic hypotension to which the shed blood is finally returned, still develops profound shock and dies with a pale ischaemic visceral mesentery and an engorged bowel submucosa. Measurement of the individual organ blood flow during shock shows that the splanchnic organs suffer profound decreases in arterial and portal venous blood flow.

(Fig. 17.) A similar pattern of ischaemic visceral anoxia can be produced by prolonged infusion of noradrenaline or metaraminol. In shocked man the histological hallmark of capillary stagnation (engorged congested capillaries, dilated arteriolar sphincters and constricted venules) is most marked in the lungs and kidneys, though changes in the bowel also occur. One effect of visceral ischaemia is to render the bowel barrier more permeable to bacteria and introduce a septic element to the shock. Hence, experimentally, germ-free animals withstand haemorrhage shock better than control animals.

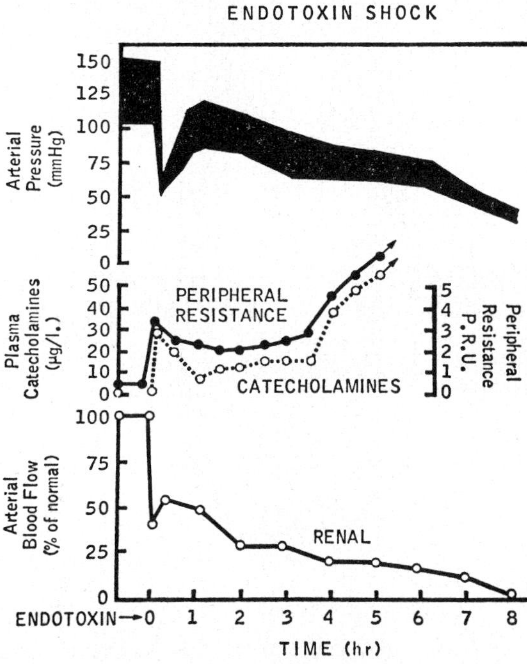

FIG. 17 Haemodynamic effects of shock

Haemodynamic Factors in Shock

There are three fundamental haemodynamic causes which may give rise to shock.

1. cardiac failure
2. loss of blood or plasma volume, and
3. peripheral pooling due to such causes as toxaemia, anaphylaxis or adrenergic withdrawal.

A low cardiac output and stroke volume accompany the state of shock. The fall in cardiac output occurs either because of damage to the heart or because central venous pressure is inadequate to fill the right side of the heart owing to failure of the peripheral circulation. The immediate physiological response to the lowered cardiac output is vasoconstriction of both arterioles and venules, especially those of the gut and kidneys. This helps to maintain circulation through the unconstricted carotid and coronary vessels. But this vasoconstriction is only of temporary benefit for not only does it increase the work of the heart but the impaired perfusion of the tissues leads to hypoxia and metabolic acidosis. (Fig. 15.) The continued ischaemia results in a loss of tone in the precapillary sphincters as capillaries are more under local metabolic control than adrenergic control. The post-capillary sphincters on the venous side are more resistant to anoxia and maintain their tone so that blood fills the capillary bed. The venous return is thus further reduced and shock becomes irreversible. (Fig. 16.) Blood viscosity is also increased and this leads not only to increased work for the heart but also to such complications as red cell sludging and microthrombi in capillaries and small vessels. The viscosity of blood in small vessels is inversely proportional to the rate of blood flow, hence as blood flow decreases viscosity rises. Although an increased thrombotic tendency is appropriate after acute trauma it is obviously harmful after myocardial infarction. Prolonged vasoconstriction whether due to physiological arteriolar constriction or induced by vasopressor agents is especially harmful to the liver, kidney and bowel.

Shock has many causes. Haemorrhage, trauma, bacteraemia, and primary cardiac disease are examples. Although the clinical picture and the consequences of impaired perfusion of the tissues are common to all forms of shock, the aetiology differs and remedies that are beneficial to one form of shock may not be so in another. The diagnosis of the aetiological factor may also be difficult. As more than sixty per cent of patients in shock, regardless of its cause, have increased serum transaminase and lactic dehydrogenase activity due to ischaemic injury to the liver, these enzymes are unreliable criteria for differentiating myocardial infarction from other causes of shock.

VARIETIES OF SHOCK

Shock is generally classified according to its etiology and there are seven main groups.

1. Hypovolaemic Shock

Losses of blood, plasma or water are undoubtedly the most common causes of shock. Blood loss from physical trauma and plasma loss following burns are familiar examples. Severe diarrhoea and vomiting or pyloric obstruction may lead to external losses of gastrointestinal fluid giving rise to hypovolaemia. Sometimes the loss of blood and fluid is not so apparent. The average occult loss from a fractured femur is two pints and that from a fractured pelvis three pints of blood. Peritonitis and paralytic ileus may be associated with severe loss of fluid from the circulation. The body can compensate for the loss of 20 per cent of the circulating volume but by the time 50 per cent of this volume is lost the blood pressure is unrecordable and the patient is in a profound state of shock. When this loss is rapid, acute coronary insufficiency and myocardial failure may occur quickly. When loss is more gradual compensatory mechanisms increase the plasma volume and prevent acute circulatory failure. The bone-marrow can increase its output six-fold so that whenever the loss of blood is less than 100 ml. per day increased erythropoietic activity can compensate fully, provided that adequate ingredients for blood are present. When acute loss is 75 to 1,250 ml. of blood, that is approximately 15 to 25 per cent of the circulating volume, a small increase in heart rate and a slight decrease in blood pressure are apparent. If the blood loss is more severe and of the order of 1,250 to 1,750 ml., that is 25 to 35 per cent of the circulating volume, there is a marked tachycardia of 100 to 120 per minute, a decrease in pulse pressure and a fall in systolic arterial pressure to about 90 mm. of mercury. The patient is usually restless, sweating, pale and oliguric. If the blood loss is more severe, that is between 35 and 50 per cent of the blood volume, the tachycardia exceeds 120, and the blood pressure is below 60 mm. Hg. or more usually unobtainable by the sphygmomanometer. There is extreme pallor and coldness of the extremities, the patient is mentally confused, and urine flow ceases. In acute conditions of blood loss the haemoglobin and packed cell volume are of little help in determining the amount of blood lost. When red cells and plasma are lost together the concentration of haemoglobin does not change. Over the process of time the plasma volume is restored and the haemoglobin and packed cell volume fall. This is however a relatively slow process and may take thirty-six to forty-eight hours. It is therefore essential that serial haemoglobin and packed cell volume measurements should be made. The central venous pressure measurement is a useful guide to the circulating blood volume. A more sensitive index of impaired circulation of blood is the divergence of rectal temperature from skin temperature as measured by a thermocouple on the big toe. When the circulation is impaired the core of the body is unable to lose heat so that the rectal temperature rises. The skin temperature at the same time falls owing to the generalized vasoconstriction.

Internal losses of fluid may result from sequestration in the gastrointestinal tract as in paralytic ileus, or in the peritoneal cavity or in the pleural spaces. After perforation of a viscus the accumulation of fluid in the peritoneal cavity and consequent peritonitis may lead to losses of large amounts of fluid from the circulating blood. The cause of shock following perforation is only in part related to the extra-cellular fluid loss for sepsis is an important factor. Furthermore distended loops of bowel also seclude large amounts of fluid. Acute pancreatitis is not infrequently associated with shock, as inflammatory oedema distends the interstitial spaces of the pancreas and as much as three litres of fluid may accumulate in the peritoneal cavity. After extensive burns fluid is lost into the area of injury but in addition large amounts of fluid evaporate from the surface of the burned area. With burns involving 50 per cent of the body surface, half the extra-cellular fluid may be lost. The features of hypovolaemic shock are sometimes seen in patients with features are hypovolaemic shock as sometimes seen in patients with barbiturate over-dosage. Cardiac output is low, plasma volume is reduced and arteriolar tone is well maintained. These patients have lost fluid from increased capillary permeability and from the failure of fluid intake in an unconscious patient. Depression of the respiratory centre in the patient who has taken an overdose of barbiturate or tranquillizer drugs further aggravates the tissue anoxia.

Treatment

(i) *Replacement of fluid loss*. The patient in shock with a low central venous pressure should be treated for hypovolaemia regardless of the clinical diagnosis. Blood is obviously best for the patient with gastrointestinal haemorrhage. Saline or plasma is better for the patient with severe burns and a haematocrit of more than 55 per cent. Dextran is useful for shocked patients with low central venous pressure and high haematocrit. The mere replacement of the precise volume of blood or fluid lost is often inadequate in hypovolaemic shock especially if it has been prolonged or severe, for blood is sequested in the capillaries and venules and is not available for circulation. If two litres of blood are lost and replaced immediately two litres will be adequate replacement. If however there is a delay in treatment, and shock is prolonged there may be a need for four litres. Over transfusion is rare if the central venous pressure is kept below 15 cm. of water.

The disadvantage of plasma is its ability to carry the virus of serum hepatitis and this is particularly relevant for pooled plasma. It is however now possible to obtain reconstituted dried plasma that has been treated to render it free of the serum hepatitis virus.

The administration of colloid solutions is often necessary to maintain the normal osmotic pressure of the blood. If saline is used exclusively fluid will eventually be lost into the tissues with the consequent development of oedema. Dextran is such a colloid solution. There are two varities.

(*a*) Low molecular weight Dextran. (Molecular weight 40,000.)

This has a powerful though temporary osmotic effect. It draws cellular fluid into the intravascular space and hence improves blood and urine flow. It also reduces blood viscosity by inducing a negative charge on erythrocytes causing them to repel each other. Dextran administration should be accompanied by saline to repair the loss of the fluid from the extra-cellular space.

(*b*) Large molecular weight Dextran. (Molecular weight 120,000.)

This remains in the blood longer but does not equal the osmotic effect of the low molecular weight variety. It has the additional disadvantage that it may promote disseminated intravascular coagulation which utilizes clotting factors and may precipitate a haemorrhagic state.

(ii) *Correction of acidosis.* Metabolic acidosis is usually a consequence of inadequate tissue perfusion and the resulting accumulation of the acid by-products of anaerobic metabolism. The best treatment is restoration of normal blood flow. However the acidosis itself may impair cardiac function and must be corrected before normal perfusion can be restored. The administration of 8·4 per cent sodium bicarbonate which contains 1 mEq per ml. is a convenient way of doing this. Serial acid-base estimations will be required to determine the dose.

(iii) *Drugs.* Drugs available for shock can be classified according to whether they are (a) predominantly vasoconstrictors (sympathomimetic drugs). The vasoconstrictor drugs are predominantly sympathomimetic. Primary vasoconstrictor effects are exerted on blood vessels of the kidney, the viscera and skin. In some patients in cardiogenic shock the inotropic effect on the heart may increase cardiac output but more often the cardiac output is reduced. Drugs which raise the blood pressure by vasoconstriction alone (methoxamine and angiotensin) do not increase cardiac output. If the total cardiac output remains unimproved it is doubtful if any good effect has been achieved. (b) predominantly cardiac stimulants. Other sympathomimetic drugs which are not predominantly vasoconstrictor (isoprenaline, mephentermine) are cardiac beta-receptor stimulators. (c) predominantly vasodilators.

The possible value of counteracting vasoconstriction with an adrenergic antagonist has recently been investigated. Phenoxybenzamine in combination with intravenous infusions has been shown to reduce the mortality in experimental shock and this regime has been advocated for the management of clinical shock. There are potential dangers to the use of adrenergic antagonists, for these drugs increase the size of the peripheral vascular bed and hence lower the central venous pressure. Their administration must therefore be accompanied by transfusion and by monitoring of the central venous pressure. Phentolamine (Rogitine) has a more predictable effect and a shorter duration of action than phenoxybenzamine and is therefore safer. Chlorpromazine has also been shown to be useful as a vasodilator.

(iv) *Corticosteroids.* In haemorrhage shock the main indication for corticosteroids is a suspicion of adrenocortical insufficiency. If the clinical severity of the shock is out of proportion to the volume of fluid loss, adrenal insufficiency should be suspected. Pharmacological doses of steroids improve the mortality in experimental haemorrhagic shock and possibly in clinical haemorrhagic shock as well.

2. **Cardiogenic Shock**

Failure of the heart as a pump is a major cause of shock. Although shock may occur in cardiac tamponade, dissecting aneurysm, myocarditis, terminal phases of congestive cardiac failure and pulmonary embolism it is most commonly seen as the result of cardiac infarction. It may also occur as a result of arrhythmias, especially where the irregularities are associated with extremes of bradycardia or tachycardia. Cardiogenic shock occurs in about twenty per cent of patients with myocardial infarction and has a mortality of eighty per cent. It is doubtful if newer methods of treatment over the last decade have improved this prognosis. Impaired contractility of the heart muscle is the main aetiological factor in cardiogenic shock, though reflex vasoconstriction secondary to pain and anxiety accentuates the impaired perfusion of the tissues found after myocardial infarction. Although significant reductions occur in the absence of shock, the cardiac output is lower in patients with myocardial infarction with shock than in those with uncomplicated infarction; the systemic vascular resistance is raised above normal though there is no significant difference in vascular resistance between the two groups. The central venous pressure may be low, normal or raised, the level depending on the presence of venoconstriction, the duration of shock and the occurrence of congestive cardiac failure. The circulation time is prolonged and reflects a reduction in the velocity of blood flow. Four major difficulties confront any attempt to assess the value of the various treatments recommended for shock. First the emergency measures necessary make controlled studies impossible to carry out, so that objective evaluation is difficult. Secondly haemodynamic observations are necessary to understand the physiological disturbance and permit the wisest choice of therapy, yet these are rarely available. Thirdly patients in cardiogenic shock are far from being in a steady state, so that even when measures of cardiac output and of venous and arterial pressures are available they must be interpreted with caution. Fourthly there is no satisfactory experimental model.

It is generally agreed that the promptness with which measures of combating shock are instituted is an important factor in recovery. Treatment should begin with relief of pain and allaying anxiety and these measures will reduce reflex vasoconstriction. The best drug to give is diamorphine (Heroin). It should be injected intravenously or intramuscularly because it will be absorbed poorly from the subcutaneous tissues of a patient in circulatory failure. The venous return to the heart should be aided by laying the patient flat. When bradycardia is severe atropine is often of striking benefit. In view of the arterial hypoxamia and tissue acidosis these patients are in urgent need of oxygen in high concentration. But the response to oxygen is disappointing because the shunting of blood through pulmonary vessels inaccessible to gaseous exchange interferes with the oxygenation of blood in the lungs. The metabolic acidosis requires correction just as it does after cardiac arrest. This helps to improve myocardial function, to reduce the ill-effects of tissue acidosis on the peripheral circulation, and to diminish the risk of cardiac arrythmia. To determine the amount of bicarbonate required to do this properly will require serial acid-base determinations. Patients with coronary shock are in heart failure and have a lower cardiac output than those with myocardial infarction uncomplicated by shock. Digoxin would therefore be rational treatment. In experimental animals prophylactic digitalization protects the heart from the impaired myocardial function following haemorrhagic shock and it increases survival. In man digitalis will increase the force of contraction and lower the oxygen requirement of hearts not in failure. In cardiogenic shock in man digoxin has been shown to raise the cardiac output and there is no convincing evidence that it induces arrythmia except when given intravenously too quickly.

Vasopressors are generally unsatisfactory and their prolonged use harmful. Increased aortic pressure may temporarily enhance coronary artery perfusion in patients with arteriosclerotic heart disease. The coronary blood flow in these patients depends on blood pressure because the coronary vessels are already maximally dilated. An increase in cardiac output and arterial blood pressure may follow the administration of metaraminol. In previously normotensive patients cardiac output is greatest when the arterial pressure is 70 to 80 mm. of mercury. The peripheral vascular resistance may actually decrease after the administration of metaraminol if the increase in cardiac output is proportionally greater than the increase of blood pressure. This is due to the beta adrenergic effects on the heart exceeding the alpha adrenergic effects on the arterioles. If the major effect of the vasopressor drug is on the heart and venous pool and not on the arterioles the result will be beneficial. If larger amounts of metaraminol are used and an arterial pressure exceeding 90 mm. of mercury is achieved the cardiac output falls and this is associated with a marked increase in the systemic vascular resistance. The elevation in blood pressure is achieved by intense vasoconstriction but at the price of a reduction in cardiac output. Maximal improvement in blood flow appears to require a systolic pressure about 30 mm. less than the patient's normal. However preoccupation with blood pressure is dangerous for it is not the pressure itself that is important but rather the perfusion of the tissues. Arterial pressures of 50/40 mm. of mercury may occur in normal persons with no reduction in cardiac output if the systemic circulation is widely dilated. Conversely if the arterioles are constricted a high diastolic blood pressure with a large pulse pressure may be associated with a very low cardiac output. In cardiac by-pass operations in a vasodilated patient good perfusion is possible with an intra-arterial pressure of 35 mm. of mercury provided the rate of flow of blood approaches the estimated requirement for the body surface. It is however only fair to say that this is continuous pressure and not pulsatile pressure. In the treatment of cardiogenic shock a pressor response does not mean relief of shock and the cuff pressure is often a misleading measure of intra-arterial pressure. Vasopressor drugs act primarily on visceral vessels to increase peripheral resistance and they profoundly decrease the flow of blood through these organs. The efficiency of an already weakened heart is further depressed by the increase in total peripheral resistance, by metabolic acidosis and by a decreased venous return resulting from the impaired perfusion of tissues. However reports have appeared from time to time indicating that the outcome of cardiogenic shock can be improved by vasopressor agents. There seems little doubt that vasopressors may be of benefit occasionally but their prolonged use is positively harmful. Both noradrenaline and metaraminol enhance myocardial contractility and this effect on cardiac muscle is probably responsible for their occasional benefit. Drugs that are pure vasoconstrictors increase vascular resistance but decrease cardiac output. Angiotensin has no stimulant effect on cardiac muscle and as it constricts coronary vessels should never be used. The possible value of antagonizing vasoconstriction with chlorpromazine or with an adrenergic antagonist has recently been investigated (p. 169). In cardiogenic shock induced in experimental animals survival was considerably increased by phenoxybenzamine and low molecular weight dextran but not by noradrenaline. Phenoxybenzamine and noradrenaline together also gave good results but no better than phenoxybenzamine alone. Phenoxybenzamine has recently been advocated for the treatment of cardiogenic shock in man. However as this drug increases the size of the vascular bed it should be accompanied by transfusion and by monitoring of the central venous pressure. The natural anxiety to avoid transfusion in patients with reduced cardiac output is possibly over-emphasized and phenoxybenzamine actually reduces the central venous pressure in patients with pulmonary oedema. It is too early to recommend adrenergic antagonists as routine treatment for cardiogenic shock. However vasopressor drugs have done little to improve the mortality and their prolonged use is undoubtedly harmful. Phenoxybenzamine will receive increasing attention though further work will be needed to establish its true value.

3. **Bacteraemic Shock**

Bacteraemic shock is usually due to invasion of the blood stream by gram-negative bacteria and it occurs most frequently in elderly men with genito-urinary infection. Frequently catheterization or other instrumentation precipitates the bacteraemia. The common organisms are Esch Coli and Proteus. Friedlander's bacillus and Pseudomonas Pyocyanea are occasionally responsible. It occasionally occurs as a complication of cholecystitis or cholangitis and sometimes as a complication of septic abortion in younger women. It is a serious condition as fifty per cent of the patients die within forty-eight hours. Approximately twenty-five per cent of patients with gram-negative bacteraemia develop clinical shock and this type of shock does not occur unless the blood stream has been invaded. Except for septic abortion bacteraemic shock is rarely observed in patients under the age of forty. Circulatory collapse also occurs in staphylococcal, pneumococcal and clostridial septicaemia and also in viraemia. Circulatory collapse in gram positive infections is usually due to local oedema of sufficient magnitude to produce intravascular fluid loss.

When gram negative bacteria, which normally reside in the gastro-intestinal tract, invade the blood stream bacteraemia occurs but the complication of shock is chiefly observed in old patients and pregnant women. The term 'vasomotor collapse' was once popular for this variety of shock as it was wrongly assumed that the arterioles were paralysed by direct effect of the bacterial toxins. However it is now recognized that there is an increase in peripheral vascular resistance so that the hypotension is not due to vasomotor collapse. Central venous pressure is normal or even low demonstrating that shock is not due to cardiac failure, and the plasma volume is normal. Thus, although experimentally myocardial contractility may sometimes be impaired in septicaemic states, myocardial damage has little part to play in the aetiology of bacteraemic shock in man. The mechanism of bacteraemic shock is best explained by the selective removal of large volumes of blood from the active circulation and by its sequestration in inactive venous pools. Experimental studies on endotoxin shock suggest that the venous pooling is due to an intense immunological reaction between the endotoxin released from the gram-negative bacteria and circulating antibody, producing an anaphylactic type of reaction. It is an immunological event for complement is fixed and histamine is released. Pooling of blood within the venous system with a consequent reduction of cardiac output is the haemodynamic mechanism. Arteriolar constriction is increased so that this shock is not due to vasomotor collapse. In the dog the part of the venous system where pooling occurs is the viscera although in man this is probably not the area responsible.

The treatment of bacteraemic shock should therefore be aimed at restoring an effective circulating volume and this requires fluid replacement. Fluid replacement should be controlled by monitoring the central venous pressure. If the pressure rises to more than 12 cm. of water intravenous fluids should be stopped. As a result of liver cell anoxia the serum transaminase levels are raised in two thirds of patients and as poor coronary perfusion may precipitate electrocardiographic changes of ischaemia the differentiation from cardiogenic shock is important.

The treatment of the infection is a matter of urgency. The choice of antibiotic cannot await bacteriological culture of organisms. Kanamycin is the most useful drug as gram negative organisms are rarely resistant to this antibiotic. Cephaloridine is safer but resistant organisms occur and by the time resistance is known it may be too late to control the infection. Kanamycin by intramuscular injection in a daily dose of 15 mg./Kg bodyweight should be given initially, but if the urine flow is reduced the dose should be less. In infections known to be due to Pseudomonas, carbenicillin, colistin or polymyxin should be used. Kanamycin is the most effective though a toxic drug. Once sensitivities of the organisms are known a less toxic antibiotic should be selected if appropriate—such as cephaloradin or ampicillin. Vasopressor drugs should be used and metaraminol intramuscularly in doses of 5 to 25 mg. is appropriate. No attempt should be made to raise the blood pressure more than 20 mm. of mercury below the normal systolic pressure for the patient. Metaraminol is preferable to noradrenaline as it does not cause local injury to tissue. A dose of 200 to 300 mg. per litre of saline by intravenous infusion is usually adequate, or 5 to 25 mg. by intramuscular injection, the dose being governed by the blood pressure response. There is evidence that metaraminol mobilizes blood in venous pools and increases venous return both in animals and in man. Persistence with vasopressor drugs in the absence of any clinical response is unwise, as excessive vasoconstriction will further compromise effective blood flow. A beta adrenergic stimulator such as isoprenaline may be useful by increasing the cardiac output. Acidosis should be corrected with sodium bicarbonate to bring the pH towards normal as this may improve cardiac function (p. 170). As the transport of oxygen is disturbed it is advisable to give 100 per cent oxygen.

Corticosteroids have been advocated to suppress the systemic reaction to endotoxins. There is general agreement that steroid therapy should be given in overwhelming infections or in associated circulatory failure. Nevertheless it is difficult to produce any conclusive evidence that a favourable response can be ascribed to the hormone treatment as the desperate nature of the situation demands that many other measures, such as pressor agents, oxygen and cardiac stimulants must be given in addition. The clinical impression however remains that corticosteroid therapy has saved the lives of many patients with peripheral circulatory failure, and also by buying time in overwhelming infections it has enabled life to be prolonged until the antibiotics could have their effect. The haemodynamic effects of corticosteroids are however probably more important than the suppression of the systemic reaction to endotoxin, because in large doses they increase cardiac output and decrease peripheral resistance. Prednisolone 100 mg. six hourly is advocated for a maximum period of five days.

The management of circulatory shock in bacteraemia therefore includes:

(i) Blood culture.

(ii) Kanamycin administered systemically until the bacterial sensitivities are known.
(iii) Intravenous fluids.
(iv) Prudent use of vasopressor drugs.
(v) Corticosteroids.

4. **Anaphylactic Shock**

Hypersensitivity is an abnormal immunological response following previous exposure to an antigenic substance. It is not only the antigen-antibody reaction that is relevant but also the special characteristics of the individual in whom the anaphylactic reaction occurs (p. 82). Hypersensitivity reactions may be immediate due to circulating antibody, or delayed due to cell bound antibody. The immediate response includes urticaria, asthma, and anaphylaxis. The consequences are really immediate, appearing within a few seconds after an intravenous challenge. Foreign proteins were frequent causes when antisera were in common use. These antisera were prepared from horses and contained foreign serum. Drugs are now the common causes. The drugs responsible include penicillin, sulphonamides, streptomycin, procaine, iodides including contrast media used in diagnostic radiology, and acetylsalicylic acid. Predisposing factors are relevant. Heredity is important for patients with atopy are particularly prone to anaphylactic reactions. Topical applications are more likely to sensitize the patient than systemic injection, and oral administration is the least likely.

Shock in anaphylaxis is precipitated by the presence of antibody due to previous contact with the antigen. Though some of the antibody is circulating gamma globulin, some is attached to the cells and it is the antibody attached to body cells that is responsible for the anaphylactic reaction. Several unrelated vasoactive compounds are liberated from the cells due to damage by the immunological reaction. Histamine, serotonin, slow reacting substance, and bradykynin are the main agents culpable. These substances cause intense vasodilatation and increase capillary permeability. They also cause contraction of bronchial and visceral smooth muscle. There is thus seclusion of large volumes of blood in venous pools and an actual loss of intravascular volume due to exudation and angioneurotic oedema.

The management of anaphylactic shock demands

(i) *The prompt administration of adrenaline*. It is given for its vasoconstrictor, and for its relaxant effect on smooth muscle. A dose of 0·5 ml. of a 1/1,000 solution should be given intramuscularly or alternatively 0·1 ml. of a 1/1,000 solution diluted in 10 ml. of saline injected intravenously. Noradrenaline, metaraminol and ephedrine are other useful sympathomimetic drugs. Aminophylline may be helpful if bronchospasm is present.

(ii) *Antihistamine preparations* such as diphenhydramine (Benadryl) should be given.

(iii) *Anti-inflammatory drugs* such as the corticosteroid hormones may be indicated.

(iv) *Treatment of hypoxia.* In this form of shock the patency of the airway is of special importance. Laryngeal and bronchial oedema are often present and tracheostomy may be indicated.

The blood vessels and visceral smooth muscle are the two main targets of the anaphylactic reaction. Dilatation of arterioles and venules precipitates an increase in capillary permeability. The smooth muscle of the bronchi and gut contract. Species differences exist for guinea pigs die of asphyxia from bronchial constriction, and dogs die of shock due to hypovolaemia from vomiting and diarrhoea. In man respiratory inadequacy or circulatory failure and shock are the clinical manifestations. Oedema of the respiratory tract is often more responsible for obstruction than bronchial constriction. The onset often takes the form of tingling of the tongue, face or head which is followed by tightness of the chest, precordial pain and dyspnoea. Epigastric pain, nausea and vomiting may occur and coughing, wheezing and oedema of the face and pharynx are frequent. Circulatory failure with the classical features of shock develop, and death may occur within fifteen minutes of the onset of symptoms.

There is little opportunity for haemodynamic observations in the human subject with anaphylactic shock, but in experimental animals a decline in central venous pressure due to pooling of blood in vasodilated areas of the venous circulation (precipitated by the release of vaso-active substances) leads to a fall in cardiac output and hence in arterial blood pressure. Loss of plasma due to capillary exudation aggravates the fall in circulating blood volume. Anoxia may also occur due to obstruction of the airways from spasm and oedema. The fatal event in anaphylactic shock is often respiratory failure due to the increased bronchial secretions. Oxygen should be given and positive pressure respiration may be required. Adrenaline however is the most important therapeutic measure and should be given immediately. Prevention is an important aspect in the treatment of anaphylaxis. Patients with atopy should be kept under close observation after the administration of drugs likely to produce anaphylaxis. Clear records of patients with hypersensitivity should be made on the notes. Unnecessary drugs should be avoided especially in patients with atopy.

5. Neurogenic Shock

This form of shock occurs when the autonomic nervous control mechanisms which are responsible for maintaining arteriolar resistance, venous return and cardiac output are impaired. It may result from transection of the spinal cord or from the administration of ganglion blocking drugs and sympathetic antagonists used in the treatment of hypertension. Although this form of shock may be considered to be due to vasomotor collapse, the cause of the shock is not so much the loss of arteriolar tone as the expansion of the venous bed. There is in effect a disproportion between vascular volume and vascular capacity. Although the intravascular volume is normal, the size of the vascular bed, particularly the venous capacitance system, is greatly expanded and the normal blood volume is insufficient to maintain the venous return. This form of shock is of special importance to the anaesthetist for most anaesthetic agents decrease myocardial contractility and dilate the peripheral vascular bed.

6. Shock from Vascular Obstruction

Any obstruction to the main flow of blood will inevitably compromise effective circulation. This situation is seen after pulmonary emboli, which may by reducing blood flow through the lungs reduce the filling of the left atrium and hence the cardiac output. Similarly cardiac tamponade whether due to pericardial effusion or constrictive pericarditis will reduce the cardiac output and effective circulation. These are the commonest causes of partial obstruction to the flow in the central circulation (i.e. heart and pulmonary vessels) and the resulting hypotension is due to reduced cardiac output. This form of shock is similar to cardiogenic shock.

7. Shock due to Endocrine Failure

The integrity of the circulation is dependent upon a number of circulating hormones and the circulatory reaction of shock is activated by a number of endocrine responses. In shock the adrenal cortical production of cortisol is increased and this is associated with raised levels of plasma cortisol. The catechol amine production of the adrenal medulla is increased as well as that produced by the sympathetic nervous system. The renin-angiotensin system is activated due to the reduction of renal blood flow and this leads to increased aldosterone production. Sodium is therefore retained in an effort to increase the circulating blood volume and restore homeostasis. Anti-diuretic hormone production by the posterior pituitary is also increased in a similar effort to restore homeostasis. Erythropoietic hormone production also rises.

Clinical shock is a complication of certain endocrine disorders. It may be a feature of both thyroid crisis and myxoedema coma. In the former the increased demands for cortisol produce a relative adrenal insufficiency and excessive sweating predisposes to hypovolaemia. In myxoedema coma shock is associated with reduced oxidative metabolism and secondary adrenal suppression. In phaeochromocytoma the intense vasoconstriction, especially of the venous system, reduces the intravascular volume and in addition there may be exudation through the capillaries due to the increased venous tone. In meningococcal septicaemia bilateral adrenal haemorrhage may precipitate the Waterhouse-Frederichsen syndrome of acute adrenal failure. This is however an extremely rare cause of septicamic shock and in most patients with bacteraemic shock the plasma cortisol levels are raised.

Endocrine shock is commonly due to cortisol deficiency. This is rarely the result of adrenal haemorrhage but is more commonly due to inadequate replacement therapy in patients with hypopituitarism or primary adrenocortical failure or in patients who have received prolonged steroid therapy. Cortisol is necessary for normal cardiovascular function and patients in an Addisonian crisis are in shock. The treatment of endocrine shock is that of the primary disease except in cases where loss of intravascular volume (e.g. phaeochromocytoma, thyroid crisis) is contributory when fluid replacement is urgent.

Selected Bibliography

DIETZMAN, R. H., MANAX, W. G. and LILLEHEI, R. C. (1967 Shock: Mechanisms and Therapy. *Canad. Anaesth. Soc. J.* 14, 276.

HARDAWAY, R. M. (Editor) (1968) *Clinical Management of Shock*. Thomas, Springfield.

MACLEAN, L. D. (1966) The Clinical Management of Shock. *Brit. J. Anaesth.* 38, 255.

Symposium on Shock (1968) *Brit. J. Hospital Medicine* 1, 300.

VIII

The Investigation of Adrenal Function

A wide variety of laboratory tests have recently become available for assessing adreno-cortical function. Some of these are simple and can be performed by most laboratories; others are exacting and require an experienced biochemist and elaborate facilities. Indirect methods such as the water excretion test and the eosinophil depression test have been replaced by measurements of the products of cortisol metabolism excreted in the urine. More recently direct measurements of the prevailing concentration of plasma cortisol and of the cortisol secretion rate have allowed more precise examination of the state of adrenal activity.

The adrenal cortex secretes three hormones (1) cortisol (or hydrocortisone), (2) aldosterone, (3) androgens (the most important of which is androstenedione). Theoretically some measure of the prevailing concentration or metabolite excretion of any of these hormones might be used as an index of adrenal activity. In practice adrenal function tests are based on cortisol production. Aldosterone is technically difficult to measure for it requires chromatographic methods and its daily production is only one-hundredth that of cortisol. Furthermore its production by the adrenal cortex is largely independent of pituitary control so that when adrenal failure is secondary to pituitary disease, aldosterone production is relatively unimpaired and so poorly reflects adrenal cortical activity. Adrenal androgen production is largely under pituitary control although in the male the testicular component is unaffected by adrenal disease. The methods for determining androgens, such as the 17-oxosteroids, are however crude and non-specific. Furthermore cortisol is the most important of the adrenal hormones for it is essential to life and it is the adrenal ability to produce cortisol about which we are most concerned. Cortisol is the principal member of the group of steroids called 17-hydroxycorticosteroids.

Measures of adrenal activity at any given time are not an index of adrenal ability or capability. What we are trying to measure in a test of adrenal function is any damage to adrenal functional ability. Most adrenal function tests however usually measure the degree of activity of the adrenal cortex at the quiescent moment of the test. What we really require is to determine adrenal activity before and after the administration of agents which are capable of stimulating the normal gland. The normal adrenal response to stress is to increase its output up to ten-fold and the most important evidence of adrenal failure is an inability to increase activity when stress demands it. Unless the degree of cortical failure is severe it may compare favourably with the quiescent phase of adrenal rhythm and unless the adrenal is put under stress its failure to respond may pass unnoticed.

I vividly recall a patient who came up to hospital with haematuria. Prior to this she had not suffered any symptoms of sufficient severity to take her to her practitioner. Because she attended a surgical out-patient department was she cystoscoped. As she was dressing after this investigation she fainted. She immediately became a medical problem and I was asked to see her. Her standing blood pressure was 60/40, the skin showed evidence of pigmentation so that a diagnosis of Addison's disease seemed probable. She had indeed been lethargic for some months but had attributed this to the demands of three young children. She had lost some weight but being somewhat vain did not complain about this. She was admitted to the ward for investigation but within two hours was unconscious in a full Addisonian crisis. This case illustrates how a patient with adrenal insufficiency may have adequate function to permit normal daily activity but once faced with the challenge of a stress such as in this woman that of a urinary infection and cystoscopy, an adrenal crisis can be precipitated rapidly. Tests of adrenal function must be able to measure the response to stress if they are to be of real value.

There are four types of tests of adrenal function.

1. Measurement of the actual amount of cortisol produced. This is called the cortisol secretion rate.

2. The prevailing plasma concentration of cortisol.

3. The amount of the products of cortisol metabolism excreted in the urine.

4. Indirect tests such as (a) water excretion test. (b) eosinophil depression test.

CORTISOL SECRETION RATE

Although this is the most accurate measure of adrenal function it is also the most laborious and involves isotopic and biochemical determinations. The basic principle is the determination of the degree of dilution of administered radio-active steroid by the non-radioactive steroid secreted in the body. If urinary excretory products are measured the secretion rate for a 24 hour period may be calculated. Cortisol labelled with Carbon-14 or alternatively tritium (H3) is given and the concentration of radioactivity measured in a metabolite, such as tetrahydrocortisol, in the urine. Knowing the total excretion of tetrahydrocortisol as well as the amount of radioactive tetrahydrocortisol it is possible to calculate a secretion rate for cortisol. The cortisol secretion rate is about 7–30 mg. per day in normal persons, 20–40 mg. a day in pregnancy and 35–420 mg. a day in Cushing's syndrome.

THE URINARY EXCRETION OF THE METABOLIC PRODUCTS OF CORTISOL

Measurements of the excretory products of cortisol are made on a 24 hourly collection of urine. Three types of study may be made on these metabolites.

1. The basal excretion.

2. The excretion after stimulation with corticotrophin or metyrapone.

3. The excretion after suppression of the pituitary by the administration of exogenous steroids. Dexamethasone and other steroid analogues suppress pituitary corticotrophin production and prevent endogenous production of cortisol and androgens by the adrenal cortex. They do not contribute themselves significantly, in the doses used, to the urinary steroids.

All the hormones of the adrenal cortex are steroids. Over forty different steroids have been isolated from adrenal glands but most of these are precursors or metabolites of active hormones. All steroids have a common molecular structure made up of 17 carbon atoms and differ only in the nature and position of the radicals attached to these carbon atoms. Cortisol has four additional carbon atoms attached to this nucleus and is therefore known as a C_{21} steroid (Fig. 18.) The mineralo-corticoids such as aldosterone and deoxycortone acetate are also C_{21} steroids. The androgens have only 19 carbon atoms and are therefore called C_{19} steroids.

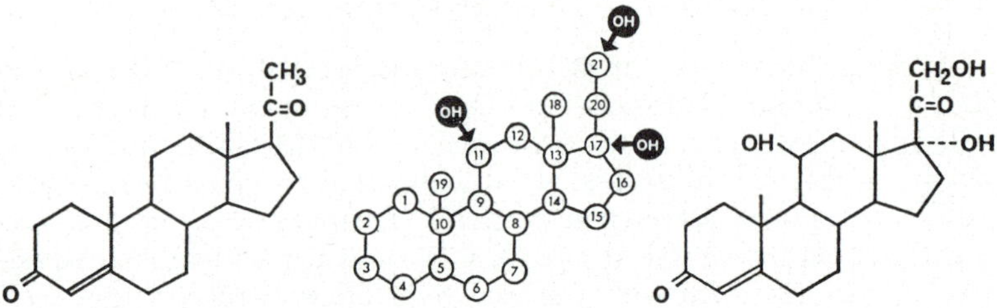

FIG. 18 Diagrammatic representation of the biosynthesis and structure of cortisol

17-oxosteroids (ketosteroids)

The 17-oxosteroids are so-called because they have an 'oxo' (=0) group at the C_{17} position. Their urinary excretion is the commonest measure of adrenal function and undoubtedly the least valuable. The 17-oxosteroids are estimated by the Zimmerman colour reaction. The normal urinary excretion is 9 to 24 mg. per day (mean 14) in males, and 5 to 18 mg. a day (mean 8) in females. In both sexes the 17-oxosteroid excretion varies with age, being low before puberty and reaching its highest levels in the second decade. The 17-oxosteroid excretion is not an accurate chemical analysis and is subject to interference by drugs in the urine. Indeed various non-specific interfering substances may comprise a large part of the material assayed by this procedure.

Adrenal androgens are excreted as 17-oxosteroids. Only a small proportion of oxosteroid in the urine comes from the metabolism of cortisol. The most important adrenal androgen is androstenedione. In the female it is responsible for (a) the development of axillary and pubic hair; (b) the stimulation of sebaceous glands; (c) protein anabolism and growth; and (d) skeletal maturation. The rate of production of adrenal androgens is controlled by pituitary ACTH but it is not the only controlling factor. There is good evidence that another pituitary hormone augments the effects of ACTH on adrenal androgen production, but this androgen-stimulating hormone has not been identified. The male has an additional source of androgen production. Testosterone is the major androgen from the testis though androstenedione is secreted here too. Indeed Δ^4 androstenedione is readily converted into testosterone. Testosterone is metabolized in exactly the same way as androstenedione so that it is also excreted as 17-oxosteroid. In the female a small amount of testosterone and androstenedione arises from the ovary and contributes to the urinary 17-oxosteroid. This is because oestrone is produced from progesterone through androstenedione, and oestrodial through testosterone. Rarely is this contribution to the 17-oxosteroid important but potentially in ovarian disorders it may give rise to significant excretion. The various oxosteroids derived from these major androgens have different colour values and there is unfortunately no correlation between their contribution to the Zimmerman colour and their androgenicity. Indeed in the male the production of testosterone, which is the most potent androgen, contributes as little as 3 mg. a day to the urinary excretion of 17-oxosteroids. In certain disorders of the ovary such as arrhenoblastoma the production of testosterone may increase from a normal female level of 0·8 mg. per day to the male testicular production rate of 7 mg. a day and cause severe virilization, and yet the urinary 17-oxosteroid excretion only increases by 3 mg. a day. As both eunuchoidal men and virile women may have apparently normal values it is a poor assay of individual androgen status.

In the female a low figure indicates low production of adrenal androgen but one cannot assume that the adrenal production of cortisol is similarly affected. Indeed there is frequently a dissociation of function, particularly in chronic debilitating diseases, where the concentration of plasma cortisol remains normal and the 17-oxosteroid excretion is reduced. Although high levels of oxosteroid excretion are found in association with many virilizing syndromes and in some patients with Cushing's disease, virilization may occur with normal oxosteroid excretion especially if testosterone is the androgen being secreted. Some of the metabolites of progesterone also give the Zimmerman colour reaction so that the 17-oxosteroid excretion normally rises in late pregnancy.

In summary, a low 17-oxosteroid excretion is not certain evidence of adrenal insufficiency but a normal level makes it improbable. A normal level does not however exclude hyperfunction of the adrenal cortex and indeed the oxosteroid excretion is often normal in Cushing's syndrome. High levels indicate increased androgen production which is most probably of adrenal origin. High levels do not mean increased cortisol production, indeed in congenital adrenal hyperplasia high oxosteroid excretion is associated with impaired cortisol synthesis. Although androgens are produced by adrenal, testis and ovary only the adrenal androgens are increased by ACTH.

17-oxogenic or ketogenic steroids

Cortisol is not metabolized by peripheral tissues but appears to attach itself to the tissues and it then subsequently returns to the blood stream. As it passes through the liver a proportion is extracted and inactivated. These conjugates (glucuronides) are soluble in water and are not bound to plasma proteins. They are therefore excreted by the kidney. Some free plasma cortisol is filtered by glomerular filtration but ninety per cent of it is reabsorbed. The urinary 17-hydroxycorticosteroids are the metabolites of cortisol and also of its inactive precursors. Thus elevated levels do not necessarily indicate increased production of cortisol but may signify a block in its synthesis.

There are two techniques in common usage for determining the urinary metabolites of cortisol and they do not measure the same chromogens. The term 17-oxogenic steroid implies that these compounds can be converted by chemical oxidation into 17-oxosteroids. This is done by oxidation of the side chain at C_{17} position giving rise to steroids which can be measured by the Zimmerman reaction for 17-oxosteroids. The steroids measured are cortisol, cortisone (and their tetrahydro derivatives) and pregnanetriol which is an excretory product of 17-hydroxyprogesterone. Pregnanetriol must not be confused with pregnanediol which is a derivative of progesterone. The oxogenic steroid is not quite synonomous with the 17-hydroxycorticosteroid for these latter steroids also include the metabolites of corticosterone which are not measured in the oxogenic steroids. In practice however these two methods give closely similar normal values. All these steroids can be estimated individually but most laboratories have neither the time nor the facilities for doing this.

In Britain the Norymberski method for estimating the oxogenic steroids is usually followed. This involves the inactivation of the 17-oxosteroids in the urine by reduction with sodium borohydride and then converting the 17-hydroxycorticosteroids to 17-oxosteroids and measuring these by the Zimmerman colour reaction. In order for a steroid with a side chain to be converted into a 17-oxosteroid, a hydroxyl group must be present in the carbon-17 position as occurs in the 17-hydroxycorticosteroids (Fig. 18.) In America the Porter-Silber method is used. This is a direct colour reaction with phenylhydrazine produced by the 17-hydroxycorticosteroids. As the presence of a hydroxyl group on the C_{17} position is necessary for this reaction the steroids are called 17-hydroxycorticosteroids.

The shortcomings of all determination of urinary excretion is that they do not reveal the level of cortisol in body fluids. Obesity increases the urinary excretion of 17-hydroxycorticosteroids but the plasma levels are normal. In hyperthyroidism the urinary hydroxycorticosteroids may be twice normal because of the rapid turnover of cortisol whereas the blood levels are not raised. It is thus necessary to obtain plasma levels in order to decide whether a patient's tissues are being exposed to elevated levels of cortisol. Furthermore in many patients with Cushing's syndrome the urinary hydroxy-corticosteroid excretion lies within the normal range. Indeed it has been shown that whilst there is some correlation between the urinary 17-oxogenic steroid excretion and the cortisol excretion rate when cortisol is being secreted in greatly excessive amounts, there is no correlation at all when the cortisol secretion rate is normal or only slightly increased. Similarly urinary 17-hydroxycorticosteroids are significantly reduced below normal in only a minority of cases of

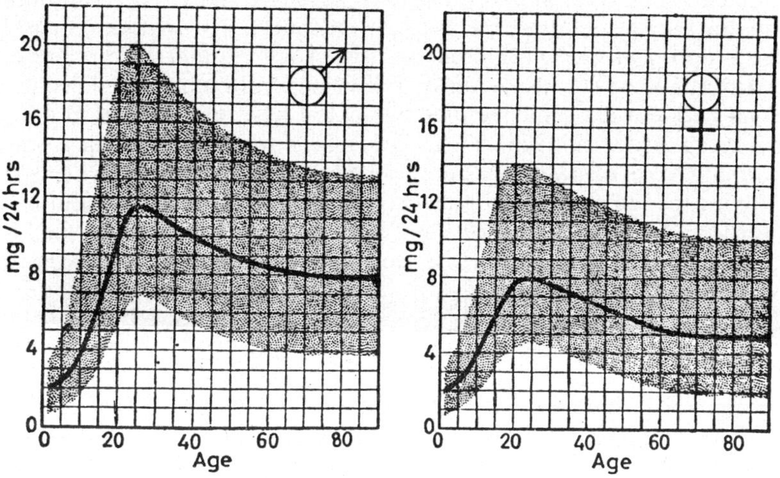

FIG. 19 The urinary oxogenic steroids in (*a*) males (*b*) females according to age

adrenal insufficiency. Stimulation tests are therefore essential if a diagnosis is to be made before the disease is far advanced.

The normal level of urinary oxogenic steroids for males is 8 to 20 mg. a day (mean 11) and for females it is 6 to 18 mg. (mean 9). In both sexes it varies with age being low before puberty and reaching its highest levels in the second decade. (Fig. 19.)

In summary the 17-hydroxycorticosteroids only give subnormal values in the more severe cases of adrenal insufficiency. In the majority of patients with adrenal insufficiency the urinary hydroxy-corticosteroids lie in the lower part of the normal range. Many patients with Cushing's syndrome will also give results within the normal range.

The ACTH *Test*

The most important procedure in the diagnosis of primary adrenocortical insufficiency is the ACTH test. This assesses the degree of adrenocortical reserve and may be used to distinguish primary adrenal insufficiency from hypopituitarism which is characterized by lack of pituitary corticotrophin. The ACTH test is also useful in determining the degree of adrenocortical suppression in patients who have been treated with large doses of corticosteroids. It may also be valuable in detecting those cases of Cushing's syndrome due to an adrenal tumour for tumours are usually unresponsive to corticotrophin.

The measurement of urinary 17-oxosteroids after ACTH is both insensitive and inappropriate as an indication of increased cortisol secretion and the 17-hydroxycorticosteroids should be preferred. Maximum ACTH stimulation following intramuscular injection increases the oxogenic steroids two and a half times. After 20 units of cortrophin zinc intramuscularly six hourly for two days the urinary 17-hydroxycorticosteroid excretion rises to 46 to 110 (mean 70) mg. per 24 hours during the second twenty-four hours of administration. After ACTH gel 20 units twice daily for four days the 17-oxogenic steroid excretion rises to levels of 40 to 90 mg. per day in normal subjects.

The plasma corticosteroid levels may also be followed after ACTH and these are considered later.

Suppression Tests

The administration of 0·5 mg. dexamethasone six hourly will inhibit the release of ACTH from the pituitary and suppress the normal adrenal to low levels of activity on the second day of administration. The urinary hydroxycorticosteroids should fall to approximately ten per cent of the pre-treatment level. In the doses required to do this the dexamethasone itself does not give rise to sufficient metabolites to interfere with the urinary steroid assays. This suppression of adrenal activity does not occur in patients with adrenal tumours as these function independent of pituitary control. Patients with adrenal hyperplasia show partial resistance to dexamethasone suppression. Small doses of dexamethasone such as 0·5 mg. four times daily may have little effect but larger doses of dexamethasone such as 6 to 8 mg. daily will suppress the hyperplastic adrenal gland. The failure of normal suppression is valuable evidence of the probability of Cushing's syndrome. Complete failure to suppress on higher doses suggests the presence of an autonomous tumour which is not under the influence of endogenous ACTH although this is not entirely reliable. The plasma cortisol of a normal person will fall to less than 6 mcg. per 100 ml. after forty-eight hours on 0·5 mg. dexamethasone four times daily.

Specific enzyme inhibition (*Metyrapone*)

The principal use of the metyrapone test is in the diagnosis of hypopituitarism. Pituitary ACTH will normally be increased when adrenal cortical activity diminishes. This ability to produce ACTH beyond the usual requirements is called the pituitary reserve. Specific inhibition of cortisol synthesis by metyrapone lowers the blood corticosteroid level and this normally results in increased ACTH production. Metyrapone inhibits the enzyme 11-beta-hydroxylase which catalyses the conversion of desoxycortisol into cortisol. (Fig. 1.) The immediate precursor of cortisol, called 11-desoxycortisol, is increased and its urine metabolites appear as 17-hydroxycorticosteroids. The quantity of the precursor produced is proportional to the dose of metyrapone and hence the completeness of the enzyme block. A dose of 750 mg. four hourly by mouth for twenty-four hours is required to inhibit this final hydroxylation of cortisol, and it is not necessary to give metyrapone for longer than 24 hours. A daily dose of 4·5 g. of metyrapone has been shown to produce 95 per cent inhibition of the enzyme system. Although there is wide individual variation, a normal response is characterized by at least the doubling of the urinary oxogenic steroids, or by an increase in excretion of more than 10 mg. per day. The increase in steroid excretion is usually greatest during the day after the drug is given. Patients with poor adrenocortical function may show signs of acute adrenal insufficiency during the test. If an impaired response is found an ACTH test should be done to ensure that the adrenal gland is able to respond to ACTH. Chlorpromazine, oestrogens, anabolic steroids and phenyl hydantoin depress the response to metyrapone.

Plasma corticosteroid determinations are not helpful with the metyrapone test as the precursor of cortisol (11-desoxycortisol), which accumulates as a result of the enzyme block, does not fluoresce.

URINARY CORTICOSTEROID (CORTISOL)

The urinary cortisol is a better indicator of increased cortisol secretion than either the hydroxycorticosteroid or oxosteroid excretion. Although only 0·5 per cent of the cortisol produced by the adrenal cortex is normally excreted unchanged in the urine, when increased quantities are produced a greater proportion exists unbound to plasma proteins and therefore available for glomerular filtration. Although the determination of urinary cortisol requires paper chromatography the fluorescence of free corticosteroids in the urine is a simple and useful test for adrenal over-activity. The normal range is 78 to 372 mcg. per day. Synthetic steroids do not fluoresce but mepacrine and spironolactone interfere with the fluorescence.

PLASMA CORTICOSTEROID (CORTISOL)

Cortisol fluoresces in strong sulphuric acid solution. This can be measured with a fluorimeter, and requires only 2 ml. of plasma for each determination. The estimation measures both free and protein-bound cortisol. Corticosterone also produces this fluorescent reaction but the amount of corticosterone in human blood is normally so small as to be of no significance. The term plasma cortisol, though established by common usage, is not strictly accurate and the word plasma corticosteroid should be used to describe the circulating fluorescing steroids. None of the synthetic analogues of cortisol such as prednisolone and dexamethasone fluoresce.

There is a large circadian rhythm in the plasma corticosteroid concentration of normal subjects due to the diurnal rhythm in the secretion of ACTH by the pituitary gland. This means that the time at which blood samples are taken is important. The highest levels are between 6 a.m. and 8 a.m. the normal range being between 7 and 26 mcg. per 100 ml. (mean level 14 mcg./100 ml.). It falls progressively during the day reaching the lowest levels at mid-night when the concentration of plasma corticosteroid does not normally exceed 8 mcg. per 100 ml. (mean level 3 mcg./100 ml.). If one is suspecting adrenal insufficiency the best time to take a sample is in the morning. If one is investigating adrenal over-activity the best time to take a sample is at midnight as the diurnal rhythm disappears early in Cushing's disease, and the level in the evening sample is high. Indeed morning levels of plasma corticosteroid are within the normal range in nearly one half of these patients. In patients with Cushing's syndrome the midnight concentration exceeds the normal upper limit of 8 mcg. per 100 ml. The disappearance of this circadian rhythm is the earliest biochemical manifestation of Cushing's syndrome. The other important biochemical disturbance is the failure of dexamethasone to suppress pituitary corticotrophin production and hence the adrenal secretion of cortisol. In a normal individual 0·5 mg. dexamethasone 6 hourly will suppress the plasma corticosteroid concentration to less than 5 mcg. per 100 ml. but this degree of suppression does not take place in Cushing's syndrome.

Approximately 95 per cent of the plasma cortisol is bound to a specific alpha-globulin called transcortin which is the cortisol binding plasma protein. Thus only 5 per cent is in solution and freely diffusible into body fluids, and this is the biologically active portion. Under normal circumstances these two are in balance. However during pregnancy or in patients on oestrogens (oral contraceptives too) the amount of transcortin may increase fourfold although the free, and hence biologically active, cortisol remains unchanged. This means that plasma corticosteroid as determined by this test will be raised often to twice the normal value in the latter half of pregnancy. Similarly the administration of 5 mg. of stilboestrol daily to normal subjects more than doubles the amount of binding protein. A similar situation applies to the thyroxine binding globulin and accounts for the raised protein bound iodine in patients who are pregnant or on oestrogens.

The analogues of cortisone do not fluoresce so they can be used for suppression tests and will not interfere with the fluorescent reaction. The urinary cortisol excretion is of value in the diagnosis of Cushing's syndrome but is of limited help in the diagnosis of adrenal insufficiency where plasma methods are more helpful. Because of protein-binding a five-fold rise of plasma corticosteroid will lead to a twelve to twenty-five-fold increase in the unbound corticosteroid and this is available for glomerular filtration and urinary excretion.

Tests of Adrenal reserve

Normal basal levels of plasma corticosteroid and urinary steroid excretion may occur in patients who develop acute adrenal insufficiency when subjected to stress. This is because they have no adrenal reserve. It is therefore important to be able to measure the stress response. There are three main mechanisms which control the pituitary secretion of ACTH and hence the adrenal secretion of cortisol.

1. *Neurohormonal*. This is concerned with the rapid response to external environmental changes and increased blood levels of ACTH can be demonstrated within two minutes of a stimulus. A wide variety of emotional, metabolic, and sensory stimuli result in adrenal stimulation. This is the reflex arc of the response to stress which is largely activated by pain and shock.

2. *Humoral*. This is concerned with the slower adjustments to changing blood levels of adrenal cortical hormones. Any fall in circulating cortisol results in increased production of corticotrophin, which can usually be detected within a few hours. Conversely the

administration of corticosteroids suppresses corticotrophin release and hence adrenocortical activity.

The stress mechanism overrides the feed-back control and is mediated by a polypeptide hormone called corticotrophin releasing factor. This is secreted by the hypothalamus into the hypothalamic-hypophyseal portal veins and controls the secretion of ACTH from the anterior pituitary. The stress response involves higher centres than the hypothalamus. (Fig. 20.)

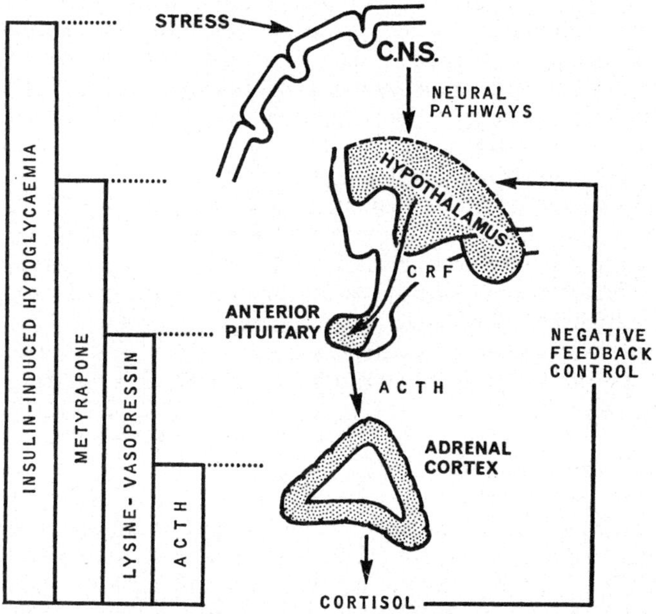

FIG. 20 Diagrammatic representation of the stress response and the point at which various tests of hypothalamic-pituitary-adrenal function focus

3. *Circadian rhythm.* The adrenal production of cortisol varies cyclically throughout the twenty-four-hour period. The circadian rhythm is due to variations in ACTH levels which are maximal in the morning and fall to low levels at midnight. This rhythmical production of ACTH persists even in patients with adrenal insufficiency. It is under the control of the higher central nervous centres in the cerebral cortex and the limbic system and it only disappears in patients with chronic impairment of consciousness due to brain damage. The limbic system is the emotional centre of the brain. It consists of the hypothalamus, the anterior thalamic nuclei, the

hippocampus and the reticular formation of the brain stem and their interconnecting fibres. It is sometimes called the reticular activating system because of the contribution of the reticular formation of the brain stem. Impulses from the reticular activating system stimulate the hypothalamus to secrete corticotrophin releasing factor which in turn controls the pituitary secretion of ACTH. The afferent stimuli are less well understood. The enhanced activity of the pituitary-adrenal axis in the morning is not a response to light or to the erect posture, as blind and supine individuals have a normal diurnal rhythm. It is probably a reflection of the pattern of the sleep and activity cycle of human life. Reversing the sleep rhythm will alter the diurnal pattern of adrenal cortisol production, although it may take several days of altered sleep rhythm to have any effect on the pattern of adrenal cortisol production.

The administration of ACTH will test the ability of the adrenal to respond to corticotrophin stimulation, but gives no indication of the ability of the pituitary to secrete ACTH. The administration of lysine vasopressin which has an action similar to the corticotrophin releasing factor will test the ability of the pituitary to release ACTH. The lysine-vasopressin test will however be normal in patients with hypothalamic dysfunction. The administration of metyrapone (p. 187) assesses the integrity of the humoral feed-back mechanism which involves hypothalamic, pituitary and adrenal function. Insulin induced hypoglycaemia however tests the integrity and reserve capacity of the entire stress response, which includes the cerebro-hypothalamo-pituitary-adrenal axis. This has become the main test of the stress response. The lysine-vasopressine test has only limited application and is not without risk and will therefore not be discussed further.

The most satisfactory method of assessing the adrenal response to corticotrophin stimulation is to measure the plasma corticosteroid response to tetracosactrin (synacthen). Tetracosactrin is a synthetic ACTH polypeptide. It is rapidly absorbed from the intramuscular route and a single intramuscular injection of 250 mg. in the morning (equivalent to 25 units ACTH) will raise the plasma corticosteroid to 31 mcg. per 100 ml. or increase the level by a mean of 17 mcg. per 100 ml. (range 8 to 27 mcg. per 100 ml. thirty minutes after the injection). A rise of less than 8 mcg. per 100 ml. is evidence of primary adrenocortical failure. Occasionally the response is delayed and it is advisable to take a sample at sixty minutes as well as at thirty minutes after the injection.

The plasma corticosteroid level may be followed after ACTH. Using a single intramuscular injection of 50 units of ACTH gel, plasma levels reach 19 to 108 (mean 45) mcg. per 100 ml.

In Addison's Disease the adrenal is completely unresponsive to ACTH even though the resting plasma levels of corticosteroid and the urinary excretion of metabolites may be within normal limits. In patients with hypopituitarism the response is frequently subnormal and it varies with the degree and duration of secondary adrenocortical atrophy. In doubtful cases ACTH gel 20 units twice daily should be given for a few days and the urinary 17-hydroxycorticosteroids or plasma cortisol monitored.

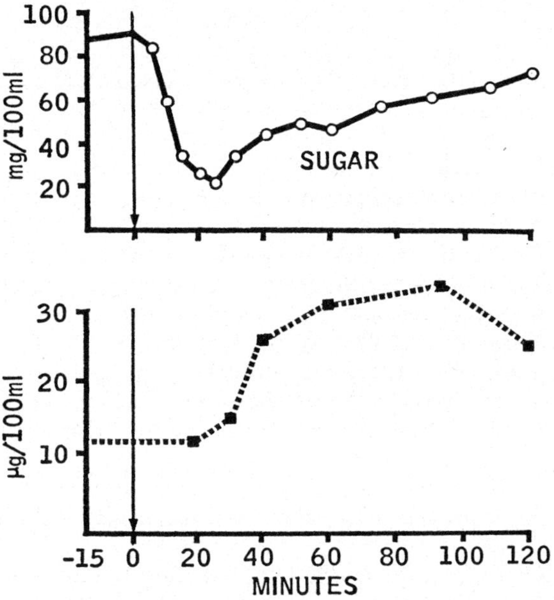

FIG. 21 The normal plasma cortisol response to insulin-induced hypoglycaemia

Insulin-induced hypoglycaemia

The basis of this test is the determination of the plasma corticosteroid response to the stress of hypoglycaemia. It is difficult to select the correct dose of insulin to produce adequate hypoglycaemia without running the risk of inducing severe hypoglycaemia. It is usually necessary to lower the blood glucose level to less than 40 mg. per 100 ml. before there is a significant rise in plasma corticosteroid. Hypoglycaemia is usually induced by the intravenous administration of 0·15 unit of insulin per kg. body weight. In malnourished patients or those with clinical evidence of hypopituitarism, 0·1 of a unit of insulin per kg. will cause an equivalent fall in blood sugar. As hypoglycaemia is the stress, it is essential to measure the blood sugar as well as the plasma corticosteroid response to the administered insulin. Blood should therefore be taken before and at 30, 60, 90, and 120 minutes after the dose of insulin. Patients with adrenal insufficiency are sensitive to insulin and a physician should be present throughout the test ready to give glucose intravenously if hypoglycaemia should be severe. A typical response is shown in Fig. 21. If adequate hypoglycaemia is achieved (blood sugar less than 40 mg. per 100 ml.) the plasma corticosteroid will rise by amounts ranging from 6·5 to 18·5 mcg. per 100 ml. with a mean value of 12·8 mcg. per 100 ml. The degree of adrenal stimulation achieved is equivalent to that of ACTH in a dose of 10 units per hour.

PLASMA CORTICOSTEROID

Normal morning plasma concentration	7 to 26 (Mean 14) mcg. per 100 ml.
Midnight plasma concentration	Less than 8 (Mean 3) mcg. per 100 ml.
Normal *rise* in plasma corticosteroid one hour after intramuscular injection of 250 mcg. tetracosactrin (Synacthen)	More than 8 mcg. per 100 ml.
Level to which plasma corticosteroid is normally suppressed after 0·5 mg. Dexamethasone 6 hourly	Less than 5 mcg. per 100 ml.
Normal *rise* in plasma corticosteroid after insulin-induced hypoglycaemia (Blood sugar less than 40 mg. per 100 ml.)	6 to 18 (Mean 13) mcg. per 100 ml.

INDIRECT TESTS

Waterload test

Cortisol is essential for the renal excretion of water. If there is a deficiency a waterload cannot be excreted adequately and this failure to excrete water will be corrected by the administration of cortisol. A waterload (20 ml. per kg. body-weight) is taken by mouth over a period of fifteen minutes after an eight hour fast.

Urine is collected for four hours. In healthy people eighty per cent of the waterload is excreted within four hours whilst in adreno-cortical insufficiency less than sixty per cent is excreted. Water excretion is also impaired in liver disease, renal disease, hypothyroidism and if the patient is dehydrated. However in only adreno-cortical insufficiency will this failure to excrete water be corrected by giving 50 mg. of cortisone acetate two hours before the test. This is a valuable screening test.

Eosinophil count

In adrenal insufficiency the blood eosinophil count rises. Thorn devised a test, in which the fall in blood eosinophils was observed four hours after the intramuscular injection of 25 units of ACTH. Normally this fall exceeds fifty per cent of the initial figure but will not occur in primary adrenocortical insufficiency. This test has little clinical application because more precise measures of adrenal function are available today.

Selected Bibliography

COPE, C. L. (1972) *Adrenal Steroids and Disease*. 2nd Ed. Pitman Medical Publishers.

GREENWOOD, F. C. and LANDON, J. (1966) The Assessment of Hypothalamic-Pituitary Function in Endocrine Disease. *J. Clin. Path.* 19, 284.

JAMES, V. H. T. and LANDON, J. (Editors) (1968) *The Investigation of Hypothalamic-Pituitary-Adrenal Function*. Cambridge University Press.

JORGENSEN, M. (1957) The Urinary Excretion of Ketogenic Steroids. *Acta. Endocrinol.* 26, 424.

LANDON, J., WYNN, V. and JAMES, V. H. T. (1963) Adreno-cortical Response to Insulin-Induced Hypoglycaemia J. End. 27, 183.

PRUNTY, F. T. G. (1966) Androgen Metabolism in Man. *Brit. Med. J.* 2, 605.

IX

The Function of the Thymus

The thymus gland is now established as a vital part of the immunological system. The acquisition of knowledge of this gland is recent. In 1960 at a symposium on cellular aspects of immunity the thymus was not even considered. Since then a great deal of information has been acquired by observations on the immunological deficiencies of thymectomized mice and on the methods of restoring immunological competence to these animals. Over the last few years studies on the clinical syndromes associated with thymic disease in man have made their contribution.

The thymus is now known to be the site of the primary proliferation of those lymphocytes which will be responsible for most of the immunological activity of the body. Its activity is greatest in the neonatal period but is taken over by other lymphoid organs in later life. Stem cells from the bone marrow differentiate into the precursors of immunologically competent cells (immunocytes) within the thymus. In addition the epithelial cells of the thymus secrete a hormone called thymosin, which provides the stimulus for lymphocyte production within the thymus and which confers on lymphocytes elsewhere in the body the capacity to respond to antigenic stimulation. This review of the function of the thymus will begin with an account of the structure of the gland. It will be followed by a summary of the information acquired by animal experiments and it will conclude with a comment on the clinical syndromes in man that are associated with abnormalities of the thymus.

Structure

The thymus is a bi-lobed organ which develops from branchial endoderm, and which is situated retrosternally in the anterior mediastinum. In 20 per cent of individuals ectopic thymic tissue may be present in the neck or in the chest and this is an important point when assessing the results of thymectomy. By the end of the second intra-uterine month the epithelial nature of the thymus is evident and lymphocytes make their appearance shortly afterwards. The thymus consists of a cortex and a medulla. The medulla grows from a down growth of the epithelium of the third and fourth branchial clefts whereas the cortex originates from lymphoid cells which have invaded the epithelial thymus from adjacent mesenchyme and thereafter proliferate within the thymus. The thymus is the first organ in which lymphocytes can be identified in vertebrates. It grows rapidly in utero but the maximum weight is not achieved until puberty, after which much of its parenchyma is replaced by fat. This process of involution is increased by stress, starvation and chronic illness. However, the thymus never completely disappears and biopsy specimens taken at thoracotomy in elderly subjects contain significant amounts of functional thymic tissue.

Thymic tissue consists of two main cell types: the small lymphocyte (thymocyte) and the epithelial (reticular) cell. The dense cortex is packed with lymphocytes and is surrounded by a continuous outer layer of epithelial cells. It is an area of intense lymphopoeisis and the rate of production of new cells is five times greater than that in lymph nodes and other lymphoid tissues. The medulla is more loosely cellular and consists of a reticulo-epithelial stroma which contains far fewer lymphocytes than the cortex; it also contains epithelial cells and Hassal's corpuscles. The thymus is thus basically an epithelial cell sponge in which lymphocytes are embedded. Though the thymus is undoubtedly a lymphoid organ it differs from other lymphoid tissue both structurally and functionally. It has a cortex and medulla but it contains few plasma cells and no lymph follicles with germinal centres. The germinal centre is the histological hallmark of antibody production and this suggests that though the thymus is the site of intense lymphopoeisis it is incapable of antibody production.

Thymic Lymphopoiesis

The inability of the thymus to produce antibody is due to the immaturity of its lymphocytes which lack immunological competence, rather than to a failure of antigen to penetrate the thymus. It has indeed been demonstrated in experimental animals by labelling antigens with radioactive isotopes or with fluorescent dyes that antigens can pass the so-called blood-thymus barrier. Antigenic stimulation is not the stimulus to thymic lymphopoiesis and it would seem that this stimulus arises within the thymus itself. Indeed, lymphopoiesis is as intense in the animal kept in a germ-free environment as in one under normal circumstances, and partial thymectomy does not produce any compensatory hypertrophy or change in the lymphopoietic activity of the remaining thymic tissue. Similarly when the thymus gland is grafted from one animal to another, the size and lymphopoietic activity of the grafted gland is not inhibited by the presence of the recipient's own thymus or by the presence of any additional grafts.

The contribution of the neonatal thymus to lymphocyte production is disproportionate to the size of the gland. In the mouse the thymus is only 15 per cent of the lymphoid mass but it produces 60 per cent of all new lymphocytes. It is not certain what happens to the lymphocytes produced in the thymus. By labelling thymic cells with a radioactive marker it is known that some cells certainly go to the spleen and lymph nodes. But only a relatively small proportion, probably of the order of 10 per cent, of the new cells produced in the thymus emigrate to other lymphoid tissues. It seems that a large proportion of thymic lymphocytes disintegrate in situ after a short life of three days.

The lymphocyte and the immune response

There are two distinct propulations of lymphocytes, one dependant on the presence of the thymus ('T' lymphocytes) and the other independant of the thymus ('B' lymphocytes). Both are concerned with immune responses. They differ in their distribution and in their life span. The former contribute the greater part of the recirculating pool of lymphocytes and have a long life, whilst the latter are more restricted to lymphoid tissue and have a short life. The thymus dependant lymphocyte is a cell which in the absence of antigenic stimulation circulates through the blood, lymph node and back into the circulation again over a period of more than ten years. It performs a policing role awaiting recognition of foreign material which it is able to identify as such. It reacts by multiplication and transformation and these are the ingredients of the immune response. The recognition of antigen by these lymphocytes is mediated by antibody synthesized in the cell and bound onto the surface membrane. The receptor on the surface of the lymphocyte thus has a molecular configuration similar to that of the receptor group on an antibody molecule. Such a recognition unit is probably part of the structure of the cell wall. The molecular structure of the antibody is specific to that particular clone of lymphocytes and combination with the appropriate antigen on the cell surface triggers off the immune response. The immediate response is the transformation of these lymphocytes into large blast cells. Transformation into a blast cell is a manifestation of preparation for mitosis. These lymphoblasts do not have demonstrable intracellular immunoglobulin and may develop in a variety of ways and lead to the release of soluble factors which bring about a number of the tissue changes associated with cell mediated hypersensitivity reactions.

1. They may divide further to form an expanded population of primed antigen-sensitive cells which provide immunological memory and police the circulation for many years.
2. They release a number of soluble factors which (a) increase vascular permeability (b) activate macrophages, and (c) stimulate other lymphocytes to reproduce.
3. They may co-operate with and stimulate 'B' lymphocytes to produce immunoglobulin. This co-operative function accounts for the relationship so often observed between delayed hypersensitivity and humoral antibody production.
4. They are killer cells which are cytotoxic for certain cells. This cytotoxic effect is achieved by their ability to activate complement bound to membranes.

The small lymphocyte is the commonest type of lymphoid cell circulating in the blood and lymph, and the most common cell in lymphoid tissue and in the thymus. They are derived from the large lymphocytes. Large lymphocytes transform into medium size lymphocytes and these in turn into small lymphocytes. The majority of small lymphocytes in the thoracic duct are not newly formed cells but re-circulating cells. Re-circulating small lymphocytes are immunologically competent cells with a long life span and they can initiate an immune response even if they are not actively engaged in antibody production. Both the thymus-dependent or 'T' lymphocytes and the bone marrow or bursa derived 'B' lymphocytes contain antigen sensitive cells with specific antibody on their surface. Morphologically 'T' lymphocytes and 'B' lymphocytes can not be distinguished but it has recently been shown that 'B' cells carry a heavier density of immunoglobulin on their surface whilst 'T' lymphocytes and thymocytes have much less. By using radioactively labelled antiglobulin it is possible to identify 'B' lymphocytes. Using this method it has recently been shown that 34 per cent of the circulating blood lymphocytes are bone marrow derived or 'B' lymphocytes and 45 per cent of spleen and marrow lymphocytes have a similar origin. The 'T' and 'B' cells of the blood take different routes through the lymph nodes.

It is facile to think of the immune response as simply the switching on by antigen of a specialized population of cells which will eventually synthesize antibodies. At least three types of cell are necessary but the nature of their interactions is not fully understood. These are (1) Macrophages, (2) Reactor cells and (3) Effector cells. Firstly the macrophage is required to process the antigen. The processing of antigen leads to the presentation of antigen-determinants at the cell surface and this is a pre-requisite for the stimulation of thymic dependant lymphocytes. Secondly reactor cells are required to identify the foreign nature of the antigen and to initiate the immune response. Thirdly effector cells must then actually synthesize the antibody. Both reactor and effector cells have similar histological appearances. In fact the round cells with the high nucleus to cytoplasm ratio which we describe as lymphocytes are a heterogeneous collection of cells with different origins, functions, fates and life spans. The reactor cells are cells of thymic origin with a long life span and are components of the circulating lymphocyte pool. Effector cells on the other hands are short-lived and reside predominantly within the follicular zones of the lymph nodes. Animal experiments have demonstrated that thymus derived cells identify foreign antigenic material and can initiate the production of antibody-producing cells. These antibody forming cells do not, however, originate in the thymus but in the bone marrow. It seems that cells derived from the thymus react with the specific antigen and multiply before in some way directing another population of cells derived from the bone marrow cell to produce antibody.

The thymus contains a higher proportion of actively dividing larger lymphocytes than other lymphoid tissues and the mitotic rate of its cell population is correspondingly higher. Kinetic studies using radioactive thymidine have shown that the thymus is actively engaged in lymphopoiesis and continually producing larger numbers of small lymphocytes, but it is unable to replace the full complement of stem cells necessary to maintain this high level of mitotic activity.

Antilymphocytic serum has been used to prolong survival of homografts by suppressing delayed hypersensitivity and erasing immunological memory. It is of interest that it can do this without destroying the lymphocyte, for the numbers of lymphocytes may be relatively unchanged in circumstances where the lymphocytes have lost their recognition ability.

It is little over ten years ago that the first association of the thymus with immune disturbance was reported. Since then an enormous amount of work has been done and published on the role of this gland in immunity. Our knowledge of the function of the thymus has been acquired by:—

1. **Observations on the immunological deficiencies of thymectomized mice:**
   (a) Fall in circulating lymphocytes and atrophy of lymphoid tissue.

(b) Impaired cellular immunity { increased susceptibility to infection. impaired transplantation immunity. }

(c) Increased susceptibility to carcinoma.

2. Means of restoring immunological competence to thymectomized animals:

(a) Immunologically competent cells.

(b) Thymic grafts.

3. Observations on marker chromosomes:

(a) Thymic graft becomes colonized by host cells originating from bone marrow.

(b) Host cells after residing in thymic graft emigrate out to peripheral lymphoid tissues and to circulating lymphocyte pool.

4. Clinical syndromes in man associated with pathological changes in thymus:

(a) Aplasia of thymus.

(b) Thymitis.

(c) Thymoma.

ANIMAL EXPERIMENTS

Effects of Thymectomy

It was the observation in 1962 of the effects of neonatal thymectomy in mice that first demonstrated the immunological function of the thymus. These effects were:

1. A reduction in circulating small lymphocytes.
2. Defects in the capacity to produce certain types of immune response.
3. Increased susceptibility to infections leading to early death from runt disease.
4. Increased susceptibility to carcinoma.
5. Decreased susceptibility to lymphatic leukaemia.

Immune deficiency following thymectomy

Thymectomy must be performed in the neonatal period for it to have any immediate effect on immunological function. The reason for this is that the cells which initiate an immune response have a long life. These lymphocytes develop within the thymus during the neonatal period and a pool of these cells is already present at birth. In adult mice and other animals thymectomy causes a reduction in the number of lymphocytes in the blood, lymph and lymphoid tissues but no apparent immediate immunological deficiencies result. However, when an animal thymectomized in adult life is challenged with a new antigen six or more months later there is clear evidence of immunological deficiency. Even the effect of thymectomy in the neonatal period varies with the species of animal, for the cell-mediated response will only be impaired by neonatal thymectomy in those species which have not developed a competent peripheral lymphoid system at birth.

After neonatal thymectomy in the mouse there is a fall in the number of circulating small lymphocytes, a gross reduction in thoracic duct cells and also to a less extent in the population of lymphocytes in lymphoid tissues. The number of lymphocytes in the thoracic duct falls to 1 per cent of its previous level. There is depletion of lymphocytes in all lymphoid organs. This depletion is not over all but is confined to certain specific areas of the lymph node, namely the mid-deep cortex or paracortical region. This area has been called the thymus-dependent area and is the area depleted by continuous thoracic duct drainage. Labelled thymic cells localize in this area within 24 hours of intravenous injection. Plasma cells and large lymphocytes are not reduced. The responses particularly affected by the fall in population of small lymphocytes are the delayed hypersensitivity response and the graft rejection response and it is known that both these responses are mediated by small lymphocytes. It is cellular immunity that is compromised. The humoral antibody response which is mediated by plasma cells is not seriously affected; plasma cells are not lacking and the circulating levels of immunoglobulin remain normal. Cells from the spleen of these thymectomized animals are less able to induce graft versus host disease in appropriate recipients than spleen cells from normal mice. Neonatally thymectomized mice will thus accept foreign skin grafts when grafted from three days to five weeks after thymectomy. Thymectomy in adult life does not have this effect. The immunological defect following neonatal thymectomy increases susceptibility to infections, so that organisms not normally pathogenic produce disease and the animal dies from a wasting disease called runt disease, in which overwhelming infection by saprophytic organisms is responsible for death.

The adult thymus also has some influence on the immune response. This has been shown by experiments combining thymectomy with sub-lethal irradiation, which will deplete the animal's circulating pool of immunologically competent cells. Recovery from sub-lethal irradiation is greatly impaired in adult animals which have undergone thymectomy when compared with similarly irradiated animals which have not. This suggests that the thymus has a function in maintaining immune competence throughout life.

Increased susceptibility to cancer

Neonatal thymectomy increases the incidence of chemically induced carcinoma in animals and also of the virus-induced malignant diseases. It is probable that an immunological mechanism exists for recognizing and eliminating abnormal or malignant cells arising in the body and that resistance to cancer is in part dependent on such a mechanism. A defect in cellular immune functions would therefore result in a predisposition to malignant disease. Tumours induced by viruses and carcinogens possess different antigens to the normal cells and the immunological response of the host may suppress growth of these tumours. The polyoma virus induces a variety of tumours in certain strains of mice when the virus is innoculated during the neonatal period. Neonatal thymectomy results in the development of tumours in normally resistant strains of mice and increases the incidence and variety of tumours in the strains which are susceptible to the polyoma virus. New antigens have been demonstrated in some human cancer cells and the rising incidence of cancer with age may be related to declining activity of the thymus.

Decreased susceptibility to leukaemia

In contrast thymectomy prevents the otherwise inevitable development of lymphatic leukaemia in certain strains of animals (murine). It also reduces the incidence of leukaemia induced by viruses and by irradiation. Thymic grafts restore this suceptibility to leukaemia. It is believed that the thymus provides the necessary environment in which lymphocytes in virus infected hosts can be transferred into leukaemic cells.

Restoration of immunological function after thymectomy

A good deal of knowledge has been acquired about the function of the thymus by studying the ways in which immunological function can be restored to neonatally thymectomized mice. This may be achieved by:

1. The injection of immunologically competent cells.
2. The grafting of thymic tissue.

1. The injection of immunologically competent cells. Immune responses can be restored by supplying immunologically competent cells. This can be done by injecting suspensions of cells from the spleen or lymph node. Grafts accepted by thymectomized animals will then be rejected and infections sustained will then be overcome. Suspensions of bone marrow cells are ineffective and so are foetal liver and marrow cells. Intravenously administered extracts of thymic cells are unable to restore immunological function. As pure suspensions of lymphocytes, obtained from drainage of thoracic duct lymph, are effective it seems that the successful organ suspensions owe their effect to the presence of these cells. Thymocytes are ineffective because few cells within the thymus have reached sufficient maturity to enable them to become immunologically competent.

2. Grafting thymic tissue. Thymic tissue grafted subcutaneously or under the renal capsule is able to restore immunological function to thymectomized mice. These grafts may be syngenic or allogenic. Syngenic means genetically identical, as are the tissues of an identical twin or individual members of a pure line strain. Allogenic means that the tissue is not genetically identical but is of the same species. Experiments using marked chromosomes have shown that a grafted thymus initially releases donor cells to the peripheral lymphoid tissue of the host. This method involves using histocompatible cells with a distinctive chromosome which allows donor and host cells to be distinguished. Subsequently the thymus graft becomes colonized by bone marrow cells of the host. These host cells, after residing in the thymus graft for a period, emigrate to the peripheral lymphoid tissues. Those myeloid cells proliferating in the recipient's thymus soon lose the ability to divide into other myeloid cells and acquire a new capacity to settle in the lymph nodes when injected into a second recipient.

The interesting observation in this experimental situation is that the lymphocytes responsible for the restored immunological activity are host cells that acquire competence by a period of residence within the donor thymus graft. A thymus graft depleted of lymphoid tissue by irradiation in vitro with 500 r. is also effective. If however a heavier dose of irradiation is given, such as 2,000 r., the epithelial cells are damaged and immunological competence is not restored. This suggests that thymic function is dependent upon the integrity of the epithelial cells. When the thymic implant is placed in a millipore diffusion chamber in the peritoneal cavity some degree of immunological competence is restored. As the walls of the chamber are impermeable to cells it suggests that some humoral mechanism must be responsible, and that a hormone must be secreted by the epithelial cells of the thymus which confers on lymphocytes outside the chamber the capacity to respond. It must be the epithelial cells that are responsible as the thymus tissue subsequently recovered from the chamber contains only epithelial cells and no lymphocytes. Furthermore the intra-uterine progeny of thymectomized pregnant rodents can restore immunological function to these animals. It is of interest that in these experiments although immunological competence was restored the number of lymphocytes remained depleted. This suggests that lymphopoiesis in the thymus is not synonymous with the induction of immunological competence. The nature of this thymic hormone is uncertain but recently a peptide has been isolated from the thymus and called thymosin. It causes lymphoid hypertrophy when injected into thymectomized mice.

Effects of thymectomy after the neonatal period

If older mice are thymectomized (at two months) and are then given a lethal dose of x-rays, their immunological capacity can be restored by injecting lymphoid cells. Bone marrow cells are no good unless a thymus gland is grafted, in which case bone marrow cells can differentiate within the grafted thymus to become immunologically competent cells. This suggests that the thymus may have a role in mature animals to provide for a sudden demand of new immunological patterns. When marked lymph node cells and bone marrow cells are injected together into a syngenic recipient that has been irradiated with a lethal dose of x-rays, the donor lymph node cells divide in the recipient's lymph nodes and the bone marrow cells in the bone marrow and spleen. The thymus too becomes populated but with cells that are of bone marrow origin. These myeloid cells are not immunologically competent. Eventually, however, descendants of these myeloid cells replace the donor cells of lymphoid origin with which the recipient lymph nodes are initially repopulated.

Function of thymus in adults

It has been shown that the population of small lymphocytes within the thymus is replaced every three to four days. The great majority of small lymphocytes formed in the adult thymus never leave it but are destroyed within it. Their nuclear DNA is re-utilized. It has been suggested that when a newly formed immunocyte meets a corresponding antigen within the thymus the subsequent immunological reaction results in the death of that cell, and that the reaction with self antigens within the thymus accounts for the large numbers of thymic lymphocytes dying in situ. The cells that leave the thymus represent immunocytes devoid of self reactivity. This hypothesis thus maintains that the thymus not only produces immunologically competent cells but vets them for auto-immune reactivity before releasing them into the circulating pool.

Certainly it has been possible to induce tolerance to a foreign antigen by direct injection of the antigen into the thymus. In these experiments rats were given a sub-lethal dose of irradiation to render the lympho-follicular system immunologically incompetent but the thymus was shielded from the irradiation. Bovine gammaglobulin was then injected directly into the thymus and the animals were subsequently tolerant of this antigen.

The purpose of thymic lymphopoiesis in adult life remains uncertain. If the adult lymphoid system is damaged, for instance by irradiation, its anatomical and functional recovery is dependent upon the thymus. No such regeneration takes place if the adult mouse is thymectomized before irradiation and a permanent impairment of cell-mediated immune mechanism results, with a failure to reject skin grafts from different strains. Animal experiments suggest that thymectomy in adult life does eventually lead to deficient responses to new antigenic stimuli. The lymphocytes in the thymus are not themselves immunologically competent and it is not certain that competence is acquired immediately they leave the thymus. It may well be that a further period of development after reaching the lymphoid tissues is required. Furthermore, lymphopoiesis in the thymus is no guarantee of the induction of competence. The millipore diffusion experiments suggest that a hormone from the epithelial cells may restore competence to a thymectomized animal without increasing the number of depleted lymphocytes. It has been shown that there is a difference in behaviour of thymic grafts when they receive light or heavy irradiation. In both cases the graft is repopulated with host lymphoid cells and lymphopoiesis is re-established. However, only the animals receiving lightly irradiated grafts regain immunological competence. Hence the ability of thymic epithelial cells to promote lymphopoiesis may be distinct from their ability to produce immunological competence through the humoral factor.

It has been suggested that the thymus provides a site for the proliferation of cells with immunological potential. These precursor cells enter the thymus from the blood stream and are stimulated to develop along lymphocytic pathways under the influence of a thymic hormone secreted by the epithelial cells of the thymus. (Fig. 22.) Cell division within the thymus is not controlled by antigenic stimulation. The elective theory of immunity maintains that contact between antigen and mature lymphocytes stimulates the cells to divide and to produce a clone of cells responsive to that antigen. The thymus thus can provide a site where lymphocytes are not subject to clonal proliferation. It has been suggested that all new or primary immune patterns originate in the thymus and that these cells are then seeded out to the lymph nodes and spleen where they can proliferate in response to antigenic challenge. It does, however, seem that in addition a thymic hormone is required to convey on lymphocytes outside the thymus the capacity to respond to immunological challenge. It is

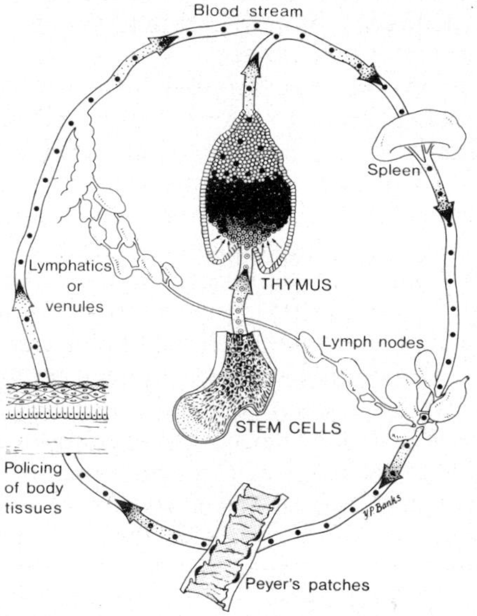

FIG. 22 Thymus gland and circulating lymphocytes

possible that a separate hormone is required to permit the transformation of lymphocytes to plasma cells so that the humoral antibodies can be produced, but this hormone is not derived from the thymus.

The control of cellular and humoral immunity

Experiments in birds suggest that cellular and humoral mechanisms of immunity are under separate control. The lymphoid system in birds can be divided into two separate morphological and functional units which are developmentally distinct. The th: nus system of cells is responsible for cellular immunity. The bursa of Fabricius controls development of germinal centres and plasma cells in peripheral lymphoid tissues and hence the production of immunoglobulins. The bursa develops as an epithelial sack budding from the dorsal region of the cloaca. Removal of the bursa of Fabricius in chickens immediately after hatching results in a selective failure of humoral antibody production. Like the thymus the bursa itself is not an antibody-producing organ and like the thymus it secretes a hormone which conveys on cells outside the bursa the capacity to make antibody (c.f. millipore diffusion chamber and the thymus). Large and medium size lymphocytes can differentiate into plasma cells which synthesize antibody. It has been suggested that the aetiology of human agammaglobulinaemia is a deficiency of a humoral factor that allows this differentiation of large lymphocytes into plasma cells. The equivalent of the bursa of Fabricius in the mammal is uncertain but it is possible that it is represented by the Peyer's patch type of lymphoid tissue in the gastro-intestinal tract. Certainly Peyer's patches are absent in human patients with congenital hypogammaglobulinaemia.

NZB Mice

Spontaneous auto-immune disease occurs in the New Zealand Black strain of inbred mice. At the age of four to six months these animals develop an auto-immune haemolytic anaemia, antibodies against cell nuclei and a nephritis similar histologically to that found in SLE. These auto-immune disorders can be transferred to normal syngenic recipients by transferring the lymphocytes of affected animals. These mice are infected from birth with a virus which can be demonstrated in lymph nodes, spleen and thymus and the disease can be transmitted by cell-free extracts from the spleen. It is believed that infection with the virus releases DNA into the circulation which results in anti-DNA antibodies. The immune complexes are deposited in the renal glomeruli causing nephritis. In the case of auto-immune haemolytic anaemia the virus probably alters a normal antigen of the red cells so that the lympho-follicular system no longer recognizes it as a self antigen and sets in motion an auto-immune reaction.

Characteristic lesions with the formation of germinal centres have been noted in the thymus of these animals. It is probable that the thymic lesion is the result of the auto-immune disease rather than the cause and indeed thymus grafts from healthy strains develop similar lesions. The thymic lesions may appear before or after the disease has become established and neonatal thymectomy does not prevent the disease, nor does a thymic graft from a different strain. Thymic grafts inserted into NZB mice develop the same morphological changes as the animals' own thymus, which suggests that the thymic changes are the result of the disease and not its cause.

Conclusion

The thymus is thus the site of the primary proliferation of those lymphocytes which will be responsible for most of the immunological activity of the body. Stem cells from the bone marrow come to the thymus where they differentiate into the precursors of immunologically competent cells under the influence of the thymic epithelial cell hormone. Developing cells which react with self antigens within the gland are destroyed and those cells that are not autoreactive migrate to the blood stream and lympho-follicular tissues where they form the circulating pool of immunologically competent lymphocytes. These cells possess the ability to identify foreign antigenic material and initiate the cellular and humoral events that characterize the immune response.

THYMIC DISORDERS IN MAN

Clinical syndromes associated with thymic disease

Over the last few years studies on the clinical syndromes in man that are associated with thymic disease have contributed increasingly to our knowledge of the thymus. Aplasia of the thymus is associated with deficiencies of immunological function. Thymitis is the term used to describe the changes of chronic inflammation which are seen in the thymus in association with certain clinical disorders. These changes include the infiltration of the thymic medulla with lymphocytes and plasma cells and the development of germinal centres. Thymitis is associated with myasthenia gravis, and similar histological changes in the thymus may be found in conditions such as systemic lupus erythematosus, auto-immune haemolytic anaemia of infancy and rheumatoid arthritis. Tumours of the thymus may be accompanied by hypogammaglobulinaemia and by disorders of autoimmunity such as systemic lupus erythematosus, myasthenia gravis, myositis, myocarditis, acquired haemolytic anaemia and erythroblastic aplasia. These associations are far too frequent to be explained by chance. Furthermore individual patients may show several of the disorders which are separately associated with thymic tumours and this strongly suggests a common aetiology.

The clinical syndromes associated with pathological changes in the thymus are tabulated below.

CLINICAL SYNDROMES ASSOCIATED WITH THYMIC DISEASE

Aplasia	(1) Congenital absence of the thymus, or pharyngeal pouch syndrome (DiGeorge's syndrome).

	(2) Hereditary thymic dysplasia
	(a) Lymphopenic hypogammaglobulinaemia (Swiss type hypogammaglobulinaemia)
	(b) Lymphopenic dysgammaglobulinaemia
	(c) Reticular dysgenesis (lymphopenia and aleucocytosis)
Thymitis	(1) Myasthenia gravis
	(2) Systemic lupus erythematosus
	(3) Auto-immune haemolytic anaemia of infancy
	(4) Rheumatoid arthritis
	(5) Chronic thyroiditis
Hyperplasia	(1) Thyrotoxicosis
Thymoma	(1) Myasthenia gravis
	(2) Myositis
	(3) Myocarditis
	(4) Erythroblastic aplasia
	(5) Aplastic anaemia
	(6) Hypogammaglobulinaemia
	(7) Systemic lupus erythematosus
	(8) Auto-immune haemolytic anaemia
	(9) Sjogren's disease
	(10) Addison's disease
Lymphosarcoma	(1) Lymphatic leukaemia
Adenocarcinoma	(1) Adrenocortical hyperplasia

Aplasia of the thymus

In the last few years investigation of the immunological deficiency syndromes associated with defective thymic function have been particularly rewarding, and the therapeutic advances achieved by transplantation of bone marrow stem cells and thymic implants have helped to differentiate the relative role of the thymus and of the bone marrow in the maintenance of immunological competence. Deficiencies of humoral immunity, that is, antibody deficiency syndromes, lead to recurrent bacterial infection, particularly by cocci. Defects in cellular immunity lead to recurrent virus infections, moniliasis, diarrhoea and wasting. Combined deficiency syndromes have features of both humoral and cellular immune insufficiency.

Disorders of the thymus are associated with defects in cellular immunity. There are two distinct deficiencies which may give rise to aplasia of the thymus and immunological incompetence. Firstly, there may be a congenital absence of the thymus due to maldevelopment. The pharyngeal pouch syndrome described by DiGeorge is due to the failure of development of structures derived from the third and fourth pharyngeal pouch endoderm and branchial cleft ectoderm—namely the thymus and the parathyroid glands. The immunological deficiency which results is similar to that produced by neonatal thymectomy in animals. In addition these children have hypoparathyroidism due to the absence of parathyroid glands. Their facies are often distinctive for the jaw is small and the ears are low-set and malformed. They present with recurrent infection and may develop progressive vaccina and prolonged varicella. In affected individuals humoral antibody synthesis and serum immunoglobulin concentrations are normal but cellular immunity is impaired. Affected children cannot reject skin allographs normally, and do not manifest delayed hypersensitivity reactions to common antigens. One child with this syndrome had a skin allograft in place for five months without even microscopic signs of rejection. Secondly, there is the 'Swiss' type of lymphopenic hypogammaglobulinaemic immunological deficiency syndrome, in which the whole of the lympho-reticular tissue is hypoplastic. This is a more serious disorder in which progressive deterioration and death have not hitherto been preventable. Although the thymus is anatomically and functionally deficient in this syndrome too, the impaired development of the thymus is not believed to be due to a primary failure of growth but is secondary to deficiencies of the bone marrow stem cells which populate the thymus and develop there along lymphocytic pathways. It seems that the thymus fails to develop because of the lack of stimulation provided by the inflow of lymphopoietic stem cells. The thymic aplasia is thus a secondary or concomitant deficiency. Correction of this disorder therefore requires administration of stem cells in addition to the implantation of thymic tissue.

There have been a number of recent reports describing the successful restoration of immunological function in infants with the pharyngeal pouch syndrome by implantation of thymic tissue. One of these children is well three years after his thymic implant. As the thymic implants were obtained from a foetus of different sex it was possible by examination of the chromosomes to observe that the restored immunological competence was due to cells of recipient origin. This suggests that implantation of the thymus had conferred on the patients lymphocytes the capacity to respond. The other point of interest is the speed with which immunological competence was restored. The normal response of the blood lymphocytes in vitro to such agents as phytohaemagglutinin was restored within four days in one case and within three weeks in another.

In the lymphopenic immunological deficiency syndrome all attempts at restoring immunological competence up to 1968 had failed. In 1968 the restoration of immunological competence was reported in an eight month old boy after giving maternal blood with foetal thymus and liver cells. Unfortunately a graft versus host reaction supervened and the patient died from a massive bilateral haemorrhagic pneumonia. In this condition it is important to replace the bone marrow stem cells as it seems that the thymic abnormality is a secondary or concomitant failure to this deficiency. Foetal cells are used in the hope that graft versus host reactions may be reduced or circumvented. Subsequent attempts using immunologically competent cells from the peripheral blood buffy coat and the bone marrow of a sibling donor have been successful.

Thymic hypoplasia with lymphopenia may occur in the presence of normal immunoglobulin levels. These immunoglobulins though quantitatively normal are functionally defective. This has been described as a lymphopenic dysgammaglobulinaemia.

Antibody deficiency diseases unassociated with thymic hypoplasia

Primary humoral antibody disorders may occur without defects in cellular immunity and without hypoplasia of the thymus. Antibody deficiency states in which hypogammaglobulinaemia is associated with defective synthesis of immunoglobulin commonly arise secondary to diseases of the lympho-follicular tissue such as chronic lymphatic leukaemia and lymphoma, or due to general systemic diseases such as renal failure. Primary hypogammaglobulinaemia in which there is no such predisposing disease is a much rarer event and when it occurs it may be:

1. Congenital sex-linked hypogammaglobulinaemia
2. Primary acquired hypogammaglobulinaemia
    (a) associated with thymoma
    (b) idiopathic.

In the sex-linked hypogammaglobulinaemia in which there is extreme deficiency of circulating immunoglobulin, cellular immunity is normal and the thymus shows no morphological abnormality. The tonsils, Peyer's patches and lymphoid tissue of the appendix are incompletely developed and devoid of plasma cells. This is also true of lymph nodes and spleen. When hypogammaglobulinaemia is associated with a thymic tumour it is probable that the peripheral lymphoid failure is of variable aetiology and that the tumour is a consequence of the immunological deficiency, perhaps reflecting efforts to compensate. Primary acquired hypogammaglobulinaemia is a rare disease and it has been estimated that a thymic tumour is present in 10 per cent of cases. IgG and IgA levels are constantly depressed but IgM concentrations are variable. In some cases the thymoma has preceded the development of hypogammaglobulinaemia whilst in other instances the two conditions have been detected together. No benefit results from removal of the tumour. Rarely hypogammaglobulinaemia has been reported after thymectomy.

In the condition of reticular dysgenesis there is deficient production of stem cells in haemopoietic tissue. There is normally a common haemopoietic and lymphopoietic cell which gives rise to stem cells for erythropoiesis, granulopoiesis and immunopoiesis. In reticular dysgenesis there is a deficiency of the stem cell for granulopoiesis and immunopoiesis. It presumably arises after differentiation of the stem cell for erythropoiesis. These children have agranulocytosis, thymic hypoplasia, lymphopenia and deficient cellular and probably humoral immunity. This is a rare disorder and these children have died too young to be investigated in any detail.

Thymitis

Thymitis describes the chronic inflammatory infiltration of the thymic medulla with lymphocytes and plasma cells. These changes are similar to those that occur in the thyroid in chronic thyroiditis. A characteristic feature of thymitis is the presence of germinal centres within the gland that are histologically identical with those seen in the lymph nodes and spleen after antigenic stimulation: germinal centres are not a feature of the normal adult thymus. Thymic dysplasia, and hyperplasia of the thymus are terms that have also been used to describe these changes. There is, however, no true hyperplasia for the weight of the thymus gland is not increased in these disorders. Thymitis is therefore a more accurate description of the chronic inflammatory changes that are present.

The clinical disorders associated with thymitis are all conditions in which auto-immune mechanisms are known to play a significant aetiological role (Table 1). Many of these disorders may also be seen in association with a thymic tumour.

Thymitis and myasthenia

Thymitis is the basic lesion in myasthenia gravis. Thirty per cent of patients with thymic tumours have myasthenia gravis and 10 per cent of patients with myasthenia gravis have a thymic tumour. The thymic tumour in patients with myasthenia contains the myoid antigen which is an antigen common to both thymic myoid cells and to skeletal muscle. Even in myasthenic patients with a tumour thymitis is nearly always found in the area of thymus surrounding the tumour. It is believed that the thymoma initiates an auto-immune reaction to the myoid antigen and that sensitized lymphocytes react with the myoid cells in the thymic medulla to give the morphological changes of thymitis. It has been shown that 95 per cent of patients with thymoma and myasthenia have circulating antibodies to thymic myoid cells. The capacity of thymic lymphocytes in thymitis to transform in vitro with phytohaemagglutinin is evidence that the thymus in thymitis contains an increased population of immunologically competent cells: this immunological competence suggests that these lymphocytes have infiltrated from the circulating pool and are not thymic lymphocytes. In an analogous way many patients with a thyroid carcinoma show the changes of chronic thyroiditis in adjacent thyroid tissue. Thymitis also occurs in myasthenic patients without a tumour but the cause of this immunological reaction within the thymus is unknown.

The striking resemblance of the lymphoid hyperplasia found in the thymic medulla of patients with myasthenia gravis to that seen in the thyroid in Hashimoto's disease first suggested an auto-immune basis. The detection of circulating antibodies to skeletal muscle was subsequently discovered in the serum of myasthenic patients and an antigenic cross-reaction was found between them and myoid cells within the thymus. The beneficial effect of thymectomy further incriminated the role of the thymus in myasthenia gravis and the occurrence of transient neonatal myasthenia in the children of mothers with the disease suggested that an inhibitor of neuromuscular transmission was circulating in the blood. One of the problems was that none of the detectable antibodies reacted with the neuromuscular junction and indeed neonatal myasthenia occurred in infants whose mothers did not have detectable circulating antibodies to skeletal muscle. Nor were circulating immune complexes, such as those obstructing the renal glomeruli in nephritis, to be found at the neuromuscular junction in myasthenic patients. The problem has, however, recently been elucidated by the demonstration of a neuromuscular blocking agent called thymin in the thymus gland. Microelectrodes can now be inserted into single neural end-plates in muscle and the size of the quanta of acetylcholine released determined. Quanta of this chemical transmitter can be detected as micro end-plate potentials. When the nerve is stimulated there is a synchronous discharge of 100 to 200 of these quanta and this initiates an action-potential which leads to contraction of the muscle fibre. In myasthenia the quanta are only one fifth the normal size and despite a normal number of quanta their strength is insufficient to generate enough potential to stimulate muscle contraction. The thymus normally secretes a hormone called thymin which affects neuromuscular transmission. This hormone has been extracted from the animal thymus and has been shown to reduce the size of acetylcholine quanta in rats. Its chemical nature is not known but it is a polypeptide of small size.

The conclusion may be drawn that in myasthenia gravis an antibody is stimulating the epithelial cells of the thymus to secrete excessive amounts of thymin just as in thyrotoxicosis another antibody (LATS) stimulates the thyroid cells to produce excessive thyroxine.

Although 60 per cent of patients with myasthenia and thymitis benefit from thymectomy, others do not. The reason may be the presence of ectopic tissue, which is present in 20 per cent of normal individuals, or the fact that permanent damage may have been done to the neuromuscular junction so that removing the offending agent does not result in remission. Certainly when myelotoxic drugs cause aplasia of the bone marrow, removing the offending agent is not always accompanied by improvement in bone marrow function.

Hyperplasia of the thymus

Hyperplasia of the thymus denotes an increase in the weight of the gland. It occurs in thyrotoxicosis and chronic thyroiditis though the increase in weight is more striking in thyrotoxicosis. The hyperplasia may be partly related to the increase in circulating thyroxine, for when thyrotoxicosis is treated with anti-thyroid drugs there is a decrease in the amount of thymic tissue. In addition to the hyperplasia of the normal components of the thymus in thyrotoxicosis, infiltration with lymphocytes and plasma cells and germinal centre formation also occurs. The increase in size of the thymus has been a recognized feature of thyrotoxicosis for many years. At one time thymectomy was even recommended as treatment. Thyrotoxicosis is the most recent addition to the auto-immune diseases and the evidence for this is considered on page 000.

Thymic tumours

The common neoplasms of the thymus are called thymomas. These tumours are not entirely benign for though they rarely metastasize they often spread locally. The neoplastic change usually involves the epithelial cells only. Lymphocytes may be a feature of many thymic tumours but they appear to differ from thymic lymphocytes in one important aspect. Unlike thymic lymphocytes the lymphocytes of thymomas are immunologically competent and this suggests that they are not neoplastic derivatives of noncompetent thymic lymphocytes. Thymic tumours are of particular interest because one-third of them are associated with systemic diseases. These include myasthenia gravis, myositis, myocarditis, erythroblastic aplasia, hypogammaglobulinaemia, systemic lupus erythematosus and auto-immune haemolytic anaemia. Furthermore, the clinical disorders which may be separately associated with a thymic tumour may occur together. Thus many patients with a thymic tumour and erythroblastic aplasia will also have myasthenia gravis or auto-immune haemolytic anaemia or hypogammaglobulinaemia. Indeed the multiple occurrence in the same patient of disorders which may be separately associated with a thymic tumour suggests a common cause. It is also of interest that malignant disease in general is more likely to develop in patients who have had a thymic tumour. In fact one report suggests that 17 per cent of patients surviving five years after diagnosis of a thymoma develop cancer.

In the clinical disorders associated with a thymic tumour no predictable benefit follows the removal of the tumour: even in erythroblastic aplasia improvement is only occasional. Moreover SLE, myasthenia gravis and thyroiditis have been reported after removal of a symptomless tumour.

Over 70 cases have now been reported of the association of erythroblastic aplasia with a thymic tumour. Erythroblastic aplasia is a rare variant of aplastic anaemia in which a selective aplasia effects the red cell series alone. It occurs more commonly in association with a thymoma than without. It has been suggested that a humoral agent is released from the thymoma which depresses erythropoiesis. Such an agent has not been demonstrated but remission of anaemia following thymectomy alone has been reported in a number of instances and this suggests that the thymic tumour may in some cases be the direct cause of the anaemia.

Thymic tumours may be associated with myasthenia gravis. The relationship of the tumour to thymitis and the release of the neuro muscular blocking agent called thymin has been discussed.

The thymic tumours associated with adreno-cortical hyperplasia have a characteristic histological appearance, being composed of small carcinoma cells with little lymphocytic infiltration. These tumours secrete an ACTH-like substance which is responsible for the adrenal hyperplasia.

Auto-immunity and the thymus

The relationship between the thymus and auto-immune disease is unresolved. It has been suggested that the function of the thymus is to destroy self-reactive immunocytes and that in auto-immune disease the germinal centres in the thymus represent the proliferation of forbidden clones of lymphocytes. There is, however, no evidence for this. Indeed the spontaneous auto-immune disease of mice develops even after the thymus has been removed at birth. In the human adult thymectomy is of no benefit to associated auto-immune disease, except for certain patients with myasthenia gravis. In childhood, however, auto-immune haemolytic anaemia may respond to thymectomy even after corticosteroids and splenectomy have failed. The relationship between the thymus and auto-immune disease is confused and it is difficult to know whether the thymus is the villain or the victim of auto-immune disease.

Selected Bibliography

GOLDSTEIN, G. and MACKAY, I. R. (1969) *The Human Thymus.* Heinemann Medical Books.

HAVARD, C. W. H. (1966) Clinical Disorders Associated with Abnormalities in the Thymus. *Brit. J. Hospital Medicine* 1, 206.

Leading Article (1971) Pathogenesis of Myasthenia Gravis. *Brit. Med. J.* 2, 1.

MILLER, J. F. A. P. (1967) The Thymus—Yesterday, Today, Tomorrow. *Lancet* 2, 1299.

Symposium on the Thymus (1970) *Proc. Roy. Soc. Med.* 63, 715.

X

Aldosterone and Hyperaldosteronism

Aldosterone is secreted by the cells of the zona glomerulosa of the adrenal cortex. Cortisol is secreted by the cells of the zona fasciculata. Both these hormones are synthesized from cholesterol through progesterone but along different pathways. In the synthesis of aldosterone the progesterone molecule is first hydroxylated at the C.21 position to form 11-deoxycorticosterone. This compound is then hydroxylated at the C.11 and C.18 positions to form 18-hydroxycorticosterone which is the immediate precursor of aldosterone. By conversion of the hydroxyl group at C.18 to an aldehyde group 18-hydroxycorticosterone is converted to aldosterone. Each of these chemical reactions requires its specific enzyme. The first stage in the synthesis of cortisol from progesterone requires hydroxylation at position 17 on the steroid nucleus. The cells of the zona glomerulosa lack the enzyme 17-hydroxylase which is necessary for this reaction and hence this area of the adrenal cortex can not synthesize cortisol. The stages in the synthesis of aldosterone and cortisol from cholesterol are shown in Fig. 23. The various stimuli to aldosterone secretion act at different stages of this biosynthetic pathway, and they are illustrated in Fig. 23.

The control of aldosterone secretion

There is some natural variation in the rate of aldosterone production. This is in part due to the circadian rhythm and partly due to variations resulting from changes in posture, or secondary to menstruation or pregnancy. However there are four main mechanisms controlling aldosterone secretion.

1. The renin-angiotensin system.
2. Changes in the concentration of potassium and sodium in the extra-cellular fluid.
3. Adrenocorticotrophic hormone.
4. Changes in the sensitivity of the adrenal glomerulosa.

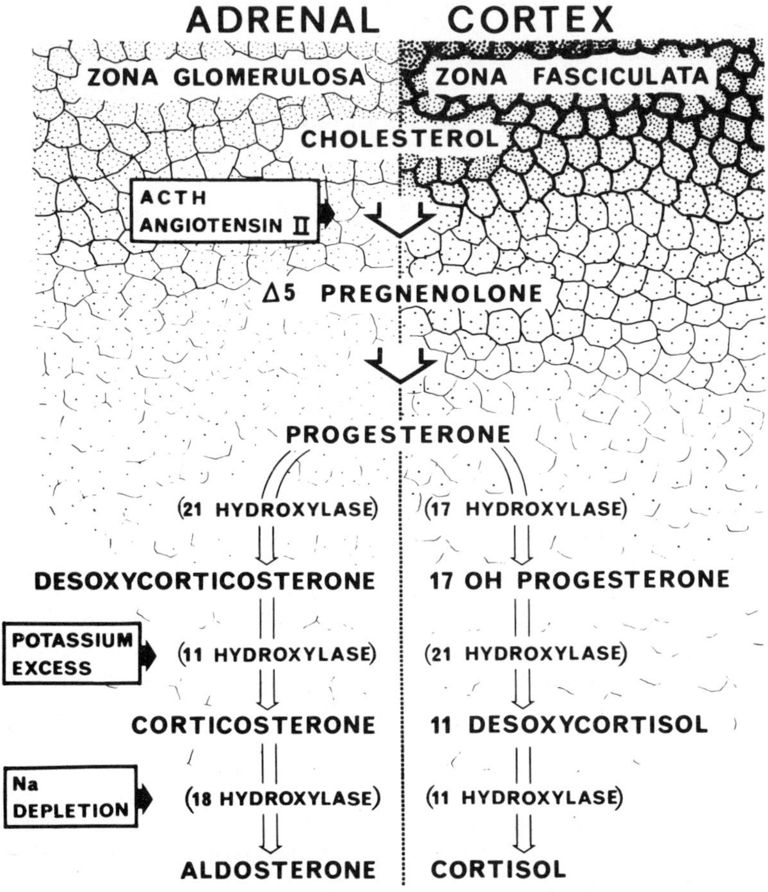

FIG. 23 Stages in synthesis of aldosterone and cortisol from cholesterol

The renin-angiotensin system

Renin is the primary regulator of aldosterone secretion. It is an enzyme elaborated in a specialized area of the nephron known as the juxtaglomerular apparatus. This area consists of the granular juxtaglomerular cells containing renin which are closely associated with the afferent arterioles of renal cortical glomeruli, and a specialized segment of the distal tubule called the macula densa which is situated at the junction between the ascending limb of Henlé's loop and the distal tubule. Each distal tubule attaches itself to its own afferent arteriole. The urine that has just passed the loop of

Henlé is hypotonic at this point and it is probable that this structure may function as an osmoreceptor detecting changes in the sodium concentration of the tubular fluid. Information on the composition of the urine is then transmitted to the juxtaglomerular cells localized at the entrance to the nephron. The control of renin secretion is also mediated by baroreceptors in the afferent arteriole, probably by the stretch in the walls of the afferent arterioles being detected by the juxtaglomerular cells. Specialized myoepithelial cells act as miniature pressure transducers, monitoring renal perfusion pressure by changes in the stretch of the afferent arterioles. A decrease in stretch of the arteriole causes the juxtaglomerular cells to release increased quantities of renin into the circulation. Conversely an increased circulating blood volume and increased stretch of the anteriole would cause the juxtaglomerular cells to inhibit the release of renin.

At all events a reduction in the effective blood volume is believed to be the main stimulus to renin production. Renin then stimulates angiotensin production and angiotensin stimulates aldosterone secretion. Aldosterone promotes the renal retention of sodium in an attempt to restore renal perfusion. A reduction in plasma volume, reduced sodium intake and a fall in renal perfusion pressure all act through a reduction of effective blood volume. Renin release is governed both by extrarenal and by intrarenal mechanisms. The intrarenal control is mediated by the chemoreceptor role of the macula densa and the extrarenal mediated by the transducer effect of monitoring renal perfusion. The extrarenal mechanisms are capable of overriding the intrarenal although in many circumstances they act synergistically.

Renin is a proteolytic enzyme that acts upon a substrate protein in the plasma to release a physiologically inactive decapeptide called angiotensin 1. This decapeptide is converted into an octopeptide angiotensin 2, by a converting enzyme in the plasma and also by its passage through the lungs. Angiotensin 2 is both a pressor agent which is more potent than noradrenaline and also the major physiological stimulus for aldosterone production by the adrenal cortex. It stimulates aldosterone production even at concentrations which do not raise the blood pressure. Figure 24 represents the stages in the renin angiotensin system.

The renin-angiotensin system is the most important regulator of aldosterone secretion and is responsible for the hyperaldosteronism that occurs in clinical disorders associated with reduced intravascular volume and impaired perfusion of the kidneys. It is also the main stimulus to aldosterone production in renal artery stenosis and in conditions associated with oedema formation. The common denominator for renin release is volume depletion: this may be induced acutely as in haemorrhage, following diuretic administration, dietary salt restriction or changes in posture, or it may exist on a chronic basis as in certain clinical disorders associated with oedema.

Potassium balance

As aldosterone plays an important part in potassium homeostasis through its effect on the distal renal tubule, it is not surprising that potassium itself has a controlling influence on the production of

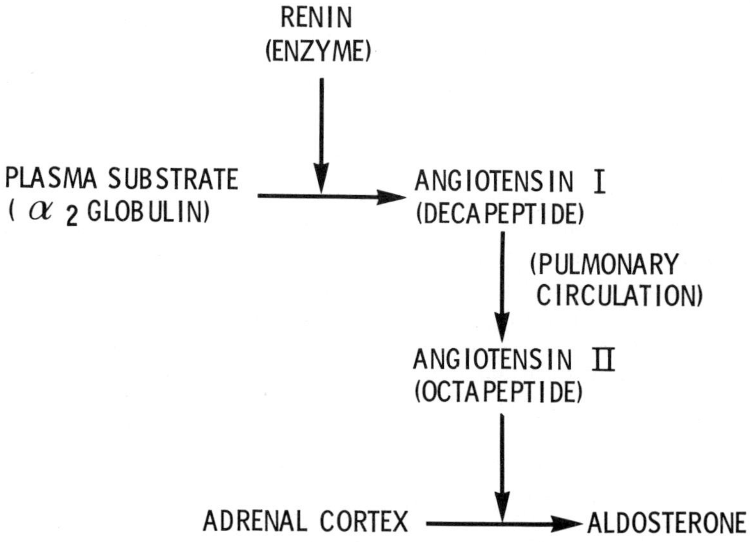

FIG. 24 The renin-angiotensin system

aldosterone. In both animals and man potassium salts stimulate aldosterone secretion. This is apparent both in vivo and when potassium is added to adrenal extracts in vitro. When a solution of potassium ions is injected into the adrenal arteries there is an immediate increase in the aldosterone levels in the adrenal veins. The effect of potassium salts is mediated by a direct action on the adrenal biosynthesis of aldosterone. Thus the administration of potassium salts increases aldosterone production and potassium restriction reduces it. As it acts directly on the biosynthesis of aldosterone its effects are not mediated through the renin-angiotensin system. This mechanism is subsidiary to the renin-antiotensin system and can be overcome by it. This is apparent from the fact that sodium depletion will induce aldosterone production through the renin-angiotensin system, even in the presence of potassium depletion. Thus the primary control of aldosterone secretion is the renin-angiotensin system, and this major mechanism is supplemented by the complementary effects of potassium on the biosynthesis of aldosterone. (Fig. 23.)

ACTH

ACTH stimulates both the secretion of cortisol and also that of aldosterone. However, the amount of ACTH required to stimulate aldosterone secretion is five times that required for the stimulation of cortisol production. Furthermore the duration of increased aldosterone secretion is transitory, for even with continued administration of ACTH aldosterone secretion returns to normal or even subnormal levels within a few days. ACTH thus plays only a minor supportive role in the regulation of aldosterone secretion. This is supported by the clinical evidence that aldosterone secretion is normal in patients with Cushing's syndrome and excess ACTH production, and that patients with hypopituitarism have normal aldosterone production. Thus the factors which control hydrocortisone production operate independently from those controlling aldosterone production. The effect of ACTH on aldosterone production is not mediated through the renin-angiotensin system but is a direct effect on the biosynthesis of the hormone. (Fig. 23.) The rate-limiting step in both the synthesis of corticosterone and cortisol is the conversion of cholesterol to pregnenolone and this is the stage in biosynthesis influenced by ACTH. (Fig. 23.)

Changes in sensitivity of the adrenal glomerulosa

There is evidence that a lowered plasma sodium concentration also has a direct effect on the adrenal biosynthesis of aldosterone. In experimental animals both angiotensin and ACTH in vivo and in vitro have more pronounced stimulatory effects when the animals are in a low sodium state. The hyperaldosteronism induced by sodium depletion is, however, largely mediated through the renin-angiotensin system and the direct effects on adrenal biosynthesis are of little clinical importance. There are probably other factors affecting the adrenal production of aldosterone but these are all secondary and subsidiary to the renin-angiotensin system.

Clinical disorders associated with hyperaldosteronism

There are three main groups of pathological disorders associated with hyperaldosteronism.

1. Diseases associated with oedema:
   - (a) Nephrotic syndrome
   - (b) Hepatic cirrhosis
   - (c) Some cases of congestive cardiac failure
   - (d) Hypoproteinaemia secondary to malnutrition or protein-losing enteropathy
   - (e) Idiopathic oedema: many of these cases are due to orthostatic reduction in renal blood flow

2. Diseases associated with hypertension:
   - (a) Primary aldosteronism
   - (b) Renal vascular disease
   - (c) Malignant hypertension

3. Disorders without oedema or hypertension.

Oedema Formation

Oedema formation is primarily the result of avid renal retention of sodium. Disorders of the heart, liver or kidney may all produce generalized oedema. The lowered osmotic pressure of the blood due to hypoalbuminaemia is the trigger in hepatic cirrhosis and nephrosis whilst in heart failure the increase in venous pressure is contributory. However the major cause of sodium retention is a disturbance in the function of the nephron resulting in an increased reabsorption of sodium.

The failure of the myocardium leading to reduced renal perfusion pressure, and hence a lowered glomerular filtration rate, can be an important factor promoting the increased tubular reabsorption of sodium in patients with congestive cardiac failure. However, the changes in glomerular filtration are not as important as changes in the rate of tubular reabsorption in determining the amount of sodium excreted in the urine. In many oedematous patients with hepatic cirrhosis and nephrosis renal perfusion is normal.

The processes of renal tubular reabsorption are under hormonal control. Patients with primary aldosteronism do not develop oedema. Yet in many oedematous states tubular reabsorption of sodium is stimulated in part by an increased rate of aldosterone secretion. There is evidence that other hormonal stimuli, probably activated by changes in the volume or pressure in other critical organs, are important factors controlling proximal tubular reabsorption of sodium.

The nephron consists of the glomerulus surrounded by Bowman's capsule, the renal tubule and a collecting tubule. There are about one million of these nephrons in each kidney. The capilliary tuft which constitutes the glomerulus is unique in that both the afferent and the efferent vessels are arterial in function. The efferent vessel continues from the glomerulus to supply the tubule where it breaks up into capillaries which are drained into the venous side of the circulation. Approximately 180 litres of cell-free and protein-free filtrate pass through the glomerulus each 24 hours. This fluid contains electrolytes such as sodium, potassium, calcium, magnesium, phosphate, bicarbonate, sulphate, chloride and water as well as the organic substances such as glucose. Whilst all the filtered glucose and half the urea are normally reabsorbed, the degree of reabsorption of electrolytes and water depends on the needs of the body.

Physiology of sodium reabsorption. Sodium reabsorption is an active cellular process requiring enzymes and energy. Less than 1 per cent of the filtered sodium, chloride and bicarbonate is normally excreted. Three sections of the nephron primarily contribute to this process.

1. *The proximal tubule.* Normally, active reabsorbtion of over 70 per cent of the filtered sodium and all of the filtered potassium takes place in the proximal tubule; chloride diffuses passively as a result of the electrical potential gradient. The osmotic force thus created promotes the passive transfer of an equivalent proportion of water. The proximal tubule is permeable to water at all times and this permeability is independent of the presence of antidiuretic hormone. Water reabsorption is thus 'obligatory'. Reabsorption of sodium at this site may vary through a wide range depending upon physiological needs such as the necessity to retain sodium in states of sodium deprivation, or in response to pathological stimuli. In the cardiac, renal and hepatic disorders associated with salt and water retention proximal tubular reabsorption may increase markedly.

On the other hand, under normal circumstances the ingestion of salt will depress sodium reabsorption in the proximal tubule to permit the excretion of excess salt and water. This mechanism is almost certainly mediated by an extrarenal hormone. It has been called the 'third factor' because it is a mechanism controlling sodium reabsorption additional to changes in renal haemodynamics and in aldosterone secretion. The reason for maintaining that it is extrarenal is deduced from animal experiments which have shown that the depression of proximal tubular reabsorption of sodium normally produced by saline infusion cannot be induced if the thoracic vena cava is first occluded.

2. *Loop of Henlé.* Thirty per cent of the glomerular filtrate is delivered as isotonic fluid to the loop of Henlé under normal circumstances.

This part of the nephron is impermeable to water at all times; although three-quarters of the remaining sodium and chloride may be absorbed at this site, most of the water remains within the tubular lumen so that a hypotonic fluid is delivered to the distal tubule. The reabsorption of sodium without water is the only means of excreting 'free water'. If this mechanism is thwarted, as for example by diuretics acting at this site, water retention may result. Furthermore, sodium reabsorption at this site provides the counter-current mechanism with its sodium ions. It is these sodium ions that render the renal medulla hyperosmotic so that in the presence of antidiuretic hormone water can be reabsorped along an osmotic gradient from the collecting ducts of the distal tubule.

3. *Distal tubule*. The greater part of the remaining sodium is actively reabsorbed in the distal tubule by three mechanisms. Water may or may not be absorbed depending upon the presence of the antidiuretic hormone.

1. Direct reabsorption of sodium with chloride.

2. Hydrogen ion exchange whereby the tubular cell actively secretes hydrogen ions into the lumen of the renal tubule in exchange for sodium ions; anions are not involved.

3. Potassium ion exchange whereby the tubular cell actively secretes potassium ions into the lumen of the renal tubule in exchange for sodium ions. As all the potassium filtered through the glomerulus is reabsorbed, the urinary potassium is derived from this process of distal tubular secretion.

Each of these processes is facilitated by physiological amounts of aldosterone and will be enhanced in states of hyperaldosteronism. The other factor affecting the activity of this cation exchange mechanism is the rate at which sodium is delivered to this portion of the nephron. In the absence of antidiuretic hormone water is not reabsorbed with sodium in this part of the nephron, thereby providing a mechanism for the excretion of 'free' water. Indeed, during diuresis the distal tubule and collecting ducts are impermeable to water. The two intracellular cations of hydrogen and potassium behave as if they were competing with each other for secretion into the urine in exchange for sodium. In conditions of potassium deficiency there is an increased distal tubular secretion of hydrogen ions and in states of potassium excess there is a reduction in the tubular secretion of hydrogen ions. Similarly, when there is a metabolic alkalosis the decreased intracellular concentration of hydrogen ions results in an increased urinary potassium loss, and in metabolic acidosis the increased intracellular hydrogen ion concentration results in an increased secretion of hydrogen ions with a corresponding reduction in potassium loss.

Tubular reabsorption of sodium in disease. In diseases which give rise to oedema an even greater proportion of the glomerular filtrate is reabsorbed in the proximal tubule and it is this excessive retention of sodium, chloride and water which is responsible for the development of oedema: the tendency for increased vascular pressure to force fluid out of the capillaries or hinder its reabsorption is of secondary importance. In cardiac disease the enhanced reabsorption of sodium is largely the result of diminished cardiac output and consequent reduction in the renal blood flow: the amount of sodium which can be filtered through the glomerulus is thus reduced. Moreover, when the renal arterial perfusion pressure is reduced cells in the juxtaglomerular region secrete a humoral agent which enhances the proximal tubular reabsorption of sodium. In nephrotic and hepatic oedema, in addition to increased reabsorption of sodium in the proximal tubule, distal tubular reabsorption is also enhanced. Both these diseases are associated with lowered levels of plasma albumin. In the former hypoalbuminaemia is due to urinary loss and in the latter to impaired synthesis. The loss of protein in the blood disturbs the osmotic retention of water within the blood vessels. As a result a significant amount of water leaves the blood and enters the tissues with a resulting decrease in effective arterial blood volume. Not only does a lowered plasma volume and osmotic pressure result, but a homeostatic mechanism is set into operation which aims at restoring an effective blood volume by renal retention of sodium. It is hampered by the loss of this fluid from the intravascular space into the extracellular tissues as oedema. Although aldosterone production is increased because of reduced renal perfusion through the operation of the renin-angiotensin system, aldosterone has little action on the proximal tubule. Other homeostatic mechanisms must, therefore, be responsible for the greater proximal tubular reabsorption in these disorders.

Reabsorption in the distal tubule is naturally affected by what has happened in the proximal tubule. Many diuretics reduce absorption in the proximal tubule and therefore more sodium reaches the distal tubule; this facilitates the exchange of both hydrogen ions and potassium ions for sodium and creates the potential hazard of developing hypokalaemic alkalosis. If glomerular filtration is reduced, more complete sodium reabsorption occurs in the proximal tubule so that less sodium reaches the distal tubule. As the distal tubule is the site where sodium may be reabsorbed without water this may impair the ability of the kidney to excrete water.

The significance of aldosterone

Enhanced aldosterone production is one of the most important factors in the development of hypokalaemia in patients with cirrhosis, nephrosis, and to a lesser extent, with cardiac disease, especially when treated with diuretics.

The excessive secretion of aldosterone is induced by a homeostatic mechanism which aims at restoring an effective blood volume by renal retention of sodium and water. In primary aldosteronism the reabsorption of sodium in exchange for potassium or hydrogen ions is enhanced: the retention of sodium expands the extracellular fluid and increases the glomerular filtration rate; more sodium is thereby presented to the distal tubule for exchange with potassium and the renal excretion of potassium is increased. Patients with primary aldosteronism do not develop oedema as the kidney, for reasons unknown, subsequently escapes from the sodium-retaining action of aldosterone, an occurrence known as the 'escape phenomenon'. It appears that once the kidney has retained 250–400 mEq. of sodium which is a quantity sufficient to expand the extracellular fluid by 2–3 litres, a new sodium balance is achieved. The natriuretic principle responsible for this escape phenomenon is believed to be the 'third factor'. On the other hand, oedema is frequently associated with secondary aldosteronism. However secondary aldosteronism is not per se the cause of oedema but it is an essential link in the retention of sodium and water required for oedema formation. In patients with oedema and secondary aldosteronism, most of the filtered sodium is reabsorbed proximally so that little ever reaches the distal tubule for exchange with potassium. Hence hypokalaemia is rarely present unless these patients are given diuretics which act proximal to this cation exchange region. The distal sites may then be presented with large amounts of sodium for exchange with potassium under the influence of aldosterone.

In oedematous patients there is a close correlation between the pre-existing degree of aldosteronism and the degree of potassium loss produced by diuretics.

Aldosterone and disorders associated with hypertension

Plasma renin levels and aldosterone secretion are both normal in most patients with essential hypertension. However, hyperaldosteronism secondary to activation of the renin-angiotensin system is characteristic of patients with malignant hypertension and of many but not all patients with hypertension secondary to renal artery stenosis. In some cases the aldosterone production may exceed the normal rate tenfold. It is probable that angiotensin is directly responsible for the hypertension that accompanies renal ischaemia. In experimental animals the blood pressure rises when angiotensin is injected and falls when antibodies to injected angiotensin develop. Primary aldosteronism in which hyperaldosteronism is secondary to an autonomous adenoma of the adrenal gland is also a cause of hypertension, and here the increased production of aldosterone is directly responsible. There are thus two types of hypertension associated with hyperaldosteronism: (i) Adrenal hypertension or primary aldosteronism which is due to an aldosterone secreting tumour of the adrenal cortex. (ii) Renal hypertension or secondary aldosteronism which occurs in a number of hypertensive disorders such as renal vascular disease and malignant hypertension. Blood renin concentrations are generally low in primary aldosteronism and high in secondary hyperaldosteronism. This promised to be a useful test to differentiate the adrenal from the renal forms of hypertension for low plasma renin and high aldosterone levels were thought to be pathognomonic of primary aldosteronism. This is now known not to be so, for low plasma renin levels may occur in 10 to 20 per cent of the hypertensive population. If in addition the sodium intake is restricted in some patients with primary aldosteronism, the plasma renin level may rise. It is thus important to know the sodium state of a patient before attempting to attach significance to a blood renin level.

Adrenal hypertension or primary aldosteronism usually presents with muscular weakness, polyuria and headache. There is associated hypertension but the elevation of blood pressure is usually only moderate and retinopathy is mild. The hypertension is nearly always benign in type and the absence of retinopathy is characteristic. It has been shown experimentally that a permeability factor which is probably identical with renin is present in kidney extracts. It is this factor which is probably responsible for retinopathy. Certainly in patients with renal artery stenosis the elevated renin levels are more common in those patients with retinopathy than in those without. Patients with renal hypertension have more severe elevation of the blood pressure and the retinal changes are worse. Cardiac and renal damage are also common.

The clinician will want to know how frequent is this condition of primary aldosteronism; which of his hypertensive patients he should investigate and how he should investigate them. The finding of adenomata in the adrenal glands of many patients with essential hypertension led to the hasty conclusion that the yield of cases of primary aldosteronism would be high. Just as glitter is not diagnostic of gold, adrenal nodules are not evidence of hyperaldosteronism. Indeed nodules are common in normotensive patients. An investigation of an estimated hypertensive population of 50,000 over a ten year period yielded only 25 cases of primary aldosteronism. It seems certain that primary aldosteronism is a rare disease and that hypokalaemia is the best guide to its presence. It accounts for considerably less than 1 per cent of all hypertensive patients.

Patients with hypertension may have lowered serum potassium concentrations for a number of reasons. They may (a) be receiving diuretics, (b) have renal vascular disease, (c) be suffering from malignant Cushing's syndrome, (d) be receiving liquorice such as in the form of carbenoxolone (Biogastrone) for gastric ulcer, or (e) be having excess DOCA or fludrocortisone. When we consider which patients to investigate for primary aldosteronism we would do well to remember that prior to the recognition of the renin-angiotensin system, the distinction between primary and secondary hyperaldosteronism could often be made with some confidence on clinical grounds. In addition to the clinical features mentioned the plasma volume is high in primary aldosteronism and the haematocrit low with a plasma sodium concentration that is usually at the upper range of normal or even elevated. In secondary hyperaldosteronism the opposite holds. The plasma volume and serum sodium tend to be low and the haematocrit at the upper range of normal. Raised aldosterone excretion can not be suppressed by a high salt diet in primary aldosteronism and this may help to distinguish the primary and secondary varieties. The best way to differentiate adrenal from renal hypertension is the spironolactone test. Aldosterone is the true cause of the hypertension in primary aldosteronism whilst it has no fundamental aetiological role in secondary aldosteronism. Removal of the source of excess aldosterone thus cures the hypertension of primary aldosteronism but it has little or no effect on the hypertension of secondary aldosteronism. Spironolactone should therefore restore the blood pressure to normal in the former but not in the latter. A dose of 100 mg. four times daily for a month has been recommended for this test. The serum electrolytes will return to normal in both primary and secondary aldosteronism.

The way angiotensin and aldosterone cause hypertension is uncertain. Both hormones increase the intracellular concentration of sodium. As sodium is largely an extracellular cation a rise in intracellular sodium will reduce the concentration gradient across the cell. A reduction of the sodium concentration gradient across the cell membrane is believed to produce arteriolar constriction which is responsible for the increased peripheral resistance of the hypertensive state.

Disorders without oedema or hypertension

There are a number of diseases in which hyperaldosteronism is present without oedema or hypertension. In these conditions the increased aldosterone production is a homeostatic response to a lowered circulating blood volume. Hyperaldosteronism is thus often a feature of blood loss, the depletion of circulating blood volume and reduced renal perfusion activating the renin-angiotensin system in an effort to retain sodium and restore the circulating blood volume. Hyperaldosteronism is also a feature of renal salt losing disorders. The later stages of chronic renal failure are often associated with salt wasting. This is largely due to the loss of sodium resulting from the osmotic diuresis induced by the high concentration of urea. The depletion in blood volume then induces hyperaldosteronism. Similarly, in chronic diarrhoea there is often a major loss of sodium through the bowel which results in a depletion of blood volume. There are also a number of psychiatric disorders such as anorexia nervosa when patients habitually induce vomiting or abuse purgatives in an attempt to lose weight. In these conditions there is a loss of body sodium and potassium. The increased secretion of aldosterone which results from the reduction of circulating blood volume aids the sodium deficiency but aggravates the potassium loss and hypokalaemia may be a striking feature of such disorders.

Selected Bibliography

CANNON, P. J. (1969) Control of Aldosterone Secretion. *Brit. J. Hospital Medicine* 2, 1344.

HABER, E. (1969) Recent Developments in Pathophysiologic Studies of the Renin-Angiotensin System. *New Eng. J. Med.* 280, 148.

LARAGH, J. H., BAER, L., BRUNNER, H. R., BUHLER, F. R., SEALEY, J. E., and VAUGHAN, E. D. (1972) *Amer. J. Med.* 52.633

Leading Article (1970) Aldosterone, Angiotensin and Hypertension. *Brit. Med. J.* 1, 769.

SPARK, R. F. and MELBY, M. C. (1968) Aldosteronism in Hypertension. Ann. int. Med. 69, 685.

Symposium on Aldosterone (1969) *Proc. Roy. Soc. Med.* 62, 1251.

WISENBAUGH, P. E., GARST, J. B., HULL, C., FREEDMAN, M. D., MATTHEWS, D. N., and HADADY, M. (1972) *Amer. J. Med.* 52.175

XI

Radioimmunoassay

In the twelve years since the development of the first radioimmunoassay, for insulin, by Yalow & Berson, this technique has been applied successfully to the assay of the majority of the pituitary, gastro-intestinal and other peptide hormones. More recently, it has also been applied to the measurement of a variety of steroid hormones. This powerful analytical tool has come to be regarded as lying within the province of endocrinology. There is no doubt, however, that the main role of this and related assay techniques will be in other disciplines. The availability of radioimmunoassays for digoxin and morphine indicates that it will revolutionize clinical pharmacology. Of still greater importance is the recent introduction of radioimmunoassays for lipoproteins and the carcinoembryonic antigen which herald a new era in medicine in which the entire population will be screened at regular intervals and treatment for a variety of diseases instituted before they have caused either signs or symptoms. Indeed, radioimmunoassay is one of a number of analytical techniques which enable one to forecast with confidence that the future of medicine lies in the laboratory rather than at the bedside.

Limitation of space necessitates that the present chapter must be confined almost exclusively to the application of radioimmunoassay in endorinology. This subject was founded as the result of the clinical acumen of physicians such as Graves and Addison. Only later did the experimental physiologist apply the classical techniques of extirpation or injection of tissue extracts in the elucidation of endocrine function. In this context some may recall the pioneer work of Schafer and his colleagues who, in the late 19th century, demonstrated the powerful effects of extracts of the posterior pituitary gland. Further advances made use of assays based on biological effects and permitted the development of extraction and purification procedures. This in turn allowed the chemical analysis of a variety of hormones. With the steroids, elucidation of structure led rapidly to the development of sensitive and specific chemical assays. Identification of the structure of the peptide hormones was delayed by the technical difficulty of amino-acid sequencing, and by the fact that their circulating levels are below the sensitivity of established chemical techniques. Until recently, therefore, determination of these hormones in biological fluids depended on bioassays of doubtful specificity, and of a complexity which rendered them unsuitable for routine use. This curtailed the investigation of their physiological and patho-physiological roles.

The study of peptide hormone physiology has been altered dramatically by the introduction of radioimmunoassay, and several fundamental advances can be attributed to its application. It should be noted that radioimmunoassay is only one branch of a technique referred to as 'saturation analysis' or 'competitive protein binding', under which heading can be included all assays in which the material studied is reacted with a specific, naturally occurring, binding protein. Such assays have been described for many of the steroid hormones, for thyroxine and for vitamin B_{12}.

The basic principles of radioimmunoassay

A radioimmunoassay depends on the ability of an unlabelled hormone to inhibit, by simple competition, the binding of labelled hormone by specific antibodies. In the following paragraphs this basic concept is explained more fully.

The combination between an antigen (such as a peptide hormone) and a specific antibody is a reversible reaction governed by the Law of Mass Action which can be described by the following equation:

$$H + AB \underset{k_2}{\overset{k_1}{\leftrightharpoons}} H{:}AB \qquad (1)$$

where H, AB and H:AB represent free hormone, free antibody and hormone/antibody complex respectively. In a radioimmunoassay, the concentrations of a labelled hormone and of its specific antibody are so adjusted that there is an excess of antigen. Thus, at equilibrium some free hormone will remain. It is conventional to refer to the antibody-bound hormone as the bound fraction (B) and that remaining unattached as the free fraction (F). Essential features of all radioimmunoassays are a procedure for separating these two fractions, followed by the determination of the percentage of labelled antigen which is bound, by means of a liquid or crystal scintillation counter.

If unlabelled antigen is added to this system, where labelled antigen is already in excess, it will compete for the limited number of available antibody combining sites. This will result in displacement of the labelled antigen from the antigen-antibody complex and, following separation, there will be a reduction in the bound fraction of radioactivity (B). This reduction is directly related to the amount of unlabelled antigen added, and it forms the basis for quantitating the amount of unlabelled hormone present. For this purpose the inhibition produced by the hormone in an unknown sample is compared with that produced by known amounts of standard unlabelled hormone.

Returning to equation (1), it is apparent that for efficient operation of the system the reaction at equilibrium must be heavily biased to the right, i.e. towards the formation of the antigen-antibody complex. This is a function of the binding energy, or K value, of the antibody, where:

$$K = \frac{k_1}{k_2} = \frac{[H:AB]}{[H][AB]} \qquad (2)$$

It is obvious that the initial concentration of labelled antigen must be comparable with the least amount of unlabelled hormone which the assay is intended to measure. Since this concentration is extremely low, and since the reaction must proceed almost completely to the formation of H:AB, an antibody with a high K value is essential. The production and analysis of such antibodies is one of the main technical problems in the development of an assay. Analysis depends on the construction of antibody dilution curves and standard curves, which will now be discussed in detail.

Antibody dilution and standard curves

Given the reagents and a method for separating bound and free hormone, the first steps in a radioimmunoassay are the construction of antibody dilution curves and standard curves.

The purpose of the antibody dilution curve is to determine the concentration of antibody required to bind 50–60 per cent of a fixed amount of labelled peptide. Doubling dilutions of the antiserum are incubated with constant amounts of labelled hormone. After incubation and separation of bound and free hormone, a graph is made of the percentage of radioactivity in the bound fraction against the dilution of antiserum. For example, when 1 nanogram (ng $= 10^{-9}$ g.) amounts of ^{125}I-human placental lactogen (HPL) were incubated with doubling dilutions of serum from a rabbit immunized with this peptide, the concentration required to bind 50–60 per cent of the label was 1:60,000.

Using this information it is now possible to construct a standard curve. Doubling dilutions of standard unlabelled hormone are prepared in a series of tubes. To each tube is added constant amounts of labelled peptide and antibody (1 ng. and 1:60,000 respectively) such as to bind some 60 per cent of the label in the absence of any additional peptide. After incubation and separation of bound and free hormone, a graph is constructed of the percentage of radioactivity in the bound fraction against the concentration of the standard unlabelled hormone. Figure 25 shows the results obtained.

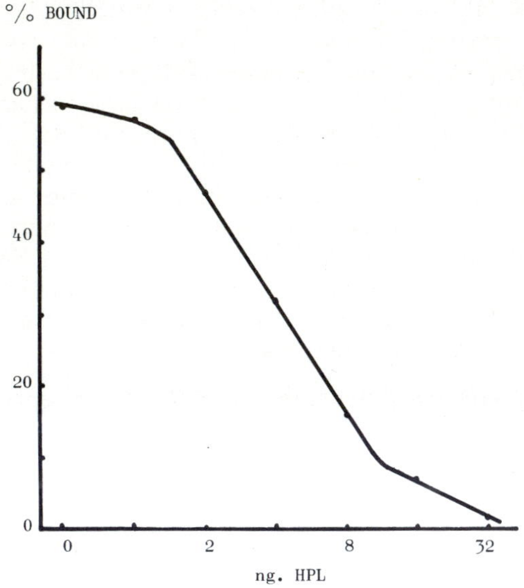

FIG. 25 Standard Dilution Curve for Radioimmunoassay

Amounts of unlabelled HPL greater than 32 ng. produce almost complete inhibition of the binding of label, while 1 ng. or less has virtually no effect. Between these points there are large changes in the amount of labelled peptide bound with successive changes in the amount of unlabelled hormone. If doubling dilutions of a plasma sample containing an amount of HPL between these limits are set up with the same concentrations of antibody and labelled hormone, then the exact amount of hormone present can be measured by comparing the inhibition produced with that of the known standards. (Fig. 25.)

Requirements for a Radioimmunoassay

The requirements include adequate amounts of the hormone; a method for labelling the hormone with a radioactive isotope; the production of satisfactory antibodies; and a technique for separating antibody-bound from free hormone. These requirements will be considered in turn.

Supplies of hormone: Ideally, highly purified hormone identical with that to be assayed should be used for the preparation of labelled materials, as a standard and for immunization. A radio-immunoassay can usually be established using only a few milligrams (mg. = 10^{-3} g.) of material and adequate amounts of most natural peptides are now available. These include human growth hormone (HGH), insulin, adrenocorticotrophic hormone (ACTH), HPL and luteinizing hormone (LH). There is also no difficulty in obtaining most of the small peptide hormones, such as oxytocin, arginine-vasopressin (AVP), lysine-vasopressin (LVP) and angiotensin I, since they are available as very pure, synthetically prepared material. By contrast, human parathyroid hormone is virtually unobtainable because it is present in only minute quantities in human parathyroid tissue. Supplies of highly purified follicle-stimulating hormone (FSH) are also extremely scarce. This, together with the difficulty (discussed later) in obtaining antisera capable of distinguishing between FSH and LH, has curtailed the development of a specific and readily applied assay for FSH.

Antibody production: As noted elsewhere, the sensitivity of an immunoassay is determined almost entirely by the affinity (K value) of the antibody used, and the production of satisfactory antisera is the most important factor in establishing a radioimmunoassay. The production of suitable antisera against the larger peptide hormones, such as insulin and HGH, seldom presents any difficulty. The majority of rabbits or guinea pigs immunized with an homogenate of the hormone in Freund's complete adjuvant (a mixture of mineral oil, detergent and killed tubercle bacilli) respond well. After a series of three to six injections at intervals of two to four weeks, the animals are bled and the serum tested by means of antibody dilution and standard curves. It should be noted that at the high dilutions at which many of the antisera are used, a few ml. will suffice for many thousands of assays. Furthermore, antisera directed against most large peptides are available commercially for those without facilities for keeping animals.

The production of antisera suitable for the assay of the small peptide hormones presents a much more difficult problem. Of any group of animals immunized with one of these hormones, only a small proportion will show any response at all, and of those which do, relatively few will produce an antiserum of sufficiently high affinity to yield a sensitive assay. A number of methods have been described for improving the chances of obtaining a good antibody, including covalent linkage of the peptide to a larger molecule such as albumin; adsorption of the hormone to microparticles of carbon or some other material so that the injected material is taken up by the macrophages and thus directly presented to the immune systems of the body; and injection of the antigen directly into the lymph nodes of the animal. However, it is still not certain whether any procedure for enhancing antibody response, other than the use of Freund's complete adjuvant, offers a significant advantage. Since the production of high affinity antisera to 'difficult' molecules seems to be almost entirely fortuitous, the best advice that can be given is to use the largest possible number of animals. Because there may be genetically determined differences in antibody production, randomly bred animals should be used unless a particular strain is known to respond well.

Separation of bound and free hormone: Numerous methods have been described for the separation of hormone bound to antibody and free hormone. The majority depend on physico-chemical differences between the peptide in question and antibody globulins. Thus advantage can be taken of the fact that antibody molecules (with a MW of about 160,000), and hence the antigen-antibody complex, are considerably larger than all hormones (the MW of HGH is only 21,500); that antibody molecules have a much slower electrophoretic mobility than most hormones; that antibody globulins tend to be much less soluble than hormonal peptides in the presence of organic solvents or high salt concentrations; and that the antibody molecule itself can be treated as an antigen, and precipitated by the use of a 'second antibody' using an antiserum to the globulins of the species in which the anti-hormone antibodies were raised. One of the most commonly used methods of separation, adsorption of free hormone to dextran-coated charcoal, depends on both size and charge, together with other properties which have not been specified.

In addition to these chemical separation methods, a number of techniques have been described in which either the antigen or the antibody is bound to an insoluble support, such as a plastic disc or particles of cellulose or Sephadex. Separation of bound and free hormone is then achieved by removal and washing of the insoluble phase. Such methods are simple and rapid, though requiring considerable technical expertize in their initial establishment.

Labelling of hormone: The sodium salts of ^{131}I or ^{125}I are universally employed for the radioactive labelling of the peptide hormones, with ^{125}I having the advantage of a longer half life (60 as compared with 8 days). In the presence of the oxidizing agent chloramine-T, iodine atoms substitute at two positions on the phenolic side chain of tyrosine residues. The reaction is stopped by the addition of a reducing agent (sodium metabisulphite). The resulting mixture contains iodinated hormone, iodinated hormone which has been damaged during the course of the procedure, and some unreacted free iodine which has not been incorporated into the peptide molecule. It is essential that the undamaged labelled hormone is freed from contamination by the other two components prior to its use. Many procedures have been described for this purpose, the most commonly used being gel filtration on Sephadex. Using this technique, which depends on differences in molecular size, peaks of radioactivity are obtained corresponding to the labelled peptide and to unreacted iodine.

The advantages and disadvantages of radioimmunoassay

Among the major advantages of the radioimmunoassay technique can be listed sensitivity, specificity, precision and speed. These are considered in the following paragraphs.

Sensitivity

In most, though not all instances, a radioimmunoassay is more sensitive than the best bioassay for a given hormone. Thus, for the peptides to which the technique is commonly applied, the most sensitive radioimmunoassays permit the detection of picogram (pg. = 10^{-12} g.) and femtogram (fg. = 10^{-15} g.) amounts of material. These amounts are dramatically small in terms of chemical and other assay procedures. A femtogram, which is one thousand billionth of a gram, represents the weight of a sufficiently small number of actual molecules for the figure to be imagined without difficulty. For instance, a fg. of oxytocin contains only 600,000 molecules, and such a level, per ml. of plasma, probably lies in the normal physiological range. By contrast, to take the example of a trace element such as iron, every ml. of plasma contains some 1×10^{16} atoms, a number which is beyond the grasp of human imagination.

The immense sensitivity of a radioimmunoassay depends on both the sensitivity of modern detectors to radioactive isotopes and the strength of the combination between an antibody and its appropriate antigen. Different antibodies vary in the strength of their reaction with antigen and thus determine the sensitivity that can be achieved. The essential point is this. To observe the competitive effect of a minute quantity of hormone, the amounts of labelled hormone and antibody used must be correspondingly small. The laws of thermodynamics dictate that at extremely low concentrations of reactants the reaction will only take place if the binding energy of the reactants is exceptionally high. This 'energy of reaction' is referred to as the 'affinity' of an antibody and its numerical value is given by the K value in the mass action equation (2) on page 000.

It should be emphasized that high sensitivity is not a requisite for all assays employed clinically. For example, circulating levels of HPL in the third trimester of pregnancy, when its measurement is of most significance, usually lie in the range 4–8 μg./ml. Since most assays for this hormone can measure ng. or pg. quantities under optimal conditions, it becomes necessary to operate the assay with a greatly reduced sensitivity. This is achieved by large increases in the amounts of labelled hormone and antibody used. Alternatively, advantage can be taken of high sensitivity by reducing the amount of plasma used. This is of special value in neonatal practice, since the μl. samples obtained by a heel prick are sufficient for some sensitive assays.

It is much more difficult to produce antisera with an affinity sufficiently high to measure the basal circulating levels of hormones such as ACTH which are in the low pg./ml. range, and impossible at present to provide antibodies for the assay of low fg. or attogram (ag. $= 10^{-18}$ g.) amounts. Thus, in order to determine the basal circulating levels of a hormone such as vasopressin, which may lie in the sub-picogram per ml. range, it is necessary to carry out an initial extraction and concentration step.

Specificity

Specificity can be the strength or the weakness of a radioimmunoassay, depending on the hormone studied. With the hormones of the posterior pituitary, oxytocin and vasopressin, radioimmunoassay is much superior to bioassay in terms of specificity, though not always in sensitivity. Thus the best available bioassays for both oxytocin and vasopressin are capable of measuring pg. amounts. Their Achilles heel is that at these extreme limits of sensitivity the biological effects of the two hormones overlap and a variety of common biological agents (such as acetylcholine and bradykinin) may produce similar effects. Radioimmunoassays have a vastly superior specificity. This is illustrated in Fig. 26, in which the standard curves produced in an oxytocin assay by either oxytocin itself or AVP or LVP are compared. To produce the same effect as oxytocin, 1,000 times the amount of vasopressin is required. In other words, if an assay of an unknown plasma sample indicated an oxytocin level of 10 pg./ml. the amount of vasopressin which would have to be present to yield the same figure would be 10,000 pg. Such levels are not achieved in any clinical or physiological situation in the human and the result can be confidently attributed to the presence of oxytocin, even in the absence of a parallel vasopressin assay.

It must be emphasized that only part of an antigen, referred to as the 'antigenic determinant', and not the entire molecule is involved in the reaction with the specific binding site of an antibody. In the case of peptide hormones each determinant consists of a sequence of some 2 to 8 amino acids which have a unique three-dimensional configuration. Even a small molecule such as ACTH (with 39 amino acids) may have more than one antigenic determinant, while larger

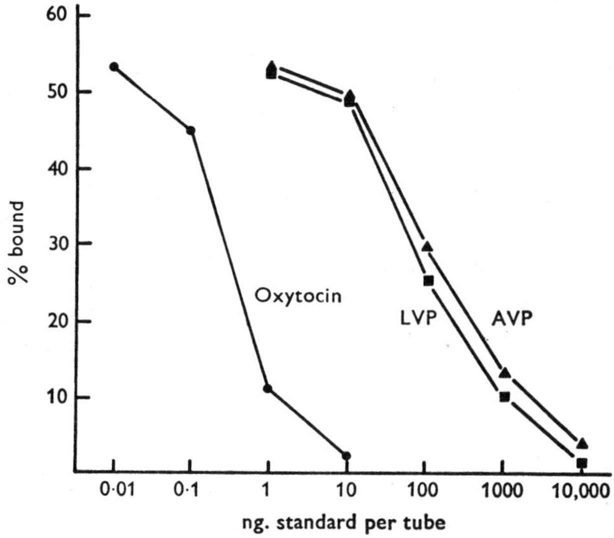

FIG. 26 Standard curves in oxytocin assay

peptides (such as human growth hormone, with 188 amino acids) have several. The specificity of radioimmunoassays is determined by the close 'fit' which is necessary for antigen-antibody binding to take place. The arrangement of the amino acids in the combining site of the antibody molecule must be such that they will complement exactly the structure of the antigen. They provide a lock which only fits one key. It will be apparent from the structures of oxytocin and vasopressin (Fig. 27) that only a small charge in configuration is required for the key no longer to fit.

The other side of the specificity coin is seen with the gonadotrophins LH and FSH. Some of the bioassays for these hormones are highly specific, but are not sufficiently sensitive to measure the levels normally encountered in plasma. The radioimmunoassays can readily measure these levels, but suffer from the major disadvantage that they often do not distinguish between the two hormones. The failure of most antibodies to distinguish between these two protein molecules results from the fact that they contain some sequences of amino acids which are identical. Equally, since the biological effects of the two hormones are so different, they possess some sequences which are quite distinct. It would appear that these biologically specific sequences are less favoured as an antigenic site than those sequences which are held in common by the two molecules.

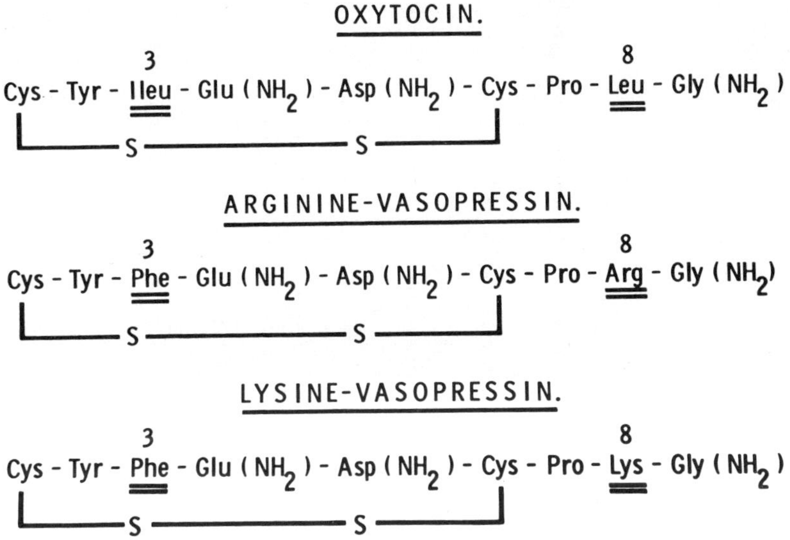

FIG. 27 Structures of oxytocin and vasopressin

Dissociation of biological and immunological activity

As noted above, the antigenic determinant of a peptide involves only part of the molecule. Since this may not correspond to the amino acid sequence responsible for the hormone's biological effects, it is apparent that a radioimmunoassay may measure biologically inactive material, including fragments of the hormone and partially denatured hormone. Thus there may be a dissociation between hormone levels determined by immunoassay and by bioassay. This is well illustrated by ACTH, which consists of 39 amino acids, numbered from the N-terminal end. The sequence 1–24 is required for biological activity, is identical in all species which have been studied, and is relatively non-antigenic. By contrast, the amino acid sequence 25–39 has no biological activity, differs according to the species of origin, and is highly antigenic. For this reason most antibodies raised against preparations of ACTH are species specific and will detect biologically inactive fragments containing the C-terminal end of the molecule. Fortunately there is usually only a small disparity between bioassay and immunoassay results.

Dissociation of immunological and biological activity is also illustrated by the plasma decay curve of oxytocin following a continuous infusion of the hormone. (Fig. 28.) It can be seen that biological activity decays more rapidly than immunological activity,

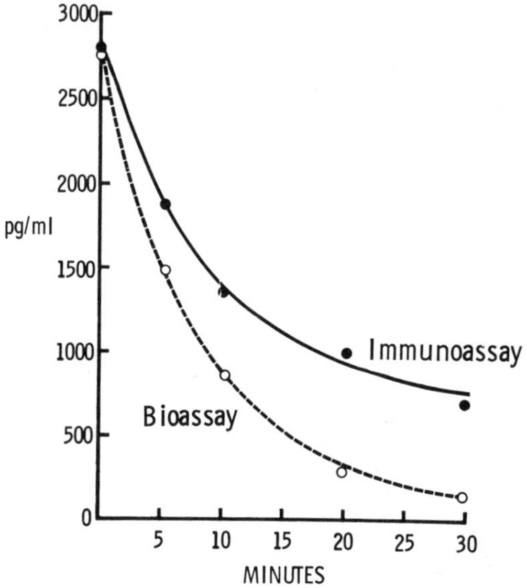

FIG. 28 Plasma decay curve of oxytocin following continuous infusion of hormone

though both curves tend to level out after the first 5–10 minutes. This dissociation can be explained by the fact that the biological activity of the molecule, but not the immunological activity, is destroyed when the ring structure of oxytocin is broken. (Fig. 27.) Since the initial action of proteolytic enzymes is to split this ring between the hemicystine and the tyrosine, the result is a more rapid destruction of biological activity.

Speed and precision

In terms of time from beginning to completion, a radioimmunoassay is often slower than a bioassay. The great advantage lies in the actual operator time involved and the ability to structure this time in an optimal manner. For instance, the dilution of samples and standards, and the preparation and addition of reagents, can be performed rapidly by an experienced technician, and in a given working day it is possible to process many more samples than with a bioassay, even though the inevitable incubation period means that the results will not be available until the following day. Furthermore, since radioimmunoassays avoid the vagaries of animal work, a degree of organization is possible which more than compensates for the longer total time taken. Finally, the ability in many cases to automate the immunoassay still further reduces net operator time, and it then becomes possible for a technician to process 400 or more samples in a working day.

Precision is another major advantage of an immunoassay when compared with a bioassay. The latter is subject to the variations encountered with any biological system, and it is the experience of most workers that published estimates of errors often represent an optimum which is difficult to reproduce in normal day-to-day practice. By contrast, the precision of a radioimmunoassay is that of chemical rather than biological procedures. Thus it is possible to reduce total error to within ± 10 per cent or less. More important, the error is likely to be a constant factor which does not vary significantly from one assay to the next.

Summary of available radioimmunoassays

Suitable assays for HGH, LH, TSH, HPL and insulin are widely available. They are all powerful immunogens, the resultant antibodies provide a radioimmunoassay of adequate sensitivity and specificity for clinical purposes, and highly purified materials are readily available. However, considerable difficulty has been encountered with some of the small peptide hormones because of their poor immunogenicity and the extreme sensitivity that is required to determine low circulating levels. Nonetheless satisfactory radioimmunoassays are available in a few laboratories for ACTH, oxytocin, LVP, AVP, glucagon, angiotensin I and II, thyrocalcitonin, gastrin, glucagon, and bradykinin.

One major advance has been the development of radioimmunoassays for steroids and other non-peptide hormones which are not themselves immunogenic. Examples include aldosterone, testosterone, tri-iodothyronine, thyroxine and digoxin. They are antigens which can combine with a specific antibody; however, they must be coupled to a larger molecule (such as albumin) in order to provoke such antibodies. A variety of chemical procedures are available for the covalent linkage of such substances to larger molecules. The method selected must not distort the structure of the hapten, since the antibodies produced will reflect the structure of the prosthetic group as it exists in the conjugate, but will be required to react with the original molecule.

As mentioned previously, radioimmunoassay is one of a number of assay techniques based on the progressive saturation of a specific-binding protein, for which the general term 'saturation analysis' has been introduced. Differences lie only in the nature of the binding material employed. Thus radioimmunoassays depend on the use of antibodies, while assays for thyroxine, vitamin B_{12} and a variety of steroids have been developed using specific plasma or tissue binding proteins.

Applications of radioimmunoassay

Radioimmunoassays have proved of especial value in the investigation of the physiology and pathophysiology of those peptides such as HGH and HPL for which no suitable bioassays have been developed. Conversely, they have contributed little additional information to that already obtained by sensitive and specific bioassays where these have been available, as for example for ACTH. Some of the many applications of the technique will be given in the following paragraphs, by reference to HPL and HGH.

Radioimmunoassay of tissue levels: The availability of radioimmunoassays has greatly facilitated the development of improved extraction and purification procedures for a number of peptide hormones. Its speed and relative simplicity has enabled several different procedures for extracting ACTH from anterior pituitary and ectopic tumour tissue to be compared. The best example of its application in this respect has been the isolation of HPL from placental tissue. Indeed, it is doubtful if anything would yet be known about this important hormone had it not been for the observation that it gave a precipitin reaction with antisera to HGH.

Radioimmunoassay of circulating hormone levels: (a) Application to physiological studies. Investigation of the metabolism of several peptide hormones has been made possible by radioimmunoassay. For example, it has been used to demonstrate that HPL is synthesized only within the syncytiotrophoblastic cells of the placenta; that it is secreted predominantly into the maternal circulation at a rate in excess of 1 g./24 hours during the third trimester, that it is rapidly removed from the circulation with a metabolic clearance rate of some 200 l./24 hours and a half life of less than 20 minutes, and that less than 1 per cent is excreted in the urine.

Radioimmunoassays have permitted studies of the physiological mechanisms which control the release of several hormones. Until 1963 nothing was known concerning the control of HGH secretion. Indeed, it was uncertain whether HGH continued to be secreted during adult life. Within a few years of the introduction of a suitable radioimmunoassay it had been demonstrated that HGH could be detected in the circulation throughout life and that a number of control mechanisms operate. Spontaneous, transient and well-marked increases in plasma HGH levels occur, especially at night; HGH secretion is suppressed by hyperglycaemia and stimulated by hypoglycaemia and by the injection of certain amino acids, including arginine, and HGH secretion increases in response to a variety of stressful situations. In addition, it has been shown that these mechanisms operate via the hypothalamus, and radioimmunoassays for animal growth hormone have been employed as the endpoint for the assay of the hypothalamic growth hormone releasing factor.

(b) Clinical applications. In terms of numbers of samples studied it is likely that the measurement of HPL may become the commonest of the endocrinological radioimmunoassays. The circulating levels of this hormone provide a sensitive indicator of placental function. Its measurement in every pregnant woman at each antenatal visit is feasible, since only a small sample of plasma is required and the technique can be fully automated. If its clinical value is fully confirmed, then the demand could be for several million assays per year, numbers far greater than the present demand for all other hormone assays.

Radioimmunoassay of basal circulating levels of HGH has proved of considerable value in the investigation of patients with suspected acromegaly and of gigantism. The finding of high values which are not suppressed (as they are in normal subjects) by glucose administration virtually proves these diagnoses. The assay has also contributed to comparison of the available forms of therapy. Thus, conventional irradiation has been shown, in general, to be without effect while proton beam therapy, cryotherapy and irradiation by local implantation of radioactive seeds usually reduces circulated HGH levels to within normal limits. The finding of undetectable values in suspected hypopituitarism or dwarfism is of much less diagnostic value since hormone levels are below the sensitivity of the assay in 50 per cent of samples from normal subjects. Use is therefore made of diagnostic test procedures such as insulin-induced hypoglycaemia, infusions of arginine and ingestion of Bovril, designed to stimulate HGH secretion. An impaired response to these stimuli is found in a variety of hypothalamic and pituitary disorders and may result from interruption of hypothalamic-pituitary vascular connections.

Other applications. Radioimmunoassay has been applied in many other fields, for example to monitor the rate of synthesis of hormones by tissue slices and cell-free systems, and for assessing the purity of synthetically prepared material. Another application can be illustrated by reference to renin. Scarcity of this material has to date precluded the establishment of a direct radioimmunoassay. However, its circulating levels can be determined indirectly by the assay of angiotensin I and II released by its proteolytic action on their substrate.

Conclusion

In this chapter we have indicated the underlying principles of radioimmunoassay and stressed that similar principles can be applied to the whole range of techniques termed 'saturation analysis' or 'competitive protein binding'. The only difference is in the nature of the binding reagent used, though in general it can be predicted that the methods depending on antibodies will replace those using other binding proteins.

To date, the main field of application of radioimmunoassay has been with hormones, at first the peptides and more recently the steroids. However, it seems certain that radioimmunoassay methods will see as large an expansion in the coming decade in such fields as cancer detection as they have in the last decade in the field of endocrinology. In addition, automation will increase their availability and their physiological, clinical and other applications.

Selected Bibliography

BERSON, S. A. and YALOW, R. S. (1964) Immunoassay of Protein Hormones. *The Hormones.* Ed. Pincus. Thimann, Astwood. Vol. 4, Academic Press. p. 557.

LANDON, J. (1968) The Basis of Radioimmunoassay with Particular Reference to Adrenocorticotrophic Hormone, *Recent Advances in Endocrinology*. 8th Ed. ed. James, Churchill. p. 240.

Various Authors (1969) A series of articles on radioimmunoassay, Brit. J. Hospital Medicine 3, Nos. 2, 3, 4, 5, 6, 7, 8, 9 and 11.

XII

Adrenergic Receptors

In recent years considerable interest has centred around the ending of postganglionic sympathetic nerve fibres and the receptors on the effector organs which they supply. Noradrenaline is the transmitter at these nerve endings, except in those fibres which supply sweat glands where it is acetylcholine.

Sympathetic nerve endings

It appears that noradrenaline is present in at least two distinct pools in the nerve ending. (Fig. 29.) Some is stored within granules, bound to tissue protein, whilst another fraction is in a diffuse form in the extragranular cytoplasm. An active transport mechanism is involved in the uptake of noradrenaline from the cytoplasm into the granules, and an equilibrium develops between the concentrations in each part. Also present in the cytoplasm is the enzyme monoamine oxidase (MAO) which metabolizes noradrenaline. Another active uptake process exists in the nerve cell membrane so that noradrenaline in the plasma and extra-cellular space is taken up into the cell and may be stored in the granules. Isotopically-labelled noradrenaline given intravenously to an animal may be demonstrated autoradiologically in the nerve endings within a short period of time. In the extracellular space the enzyme catechol-o-methyl transferase (COMT) is responsible for noradrenaline breakdown. The noradrenaline present in a nerve ending is, therefore, derived from two sources. Some is synthesized within the nerve cell from tyrosine and some is secreted by the adrenal gland and actively taken up from the extracellular space.

When a nerve impulse arrives at the sympathetic nerve ending, noradrenaline is released from the granules into the extracellular space to stimulate special areas on the effector cell called receptors. These are called 'adrenergic' as distinct from 'cholinergic' receptors, which are stimulated by acetycholine.

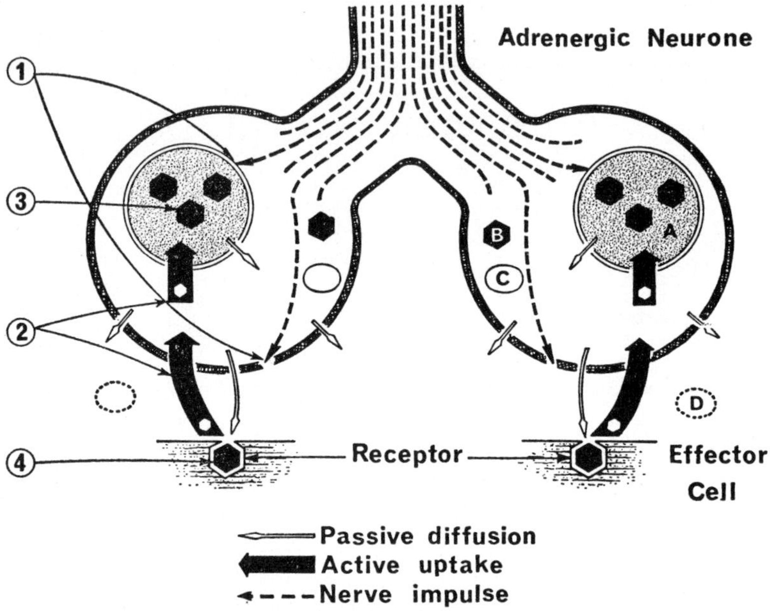

FIG. 29 Diagrammatic representation of adrenergic nerve ending and receptor

Right—A = granular pool of noradrenaline; B = cytoplasmic pool of noradrenaline; C = Monoamine oxidase; D = Cathechol-O-methyltransferase

Left—Neurone blockade by (1) prevention of release of noradrenaline from granular stores and cytoplasm, (2) depletion of noradrenaline stores by preventing uptake into neurone and into granular stores. (3) formation of false neuro-transmitter, (4) receptor blockade

It is evident that sympathetic-neurone blockade may be achieved in various ways.

1. The impulse may arrive at the nerve ending but fail to release noradrenaline. This is the mode of action of bretylium ('Darenthin') and debrisoquine ('Declinax'), and also of bethanidine ('Esbatal') and guanethidine ('Ismelin') in oral therapeutic doses.

2. The nerve ending may be depleted of noradrenaline so that there is no transmitter for the impulse to release. This is achieved by blocking uptake mechanisms so that noradrenaline is metabolized by MAO and COMT. Drugs which act in this way are reserpine and the Rauwolfia alkaloids, and also guanethidine and bethanidine in high centrations.

3. A false neurotransmitter may be substituted for noradrenaline which, when released, has a weaker or absent sympathetic action. Alpha-methyldopa ('Aldomet') probably acts in this way to form alpha-methylnoradrenaline instead of noradrenaline, but it has other actions as well.

It is important to understand that these drugs block transmission in the sympathetic neurone, and are quite distinct from those which act on the receptor site.

Adrenergic receptors

In 1878, Langley introduced the term 'receptor' to describe the molecular component of a cell which combines with a drug to initiate a biological change. Thus, noradrenaline combines with a receptor on the effector cell to produce effects recognizable as due to sympathetic stimulation. The series of events may be summarized in the figure

$$\begin{matrix}\text{Drug} & & & & & & \\ \text{or} & + & \text{Receptor} & \leftrightharpoons & \text{Drug-Receptor} & \rightarrow & \text{Effect} \\ \text{Transmitter} & & & & \text{Complex} & & \end{matrix}$$

The pharmacological actions of adrenaline are many and complex, and tend to reproduce the effects of stimulation of the sympathetic nervous system. In 1948 Ahlquist suggested that these actions could be divided into two broad groups, which might be explained in terms of two types of receptor, alpha and beta. These were originally called 'excitatory' and 'inhibitory' receptors respectively, because of their general tendencies to produce excitation or inhibition of smooth muscle activity when stimulated, but as there are important exceptions to this in both groups, it is better to refer to them simply as alpha and beta-receptors. Ahlquist studied various compounds related to adrenaline and found that their alpha-receptor stimulating potencies tended to be inversely related to their beta-receptor effects. Thus, isoprenaline was a potent stimulator of beta-receptor activity but had only weak alpha-receptor effects. On the other hand, noradrenaline had marked alpha-receptor but little beta-receptor activity. Adrenaline was a potent stimulator of both alpha- and beta-receptors. (See TABLE 1.)

Alpha-receptor activity

The alpha actions of adrenaline are most easily demonstrated by noradrenaline which possesses predominant alpha-receptor activity. The most important action is vasoconstriction of skin and splanchnic blood vessels, producing a rise in blood pressure and a reflex slowing of the heart. Blanching of the skin, and a reduction in blood flow to the gut, liver, and to the kidneys occurs. Other actions include dilatation of the pupil and relaxation of the gut smooth muscle. The sympathomimetic agents metaraminol and mephentermine are drugs with predominant alpha-receptor properties.

TABLE 1

Receptor	*Produced by*	*Blocked by*	*Main actions*
Alpha	Noradrenaline	Phenoxybenzamine	Vasoconstriction of skin and splanchnic vessels
		Thymoxamine	
		Tolazoline	Pupil dilatation
	Metaraminol	Phentolamine	Relaxation of gut
	Mephentermine		Metabolic actions
	Isoprenaline	Propranolol (DCI)	Vasodilatation of coronary and muscle vessels
Beta	Orciprenaline	(Pronethalol)	Cardiac acceleration
	(Salbutamol)	Alprenolol	Increased force of cardiac contraction
	(Isoetharine)	Oxprenolol	
		(Practolol)	Bronchial relaxation
			Metabolic actions

Beta-receptor activity

The beta-receptor actions of adrenaline are mimicked by the synthetic sympathomimetic drug isoprenaline, and include both acceleration and increased force of contraction of the heart, dilatation of coronary vessels and of arterioles supplying skeletal muscles, and relaxation of the smooth muscle of bronchi and uterus. Beta-receptor dilatation of skin vessels may be demonstrated in various regions such as the face, neck and forearm, but it is probably of little clinical importance.

Although these effects are best seen following isoprenaline, they are also readily produced by adrenaline, and even by noradrenaline if the masking affect of alpha-receptor activity is prevented by an alpha-receptor blocking drug.

Some effects of adrenaline are mediated by both alpha- and beta-receptors. Chief among these actions are the metabolic effects which raise the concentrations of blood glucose and free-fatty acids. It is probable that the conversion of glycogen to glucose in the liver is mediated by alpha-receptors, whilst that in skeletal muscle is mediated by beta-receptors.

Beta-receptors should not be thought of as a homogeneous population. Salbutamol is a beta-receptor agonist which preferentially stimulates receptors in the bronchi and peripheral vascular system, with significantly less action on the heart. Isoetharine has a similar spectrum of activity. It has been suggested that a distinction should be made between $beta_1$ receptors in heart muscle and $beta_2$ receptors in bronchial and vascular smooth muscle.

Nature of the adrenergic receptor

It is probable that the adrenergic receptor is an enzyme in the effector cell wall closely related to, or identical with, adenylcyclase. This catalysis the conversion of ATP to cyclic AMP and is therefore intimately concerned with phosphorylation of glucose and energy production, Its effects are antagonized by another enzyme, phosphodiesterase, which in turn is inhibited by drugs such as caffeine and theophylline. The stimulant property of these drugs is probably due to enhancement of adenylcyclase activity by phosphodiesterase inhibition.

Receptor blocking drugs

Sir Henry Dale first showed that ergot alkaloids prevented the increase of blood pressure but not the force and rate of cardiac contraction produced by adrenaline. It is now understood that this is because ergot alkaloids and a variety of other unrelated chemical substances selectively block alpha-adrenergic receptors but leave beta-receptors intact. Ergot has direct intrinsic vasoconstrictor activity of its own and is, therefore, not suitable for clinical use as an alpha-receptor blocking drug, but other drugs such as phenoxybenzamine are of value in conditions where excessive alpha-receptor activity may occur. Tolazaline and phentolamine are weak alpha-receptor blocking drugs, but have other and more marked pharmacological actions. For example, phentolamine has profound direct relaxant effects on vascular smooth muscle so that its hypotensive effect may well be due to this rather than to alpha-receptor blockade. All these compounds, however, have unpleasant side-effects which limit their clinical usefulness.

Thymoxamine is a more recently discovered compound with marked alpha-receptor blocking potency which offers considerable therapeutic promise.

Specific beta-receptor blocking drugs have only been known comparatively recently. The first of these compounds to be discovered was dichloroisoprenaline (DCI) which blocks the effects of isoprenaline on the heart and blood vessels. However it has so much intrinsic sympathomimetic activity of its own that it is unsuitable for clinical use. This was followed by pronethalol which had fewer sympathomimetic actions but was shown to be carcinogenic in experimental animals. Propranolol is relatively free of intrinsic sympathomimetic activity and is not carcinogenic in animals, and has been widely used both experimentally and therapeutically. It blocks the effects of exogenously administered isoprenaline and of endogenously secreted adrenaline on beta-receptors. At rest it produces a significant fall in heart rate, cardiac output and arterial systolic pressure, and it increases the systolic and diastolic diameter of the heart. The pressor response to noradrenaline and adrenaline may be exaggerated by the loss of muscle vessel dilatation. During exercize the effects of beta-receptor blockade are more marked, producing a reduction in the normal increment of heart rate, cardiac output, mean arterial pressure and left ventricular work.

Blockade of beta-receptor mediated bronchodilator tone results in an increase in airways resistance.

A variety of beta-receptor blocking drugs have recently been synthesized and are now being evaluated, and it appears that some will have more specific activity. There are some drugs which block the direct effects of isoprenaline on the heart but not on blood vessels and bronchi. Practolol is the most important of these. Others, such as butoxamine, have relatively little effect on the heart, blood vessels and bronchi, but specifically block the increase in blood glucose and free fatty acid concentrations which are produced by adrenaline. It is evident, therefore, that a simple division of adrenergic receptors into alpha- and beta-types is an oversimplification. Nevertheless, it is a useful classification, and in general terms it may still be said that the administration of adrenaline with an alpha-receptor blocking drug such as phenoxybenzamine results in the appearance of beta receptors effects, while adrenaline together with a beta-receptor blocking drug such as propranolol produces alpha-receptor effects.

CLINICAL APPLICATIONS

Sympathomimetic amines

Adrenaline and its related sympathomimetic amines have a variety of clinical applications which depend on their alpha or beta receptor stimulating properties.

Bronchial asthma. Bronchodilatation is mediated by beta-receptors. It is, therefore, reasonable to administer adrenaline and beta-receptor stimulating amines such as isoprenaline and orciprenaline in conditions such as chronic bronchitis and bronchial asthma where bronchospasm is a prominent feature. It is important to remember, however, that airway obstruction, although distressing to the patient, may not be the most important part of this disorder, and that impaired gas exchange leading to hypoxia is often present which is not improved by adrenaline or isoprenaline. In addition isoprenaline and related compounds have central nervous system stimulant effects to which patients may become habituated, and their indiscriminate use is to be discouraged. Salbutamol, with predominantly $beta_2$ actions, may be more specific in its broncho-dilator activity, and its place as an aerosol (Ventolin) in the management of asthma is being assessed. Propranolol, which blocks beta-receptor activity, may increase airway resistance and should not be given to a patient with a history of asthma or chronic bronchitis.

Shock and Hypotension. Noradrenaline and other amines such as metaraminol and mephentermine which have predominantly alpha-receptor stimulating actions are widely used in the treatment of hypotensive states and shock. This is because of their vasoconstrictive action on vessels in the skin and splanchnic areas, which produces an increase in systemic blood pressure. In recent years there has been a change of emphasis in the treatment of shock away from preoccupation with blood pressure to the increase of tissue perfusion which is the most important factor in these conditions. (See Chapter VII). The danger of hypotension and of shock lies in tissue ischaemia, particularly in the gut and kidneys. The patient is often in a state of high sympathetic activity, pale and sweating, and the administration of noradrenaline and other alpha-receptor stimulating drugs may further reduce blood flow through these organs, even though the systemic blood pressure may rise. Although the subject is still under investigation, it is probably true to say that in the presence of slight to moderate hypotension it is better to withhold sympathomimetic amines and rely on simpler methods of maintaining blood pressure, such as raising the foot of the bed. In extreme states of shock the use of an alpha-blocking drug such as phenoxybenzamine, to reduce alpha-receptor mediated vasoconstrictor tone and increase tissue perfusion may be justified and should be accompanied by patenteral fluid replacement to restore the circulating volume and maintain central venous pressure.

Anaphylaxis and hypersensitivity reactions

The release of histamine in hypersensitivity reactions may be accompanied by widespread vasodilatation and hypotension. Adrenaline opposes these effects through its vasoconstrictor action and is the drug of choice in the treatment of acute anaphylactic crises.

A large number of alpha-receptor stimulating sympathomimetic amines are used as nasal decongestants in hay fever and allergic rhinitis generally. Their effect depends on vasoconstriction of mucosal blood vessels and their use is not without hazard. The quantity of drug absorbed from local application may be sufficient to increase blood pressure, and shivering, anxiety, insomnia and nausea may occur. They may also themselves cause a 'medication rhinitis' with severe mucosal congestion and produce a condition worse than that which they were designed to treat.

Cardiac arrest and Stokes-Adam Syndrome

The cardio-stimulatory effects of adrenaline are mediated through beta-receptors, and therefore isoprenaline or adrenaline are of value in the prophylaxis and symptomatic treatment of paroxysmal cardiac arrest. Isoprenaline can be given sublingually or as a sustained-action oral tablet. Ephedrine and hydroxyamphetamine are sympathomimetic amines with both alpha- and beta-receptor stimulating actions, and may be given orally. They have a more prolonged action than isoprenaline.

Other indications. The vasoconstrictor action of adrenaline applied locally may be used to control superficial haemorrhage from skin and mucous membranes. Adrenaline is used widely in concentrations of 1:100,000 to 1:20,000 in solutions of local anaesthetics to slow absorption by producing local vasoconstriction. The hyperglycaemic action of adrenaline may be exploited in the emergency treatment of severe hypoglycaemia due to hyperinsulinism or overdosage with insulin. It depends on the presence of adequate stores of glycogen in the liver and skeletal muscle. If a single dose is ineffective it should not be repeated.

Local application of various sympathomimetic amines to the eye dilates the pupil for ophthalmoscopic examination without causing paralysis of accommodation.

ALPHA-RECEPTOR BLOCKING DRUGS

Although alpha-adrenergic receptor blocking drugs are widely prescribed for a variety of conditions, their proven value is limited to a few well-defined situations. Their place in the treatment of shock has already been discussed, and is still under review.

Phaeochromocytoma. The dangers of this condition lie in the production of:

1. Hypertension due to alpha-receptor mediated vasoconstriction of skin and splanchnic vessels by the adrenaline and noradrenaline released from the tumour.

2. Cardiac arrhythmias, particularly ventricular tachycardia and fibrillation, due to beta-receptor mediated cardiac stimulation by adrenaline. This hazard is even more possible during surgical operation if an anaesthetic agent with arrhythmic properties, such as halothane, is used.

These two effects of catecholamines produced by a phaeochromocytoma may be seen at any time before treatment, and also during the pre-operative handling of the tumour before its removal. Serious hypertension may also be produced in some of the tests used for its diagnosis, such as the histamine test which relies on the release of noradrenaline and adrenaline from the adrenal medulla by histamine, and the tyramine test in which noradrenaline is released from sympathetic nerve endings throughout the body.

An alpha-receptor blocking drug such as phenoxybenzamine is indicated in the pre-operative and per-operative management of patients with this condition. It may be administered orally until 36 hours before surgery when the intravenous preparation should be used. Phentolamine is a suitable alternative drug to use.

The arrhythmic hazards of phaeochromocytomata may be prevented by the use of a beta-receptor blocking drug such as propranolol. Once again this is given orally until operation when it should be given intravenously.

Hypertension due to a phaeochromocytoma is the principle indication for the use of alpha-receptor blocking drugs. They are also indicated in the rare cases of hypertension in patients receiving monoamine-oxidase inhibitors for depression. Such crises are provoked by sympathomimetic amines and by tyramine in cheese and other foodstuffs, and are due to potentiated noradrenaline activity at alpha-receptor sites.

Peripheral vascular disease

Although alpha-receptor blocking drugs such as tolazoline are widely used in peripheral vascular disease, it is doubtful if they are of much value. In fact there is evidence that in intermittent claudication blood may actually be shunted away from an ischaemic limb into other areas because of vasodilatation in normal vessels. Thymoxamine produces vasodilatation with an increase in skin temperature when applied locally and it may be that it will find an application in ischaemic skin disease, but this awaits evaluation.

BETA-RECEPTOR BLOCKING DRUGS

The use of propranolol in preventing arrhythmic crises from a phaeochromocytoma had already been discussed.

Cardiac arrhythmias

Propranolol not only prevents and abolishes catecholamine-induced cardiac arrhythmias, but it is also effective against many digitalis-induced supraventricular and ventricular arrhythmias. Although proporanolol is of value in some cases of atrial fibrillation, its effects are less consistent in this condition, and it cannot be considered the drug of choice. It used to be thought that arrhythmias produced by digitalis were mediated by sympathetic activity, and that their control by propranolol, like the catecholamine-induced arrhythmias, was further evidence for this. However, there is now considerable evidence that propranolol has quinidine-like actions on cardiac muscle, increasing the refractory period and reducing excitability and conduction velocity. It is probable that this action, rather than a specific beta-receptor blocking effect, accounts for its anti-arrhythmic properties. This is supported by the finding that the dextroisomer of propranolol is effective against digitalis and catechaolmine-induced arrhythmias but has little beta-blocking action compared with the racemic mixture.

Angina pectoris

Coronary vasodilatation is mediated by beta-receptor activity, and propranolol may produce a *fall* in coronary blood flow. However, the reduction in cardiac work and oxygen requirements which it produces are greater than its effects on coronary flow. It also reduces the tachycardia and the increased work of the heart associated with emotion and exercize, which often precipitate anginal attacks, and it has therefore proved to be of value in many patients with angina pectoris. Large doses may be required, in excess of those required to block exogenously administered isoprenaline, and it is possible, therefore, that other mechanisms such as its quinidine-like actions may be involved.

Hypertension

Propranolol has a significant hypotensive action which is seen when it is used alone or in combination with other anti-hypertensive drugs. It is of a similar potency to that of the thiazide diuretics. The mechanism of action is probably a fall in cardiac output due to beta-receptor blockade rather than to any change in peripheral vascular resistance. The maximum hypotensive effect is not usually seen for several weeks after starting treatment.

Aortic stenosis

In idiopathic hypertrophic subaortic stenosis, there is increased obstruction whenever myocardial contractility increases, as for example, from raised sympathetic activity associated with exercize or emotion. Propranolol reduces or prevents this, and is of value in the management of patients with this condition, reducing the frequency of anginal attacks and the dyspnoea which are so commonly associated. It also reduces the frequency and severity of dyspnoeic attack in Fallot's tetralogy by reducing constriction of the right ventricular outflow tract.

Hyperthyroidism

Many of the peripheral manifestations of hyperthyroidism, such as tachycardia, raised cardiac output, tremor and lid-retraction resemble the effects of sympathetic stimulation. In addition, patients with clinical hyperthyroidism show an increased sensitivity to adrenaline, and their response to sympathomimetic amines is reduced by treatment with antithyroid drugs or by thyroidectomy. In animals the cardiovascular and metabolic manifestations of experimental hyperthyroidism have been inhibited by interrupting sympathetic activity by high epidural block. These observations suggest that sympathetic activity may be important in mediating the peripheral manifestations of hyperthyroidism. Furthermore the therapeutic value of sympathetic neurone and receptor blocking drugs in this condition is undoubted. Reserpine and guanethidine reduce the tachycardia, palpitations and tremor of clinical and experimentally-induced hyperthyroidism, although the raised Iodine-131 uptake and serum protein bound iodine concentration are unaltered. Resperine may produce depression and guanethidine cause postural hypotension even in normotensive subjects, and these drugs are not suitable for long-term treatment. Guanethidine in the form of eye-drops may be used in the treatment of hyperthyroid lid-retraction, and will reduce the width of the palpebral fissure by 25–30 per cent. Such treatment is of particular value in patients with unilateral lid-retraction. It does not however significantly affect exophthalmus.

Propranolol reduces the heart rate and cardiac output of patients with hyperthyroid tachycardia, both at rest and after exercize, and it controls the ventricular rate in patients with atrial fibrillation. At the same time it reduces the associated tremor, sweating and anxiety, and it may even reduce the frequency of bowel action. These observations indicate that it is predominantly beta-receptor activity which is involved in hyperthyroidism. It may be that the enzyme adenylcyclase is a common site of action, for it is known to be increased in thyrotoxicosis and it also has an important role in promoting beta-adrenergic activity.

There are several situations in which propranolol may be used in hyperthyroidism.

1. *Pre-operative management.* Propranolol rapidly controls the clinical signs, and when combined with iodine therapy reduces the period necessary for preoperative preparation before thyroidectomy.

2. *Post-operative period and thyroid crisis.* Intravenous propranolol is particularly effective in the management of a thyroid crisis. It rapidly controls the psychiatric and circulatory disturbances. Although such crises are most frequently seen in the post-operative period, they may occur at other times. Propranolol should be used with great care in patients suspected of having hyperthyroid cardiomyopathy, in whom the risk of precipitating heart failure may be greater.

3. *After Iodine-131 therapy.* A period of several weeks elapses between the administration of therapeutic doses of *Iodine*-131 and the control of hyperthyroidism. During this time propranolol may be used as it exerts a more rapid and more easily regulated effect than the thiouracil compounds. It has also been used successfully in patients who developed hypersensitivity to the thiouracil drugs.

Earlier beta-blocking drugs such as pronethalol did not have this beneficial effect in hyperthyroidism and others now available such as oxprenolol, alprenolol and practolol are markedly inferior to propranolol. This is probably because they possess intrinsic sympathomimetic activity. Hyperthyroid patients are particularly sensitive to sympathomimetic drugs. Propranolol, in fact, is the only beta-adrenergic blocking drug currently available which is free from such sympathomimetic activity, and it is the drug of choice in this condition.

Anxiety

Autonomic activity, particularly of the sympathetic nervous system and adrenal medulla, is enhanced in anxiety states, and it has been shown that propranolol significantly reduces the physical symptoms of patients with these conditions. Its effects are particularly evident when cardiovascular manifestations such as palpitations and tachycardia are major symptoms but it may also relieve other autonomic disturbances such as sweating and diarrhoea. The mechanism of this anti-anxiety action is not clear. It is possible that there are beta-adrenergic receptors in the central nervous system and that propranolol exerts part of its action at this level. It is probable, however, that a large part of its effect must be exerted peripherally by preventing cardiovascular and other autonomic responses to the anxiety-producing situation, and so breaking the vicious circle which has been set up. It is important to remember that bronchial asthma is a not uncommon feature of an anxiety state, and that propranolol should NOT be given when this is present, or when there is a history of this disorder.

Other indications

Noradrenaline and adrenaline have peripheral actions on skeletal muscle function. One effect of this is to increase the tremor of patients with Parkinson's disease and hyperthyroidism. This action is mediated by beta-receptors, and may be reduced by propranolol which has therefore a place in the management of some patients with severe Parkinsonian tremor.

Unwanted effects

Although propranolol is widely used both in the investigation and treatment of a variety of disease states, its use is not without hazard. The danger in patients with a history of bronchial asthma and chronic bronchitis has already been mentioned. Practolol, with its more specific action on cardiac rather than bronchial receptors, might be expected to be safer in patients with a history of airways obstruction and preliminary clinical studies seem to have confirmed this. Other hazards of propranolol include the precipitation of:

(a) *Cardiac failure.* This is seen in patients with diminished cardiac reserve, in whom the decrease in sympathetic drive to the heart produced by propranolol results in cardiac decompensation. Cardiac failure and hypotension may develop rapidly after intravenous administration in these cases.

(b) *Cardiac arrest.* This may occur in patients with disturbances of atrio-ventricular conduction.

(c) *Potentiation of the hypoglycaemic action of insulin.* This results from inhibiting beta-receptor mediated gluconeogenesis from glycogen. At the same time it may reduce or abolish the sympathetically-produced clinical manifestations of hypoglycaemia. Propranolol should, therefore, only be used with caution in diabetic patients receiving insulin or sulphonylurea drugs.

Adrenergic receptor blocking drugs, particularly those affecting the beta-receptors are of recent introduction and their true therapeutic value has not yet been established. They have, nevertheless, already permitted more detailed study of autonomic activity both in normal and in disease states than was previously possible. It would seem reasonable that future research will be directed towards developing drugs with more specific activity on certain tissues, leading to selective receptor blockade without the unwanted effects of a general reduction in sympathetic activity.

Selected Bibliography

GRANVILLE-GROSSMAN, K. G. and TURNER, P. (1966) The Effect of Propranolol on Anxiety. *The Lancet* 1, 788.

MASON, D. T. and BRAUNWALD, E. (1967) *Mechanisms of Action and Therapeutic Uses of Cardiac Drugs.* Ed. FULTON, W. F. M. Butterworths, London.

Symposium on Beta Adrenergic Receptor Blockade. Ed. BRAUNWALD, E. (1966) *Amer. J. Cardiol.* 18, 303.

TURNER, P. (1969) *Clinical Aspects of Autonomic Pharmacology.* Heinemann Medical Books.

TURNER, P., GRANVILLE-GROSSMAN, K. G. and SMART, J. V. (1965) Effect of Adrenergic Receptor Blockade on the Tachycardia of Thyrotoxicosis and Anxiety State. *Lancet* 2, 1316.

XIII

Medical Aspects of Transplantation

The immune system functions by producing both circulating antibody and sensitized cells. In the presence of invading bacteria or foreign proteins, an immune reaction occurs which leads to destruction of the foreign material by a combined humoral and cellular attack. The humoral agent is antibody and there are at least five classes of gamma globulin to which such antibodies may belong. They are known as Ig (immunoglobulin) A, D, E, G and M. The cells involved are macrophages, lymphocytes, plasma cells and other cells of the lympho-reticular tissues.

Although immune reactions serve to protect against infection and external irritants, this is not their only function. They play a part in the local reaction to any type of tissue damage. Their reaction to breakdown products of damaged cells may help to limit the effects of local tissue destruction. Their reaction to abnormal or deviant cells may help to limit cell mutation and the origin and spread of cancer. The essence of this process is the recognition of self and the reaction to anything that is deviant or foreign.

Foreign tissue grafts are not, ordinarily, tolerated by the body and are rejected by a combination of cellular, humoral and vascular factors. Material from the graft may circulate in the host or lymphocytes from the host's blood may be carried to the graft. In either case sensitization occurs, the lymphoid cells respond to the antigenic stimulus, sensitized cells proliferate and antibody is released into the circulation. Grafts that remain unvascularized, such as corneal grafts, may be spared this sensitizing contact with the host's immunological apparatus and so provoke no response. There is a difference between the 'first set' response to a foreign graft and the accelerated rejection of a second graft from the same donor. At the first encounter most types of homograft are destroyed by the activity of infiltrating lymphoid cells. On the other hand the response to a graft of dissociated individual cells (e.g. a blood transfusion) or the 'second set' response to an organ transplant in subjects that have been previously immunized is mediated, to a considerable extent, by circulating antibody aided by complement. Finally, circulating antibody, in a previously sensitized recipient, may lead to acute vascular 'shut-down' or, if the reaction is partly suppressed by drug treatment, to the accumulation of antibody deposits on or in the vessel wall. This leads to a progressive endarteritis.

The aims of medical management are to achieve tissue compatibility in the first instance and to suppress immune rejection thereafter. Immunosuppressive drugs make it easier to induce a true immunological tolerance, a state in which the recipient fails to recognize the graft as foreign and does not react against it. Alternatively, immunosuppressive drugs make it possible for graft 'enhancement' to occur—a condition in which a graft can survive despite the presence of antibodies. In this case antibody combines with donor cells and in some way suppresses their antigenic effect. If the graft is not killed by the antibody itself it may thus be less liable to provoke a further immune reaction and less susceptible to immune destruction.

At a time when tissue transplantation is being undertaken on an increasing scale, considerable experience has been gained in the medical management of homograft patients and in the use of immunosuppressive drugs. Much that is of value here may be applied almost equally well to other immunological problems and to immunosuppression in other diseases.

DONOR SELECTION

As in the early days of blood transfusion, there is a growing recognition of the need for accurate tissue typing and cross-matching procedures. In this case the need to type both red and white blood cells presents special problems. As methods of storing viable tissues improve, banks of skin and other organs may become available and the possibility of providing a compatible donor for an individual patient should improve as better methods of tissue typing come into use. Even without these methods the results of grafting kidneys between identical twins or close relatives has shown that results of tissue transplantation are best when the genetic disparity between donor and host is minimized.

Although it is important to have ABO blood group compatibility between donor and host, a single case has been reported in which the kidney from a B+ donor was still functioning normally $3\frac{1}{2}$ years after transplantation into an A+ receipient. In fact, the red blood cells do not carry the major HL-A antigens that are concerned with homograft reactions. These antigens are carried on white blood cells as well as on other tissues and have been analyzed further with the help of serum taken from sensitized subjects—either women who have become sensitized to incompatible foetal products during a pregnancy or volunteers who have been immunized by receiving skin homografts. There appear to be 20 or more antigens which are present in different combinations in different subjects, and selected antisera are now available which will react specifically with individual antigens that are present on white blood cells and in other tissues. For convenience tissue typing is carried out by exposing the patient's white blood cells to micro-amounts of the standard antisera. Cells which contain a particular antigen are killed by the corresponding antiserum and in any particular individual the presence of several antigens can be defined. Not all of these antigens are of equal importance. In tissue matching a few 'strong' antigens are beginning to emerge which seem to matter more than others. In general, three or more discrepancies between donor and host reduce the chances of a successful graft. A single discrepancy, or even two, is accepted in practice because of the difficulty of obtaining identical tissue types for both white and red blood cell groups.

There is, in some cases, the opportunity to carry out a direct compatibility test. Lymphocytes that are grown in cell culture proliferate when they are antigenically stimulated and they can be made to incorporate isotope-labelled thymidine. This is the basis of some recent tests for drug hypersensitivity and it is also the basis of lymphocyte compatibility tests for homograft purposes. In these compatibility tests the mixed lymphocytes of prospective donor and host can be tested in two ways, first for the response of host against donor and second for the possibility of a graft versus host reaction. Although less likely to occur, this second possibility should be considered because, in animal experiments, grafted cells which survive have been shown to react against the host. A similar situation has been suspected in man in patients who develop fever and splenomegaly late after renal transplantation. Although the mechanism has not been established this has been likened to the very similar effects of graft versus host reactions in adult animals.

IMMUNOSUPPRESSIVE AGENTS

Experience with the use of immunosuppressive drugs has emphasized the biological effects of a generalized suppression of the immune response. Patients who are receiving long-term immunosuppressive treatment show an increased susceptibility to infection and eventually have an increased incidence of cancer, especially lymphosarcoma. A depression of their immune reactions may also be associated with an increased tendency to produce allergic or auto-allergic reactions, as in other types of immune deficiency. For these reasons the current search is for more selective and less toxic methods of immunosuppression.

The majority of immunosuppressive agents can be shown to inhibit the synthesis of DNA, RNA, proteins and other materials necessary for cell division. They also inhibit the processes of mitosis and prevent the proliferation of lymphoid cells. Inevitably, however, they also damage other rapidly proliferating cells in bone marrow and gut.

It is not only in homograft rejection that attempts to interfere with cell division are of importance. Interference with cell proliferation in tumours is the basis of cancer chemotherapy, and interference with the proliferation of bacteria is the basis of much of the treatment of infection by means of antibiotics. It is no accident, therefore, that antimitotic agents ranging from x-rays to antibiotics and cytotoxic drugs all have interesting properties in suppressing the immune response. Since the proliferation of lymphoid cells plays an important part in homograft rejection, any interference with this process has an immunosuppressive effect. Procedures such as thymectomy or thoracic lymph duct drainage are relatively ineffective when used alone but can add to the effect of other immunosuppressive measures.

Rapid destruction of lymphoid cells is caused by radiation, which fragments the DNA chain, and also by corticosteroids, colchicine, actinomycin and alkylating agents such as the nitrogen mustards. On the other hand, many other immunosuppressive agents produce relatively little damage to lymphoid tissue in the short term, although they may cause lymphoid atrophy when administered over long periods. These include the purine and folic acid antimetabolites, acriflavine, chloramphenicol, busulphan and anti-lymphocyte serum. Actinomycin inhibits synthesis of RNA, while chloramphenicol inhibits the synthesis of protein. Other agents interfere more subtly by substituting bogus substances within an essential metabolic pathway. In this way 6-mercaptopurine and its derivative azathioprine block purine synthesis, while fluorouracil is incorporated in an abnormally functioning nucleic acid. There are other points at which suppressive agents may act on the afferent pathway that triggers an immune response, for example by inhibiting the transmission of antigenic stimulation from macrophage to lymphocyte. Such an effect might be produced by anything which alters the permeability of cell membranes.

A study of the detailed mode of action of immunosuppressive drugs is important, because without this there can be no logic in the search for further agents or for synergistic combinations of differently acting drugs. Corticosteroids produce an anti-inflammatory effect by decreasing the permeability of cell membranes, but they also have a toxic effect on lymphocytes which is still unexplained. Much more is known about the mode of action of purine analogues, folic acid antagonists, and alkylating agents. One of the effects of 6-mercaptopurine (and of azathioprine) is to prevent the formation of inosinic acid which is the first purine to appear in the synthesis of nucleic acids. The metabolism of 6-mercaptopurine to the bogus thio-inosinic acid blocks any further conversion of this key substance.

Folic acid antagonists are able to block purine synthesis as well as protein synthesis, but their chief effect is on the synthesis of thymidylate, a component of DNA. These drugs are effective in man but are destroyed by high levels of aldehyde oxidase in the liver of some animals, so that animal trials may be misleading. Amethopterin (methotrexate) differs from folic acid in only one amine and one methyl group. It binds onto the enzyme dihydrofolate reductase and inhibits the formation of tetrahydrofolic acid. This last compound is important as a carrier of single carbon atoms in the synthesis of purines, thymidylate and several amino acids.

Alkylating agents are less specific in their effects. They form cross-links which prevent separation of the two strands of DNA and so stop the reproduction of cells. They also appear to inhibit a number of different enzyme systems. These effects occur rapidly, and there is a marked necrosis of lymphatic germinal centres within three hours of an intravenous dose of nitrogen mustard. A search for nitrogen mustards of low toxicity has led to the development of over seven hundred alkylating agents, including chlorambucil, melphalan and cyclophosphamide. The low toxicity of cyclophosphamide probably depends on the fact that the drug remains inactive until the cyclic phosphamide group is split enzymatically in the body. The success of this drug, like the success of azathioprine, may depend on the fact that it not only destroys lymphocytes but also suppresses the production of immunoglobulins.

In practice most experience with immunosuppressive regimes for the purposes of transplantation have been gained in cases of renal homografts. Since the side effects of immunosuppressive treatment can be as troublesome as homograft rejection itself, the tendency in recent years has been to use smaller doses of drugs. Prednisolone may be started on the day before operation and after high initial doses of up to 100 mg. a day or more a maintenance dose of 15 mg. of prednisolone daily is aimed at. Azathioprine in a dose of 3 mg. per kilogram per day is given as long as the creatinine clearance is above 20 ml. per minute. Evidence of commencing rejection of the kidney (see below) is an indication to raise the daily prednisolone dose to 200 mg. and to double the dosage of azathioprine for five days. The dosage of prednisolone is then reduced steadily over a period of six or seven weeks until it is restored to the maintenance level. Because of the increased sensitivity to immunosuppressive drugs which occurs in renal failure a fall of creatinine clearance to below 20 ml. per minute is an indication for halving the dose of azathioprine. Actinomycin D is of unproven value as an added agent in rejection episodes.

Anti-lymphocyte serum. Anti-lymphocyte globulin (ALG) is more selective than the immunosuppressive agents mentioned above and is able to prolong the survival of homografts very considerably in animal experiments. An antiserum raised in one species of animal against the lymphocytes of another coats, damages, agglutinates or destroys the circulating lymphocytes of the recipient. It leaves the recipient with an impaired immunological 'memory', depleted of sensitized cells and dependent mainly on circulating antibody for its residual immune responses. These circulating antibody responses may nevertheless be adequate to ward off bacterial infections, and it is an added advantage that anti-lymphocyte globulin is only mildly toxic to polymorphonuclear leucocytes.

The early preparations of ALG which were used in man were very toxic. More recent preparations, raised against thoracic duct lymphocytes, are much less likely to cause thrombocytopaenia, and haemolysis can be avoided by purifying the globulin or by absorption with red cell stroma. The pain caused by the intramuscular injection of horse globulin can be avoided by using the intravenous route, and the use of short courses of treatment lessens the likelihood of causing renal damage. Nevertheless, despite these and other measures to lessen the likelihood of anaphylaxis, ALG is essentially a cytotoxic drug, which causes cell breakdown, fever and sometimes other toxic side effects. Fortunately corticosteroids, which lessen these side effects, also potentiate the action of the drug. For the first time, controlled clinical trials are now being carried out to assess the value of this promising material, not only in transplantation but also in a variety of immune disorders.

Enhancing serum. The search for selective ways of suppressing an immune reaction still continues. It has long been known that attempts to give immunizing injections of killed cancer cells may fail to eliminate a cancerous growth and may even lead to a very rapid extension of the cancer. In animal experiments it is possible to give an antiserum to grafted tumour cells, or an antiserum to other grafted tissue, and to demonstrate that the graft is protected instead of being destroyed. It is presumed that antibody combines with antigens from the graft and that immune complexes which form may then inhibit the immune reaction. French and Batchelor have now used a similar principle to protect renal homografts in rats. By giving an enhancing serum directed against the donor's tissue they were able to obtain the indefinite survival of the grafted kidney without impairing the recipient's immune reactions in any other way. The possible application of this method in man is now being assessed and offers an exciting prospect which may not be confined to transplantation procedures.

TRANSPLANT REJECTION

There has been a steady improvement in the results of kidney homograft operations since 1963, when the human kidney transplant registry was established. Even when the results of different centres are averaged, the survival of kidneys from related donors at the end of one year has reached 87 per cent and the survival of kidneys from cadaver donors at the end of one year has reached 42 per cent. The results of many individual centres have been considerably better than this and show that good results may be maintained over a number of years. Most of these grafts, however, undergo one or more episodes of rejection, even when the donor of the kidney is a non-identical twin. Immediate rejection within the first few hours differs from the acute rejection episodes that occur later and also from the late insidious rejection which occurs months or years after transplantation. Comparable changes are seen after the transplantation of other organs, but these are modified by the nature of the tissue concerned and the length of survival. The degree of cellular infiltration, vascular change, haemorrhagic tendency and infection vary considerably in different organs.

Immediate rejection

Rejection of a kidney may occur within the first few hours after transplantation in the presence of pre-existing circulating antibodies in the recipient. This can occur when there is a major blood group incompatibility between host and donor or when the host has been previously sensitized, for example by multiple previous transfusions. Some minutes after the circulation is restored to the transplanted kidney it becomes blue and flaccid and urine production ceases. The arterioles and capillaries become distended with sludged red blood cells and microthromboses and interstitial haemorrhages occur. Later there is fibrinoid necrosis of the glomerular capillary walls and tubular necrosis or cortical necrosis may ensue. It is probable that when circulating antibodies are present in the recipient they bind to blood group or other antigens in the vessel walls of the transplant and that spasm and intravascular red cell clumping then lead to thrombosis and to necrosis of the vessel wall.

Acute rejection

In the majority of cases rejection of a renal homograft is not an all-or-nothing affair. Sudden and severe rejection episodes are easy to recognize but these are so modified by the use of immunosuppressive drugs that a much more mild and gradual process may occur which can be extremely difficult to identify.

In a classical rejection crisis the volume of urine decreases suddenly and fluid retention occurs with a weight gain which may be as much as a kilogram or more over a period of one or two days. There is fever, tachycardia and considerable enlargement as well as tenderness of the transplanted kidney. Salt retention leads to a rise in blood pressure and there is also retention of urea and a falling creatinine clearance. In the urine there may be an increased number of lymphocytes together with tubular cells and casts. A fall in the blood platelet count may occur, either as part of the rejection episode or because of an increased susceptibility to the toxic effects of drugs. In the kidney there is oedema, focal infiltration of the cortex by mononuclear cells and the presence of pyroninophilic cells in and around the small blood vessels. Restriction of the blood flow may lead to necrosis of the proximal convoluted tubules.

This pattern is slightly modified in the later stages, when the effects of circulating antibody are more in evidence. In 39 of the first 83 patients to receive renal homografts from living donors at the University of Colorado acute rejection occurred 11 days or more after transplantation. Cellular infiltration is usually less striking at this stage and there is fibrinoid necrosis of the arteriolar walls with deposits of gamma globulin, platelet aggregates and fibrin over the damaged part of the vessel walls. Some of the affected arterioles become obstructed by thrombus.

When the diagnosis of rejection is difficult needle biopsy may be of value but there is a risk of renal haemorrhage following this procedure. Fine needle aspiration carries a smaller risk and smears of the aspirate show characteristic large basophilic cells. In addition there may be an increase in the number of mononuclear cells, striking aggregates of platelets and in some cases macrophages and degenerating epithelial cells.

Treatment

Prompt treatment (see above) can reverse a rejection episode and it has been claimed that prednisolone acts by reversing the aggregation of platelets and so allowing renal blood flow to be restored and a diuresis to occur. In the earlier stages after a cadaver kidney has been transplanted ischaemic tubular necrosis provides a problem of its own. In addition to immunosuppressive therapy heparin may be of considerable value here in helping to clear the thrombi that are present in small vessels. Once fibrin has been deposited, whether as the result of post-operative tubular necrosis or of a rejection episode, the process appears to be irreversible, however, and the deposits of antibody, platelets and fibrin become covered with a new layer of endothelium and incorporated into the intima of the capillaries. Later, as organization of the mural platelet thrombi occurs, narrowing of the interlobular arteries and ischaemic changes follow.

Late Insidious Rejection

In spite of the absence of any clear cut rejection episode there may be gradual deterioration of renal function some months or years after transplantation, with proteinuria and a progressive fall in creatinine clearance. The urine does not contain lymphocytes as it does in acute rejection episodes but there are glomerular lesions within the graft, with appearances which usually resemble glomerulonephritis of the membranous type. Electron microscopy shows thickening of the basement membrane with deposits of amorphous material on the endothelial surface and fusion of the epithelial foot processes.

Although these late glomerular lesions might suggest a recurrence of the original disease in patients whose renal failure was due to glomerulonephritis similar appearances are seen in patients whose original complaint was bilateral polycystic disease, hydronephrosis or chronic pyelonephritis. These glomerular lesions correspond more frequently with the finding of incompatibility of host and graft in lymphocyte typing tests and appear to be the result of a minor degree of deposition of antibody globulin continuing over a long period. In such cases circulating antibody which reacts with capillary basement membrane may be found. These antibodies are present in the blood only in trace amounts and appear to be absorbed rapidly onto the renal graft. Fluorescent microscopy shows a fine deposit of IgM antibody on the glomerular capillary walls, accompanied in many cases by complement, IgG and sometimes fibrinogen. Should the transplant be removed surgically, further absorption of antibody onto the glomerular basement membrane is not possible and the blood level of antibody rises sharply.

Lesions which appear almost identical to those seen in man can be produced in experimental animals by injecting antibody which has been raised in other animals and is directed against glomerular basement membrane. This antibody is deposited on the basement membrane which becomes distorted and thickened as a result. A form of glomerulonephritis with a very similar immunopathology can also be seen in mice infected with the virus of lymphocytic choriomeningitis. If these animals survive the initial allergic reaction to the virus, which is the usual cause of death, they may, while excreting virus through the kidney, lay down antibody on the glomerular membrane and develop established renal disease. Suppression of the allergic reaction with antilymphocyte serum can prolong the life of these animals but at the same time allows an increase in the amount of circulating virus in the blood, a marked increase in the circulating antibody to virus, and a striking increase in the rapidity and severity of glomerulonephritic changes.

These various observations have important implications. Late immunopathological changes in the kidney may be of two main types. The first is partly cell mediated and responds to immunosuppressive drugs. The second, based on the local deposition of antibody, may become more conspicuous with the increasing success of early immunosuppressive treatment. It remains to be seen whether this second change invariably progresses or whether, by the protective barrier which it provides, it may form a basis for 'enhancement' and the long term acceptance of the graft.

Prolonged Survival

Prolonged survival after a homograft may bring to the fore the toxic influence of immunosuppressive drugs, the long term effects of insidious rejection, and also the late complications of renal or hepatic failure. Diabetes mellitus, peptic ulcer, leucopenia and hepatic damage reflect the direct toxic action of corticosteroids and of the other drugs used. Viral and fungal infections take on a virulent character in patients whose lack of resistance allows the dissemination of *cytomegalovirus*, *h.simplex*, *aspergillus*, *candida* and other agents which are so widespread in nature that no 'germ-free' environment can keep them out. Hypertension, made worse by corticosteroids, may be due initially to long standing renal disease, and this is true of hyperparathyroidism which, in long term survivors, takes on new, autonomous features.

There is no clear distinction between the histology of successful grafts and those which show progressive deterioration in their function. Biopsy studies have shown that apparently well tolerated renal transplants show oedema and cellular infiltration during the early months which does not necessarily have any direct correlation with ischaemic damage during transplantation, with the incidence of crises, or with the eventual development of vascular or glomerular lesions. These changes are no longer found after a few months, but biopsy at this stage often shows features of late insidious rejection, with interstitial fibrosis, local endarteritis and glomerular lesions. Tolerance of the kidney, in clinical terms, may be much better than these histological changes would suggest. One possibility, mentioned above, is that the deposition of a layer of antibody from the host on the vascular endothelium of the donated kidney provides a barrier against further immunological attack. Alternatively endothelium from the recipient may replace donor endothelium, especially if it has been damaged by immunological reactions. Whatever the explanation a long tolerated homograft appears to enjoy a form of protection which is not available to a second graft from the same donor. When an animal carrying a viable graft receives a second graft from the same donor immunosuppressive therapy often fails to prevent rejection of the second graft while the first is still viable.

The outcome of second grafts from the same donor in experimental animals is, by comparison, much worse than the fate of second and third *human* kidney grafts taken from *different* donors. The analysis of 85 human cases has shown that these second transplants may do as well or better than the first graft. The part played by gross tissue incompatibility in the rejection of the first graft has not been studied in these patients but there may be a considerable practical advantage in the use of material, on the second occasion, which differs genetically from that of the first graft. Now that tissue typing facilities are available the results of second or third grafts will no doubt be studied carefully, so that the importance of typing the donor can be assessed further.

Cardiac transplantation

By September 1970, 165 heart transplants had been performed, but only a third of the survivors had lived for more than three months. Problems have arisen from rejection, emboli and from platelet aggregations in the smaller coronary vessels. But the greatest difficulty, undoubtedly, has arisen from the inadequancy of supporting measures to replace the function of this organ when it fails. Methods of maintaining the donor heart after death have also been inadequate to avoid the almost desperate haste which has attended the securing and implanting of this vital organ. The essential condition of reasonable compatibility between donor and recipient has not been fulfilled in many of these cases. Postoperatively, no supportive measures have been available that compare in effectiveness with haemodialysis after renal transplantation. It is clear that considerable advances must be made before cardiac transplantation can be considered a very practical procedure. Even then, the ethical doubts that attend the transplantation of cadaver organs may not easily be dispelled for this particular viscus, since it is still, in the emotions of many people, the ancient, traditional seat of the soul.

Hepatic transplantation

Prominent among the complications of hepatic transplantation is infection, which tends to occur during rejection crises or when large doses of immunosuppressive drugs are given. Anomalous or kinked hepatic arteries may also encourage infection to localize in the affected lobe. Other complications of surgery include liver necrosis, pulmonary emboli and necrotic ulcers in the oesophagus or stomach. The problems of blood supply, drug toxicity and serum hepatitis all play some part. Despite this, five of Starzl's first 25 patients who received a liver graft have survived for over a year and one for almost two years. The ineffectiveness of conventional treatment for liver failure is underlined by the fact that 95 per cent of patients accepted by Starzl for liver transplantation died before a donor could be found.

Transplantation of the lung

Although the longest survivor with a transplanted lung has lived only ten months the problem here is not always that of rejection. There is difficulty in selecting recipients who are ill enough to be incurable by other means but who have managed to avoid serious pre-operative lung infection. It is also difficult to obtain a donor lung which is both uninfected and viable. When a single lung is transplanted some of the reflexes that are concerned with coughing and deep breathing are preserved, but some of the disadvantages that follow arise from overfilling of the vascular bed of the transplant. Nevertheless in 1972 a single lung was successfully transplanted in a patient with emphysema. Pulmonary fibrosis may, in future, offer a further indication for this form of treatment, and there is also the possibility that a lung graft could sometimes be used to replace an obliterated vascular bed, for example in advanced primary pulmonary hypertension.

THE DEVELOPING SCOPE OF TRANSPLANTATION

The transplantation of vital organs must always be limited in scope. When a living donor is concerned, the kidney is the only vital organ that can be removed with little risk to the donor. When cadaver organs are used there are difficult ethical and legal problems. These have been the subject of a Symposium of the Ciba Foundation in 1966 and are still controversial. The major obstacle to a greatly increased application of homograft procedures, however, is not moral but practical.

At present it is only in the case of renal failure that a patient can be maintained artificially by dialysis, while waiting for a homograft replacement of a vital part. The development of supportive procedures to replace the function of other failing organs is an important requirement in homograft surgery, both in the preoperative preparation of the patient and in his post-operative management in case of difficulty. So is the development of improved methods of organ preservation.

As yet it is only possible to store a limited number of tissues in a viable state for any length of time while a suitable recipient is found. Although blood cells can be deep frozen and similar methods could be used in the setting up of skin banks, progress in the preservation of other living tissues has been slow.

The immunological aspects of transplantation may also lead to new developments, and there is a good deal of current research into specific methods for inducing tolerance or 'enhancing' graft survival. Some transplantation procedures, for example those concerned with heart valves, do not require a living graft. Others, like those of cartilage and cornea, are concerned with 'immunologically privileged sites' where rejection does not occur because of the lack of a blood supply or lymphatic drainage. Future developments may exploit this, and it cannot be long before an ovum is successfully implanted into the privileged site of the uterus. Other hopeful prospects depend on improvements in immunosuppression, which might make it possible to carry out marrow infusions or other types of stem cell transfer. Marrow transplantation has so farsucceeded mainly in infants suffering from immune deficiency states, since in this case the recipient is quite incapable of rejecting the grafted cells. Foetal thymus has also been used with some success in the case of infants with immune deficiency states. These procedures demand perfect tissue matching or perfect suppression of the immune response, but if successful their scope and usefulness might be considerable. It has now proved possible to treat aplastic anaemia in this way. The haemoglobinopathies may follow, and infants with enzyme deficiencies may yet respond to the transfer of foetal liver or other stem cells. Unlike the transplantation of organs, these procedures offer an essentially simple approach, and the availability of donor material presents no major problems.

SELECTED BIBLIOGRAPHY

BILLINGHAM, R. E. and SILVERS, W. K. (1571) The Immunobiology of Tissue Transplantation. *Immunological Diseases* 2nd Ed. Vol. 1 Ed. Samter, M. Little, Brown and Co., Boston, p. 265.

CRUIKSHANK, K. and WEIR, D. M. (Editor) (1967) *Modern Trends in Immunology*. Butterworths, London.

HOLMAN, H. R. (1970) Control of Homograft Rejection. *Advances in Internal Medicine* Vol. 16. Year Book Medical Publishers, p. 265.

LESSOF, M. H. and RUSSELL, A. S. (1971) Immunity, Autoimmunity and Immunosuppression. *Progress in Clinical Medicine*. 6th Ed. Daley, R. and Miller, H. Churchill, p. 32, London.

PORTER, K. A. (Editor) (1967) Tissue and Organ Transplantation. *Symposium of the College of Pathologists* (suppl. *J. Clin. Path.*) 20, 415.

RAPAPORT, F. T. and DAUSET, J. (Editor) (1968) *Human Transplantation*. Grune and Stratton. New York.

RUSSELL, P. S., AUSTEN, K. F., FLAX, M. H. and WINN, H. J. (1969) Clinical Immunopathology of Renal Transplantation. *Textbook of Immunopathology* Vol. II Ed. Miescher, P. A. and Muller-Eberhard, H. J. Grune and Stratton, New York, p. 752.

Transplantation of Tissues and Organs (1965) *British Medical Bulletin* 21, No. 2, 97.

XIV

Bleeding Disorders and Fibrinolysis

The bleeding disorders are comprehensively reviewed in a number of excellent monographs and a systematic consideration will not be attempted here. Rather it is proposed to emphasize recent advances in physiology, pathogenesis and treatment and to concentrate on points of practical importance.

PHYSIOLOGY OF HAEMOSTASIS

The function of the haemostatic mechanism is to prevent blood loss from intact vessels and to stop excessive bleeding from severed vessels. The mechanism by which blood loss is prevented from intact vessels is uncertain but the structural integrity of the vessels and the presence of normal platelets are necessary for this function.

Arrest of bleeding following trauma is controlled by three interrelated factors. These factors are the reaction of the blood vessels to injury, the formation of a platelet plug at the site of injury, and blood coagulation. A simplified scheme of normal haemostatic mechanism is shown in Fig. 30. When a blood vessel is severed the vessel constricts, blood is shed and the processes of platelet adhesion, platelet aggregation and blood coagulation are initiated. Platelets adhere to the subendothelial connective tissue and to the basement membrane, release ADP and then aggregate under the influence of ADP to form an unstable platelet plug. This stage of platelet aggregation takes place within seconds of injury. The unstable plug is eventually stabilized by fibrin which forms at the final stage of blood coagulation. The fibrin component of the haemostatic plug gradually increases in amount as the platelets undergo autolysis and after 24–48 hours the haemostatic plug consists almost entirely of fibrin. The fibrin is then gradually digested by the fibrinolytic system and the defect in the wall of the vessel is covered with endothelium.

The processes of platelet adhesion and aggregation, blood coagulation and vessel constriction are closely interrelated. Thus (1) vasoactive substances which cause vessel constriction are released when platelets come in contact with connective tissue; (2) platelet aggregation accelerates blood coagulation by making available platelet phospholipids (platelet factor 3); and (3) thrombin, an enzyme which is produced during blood coagulation, not only converts the soluble protein fibrinogen into the insoluble gel fibrin, but it causes platelets to release ADP and therefore produces further aggregation.

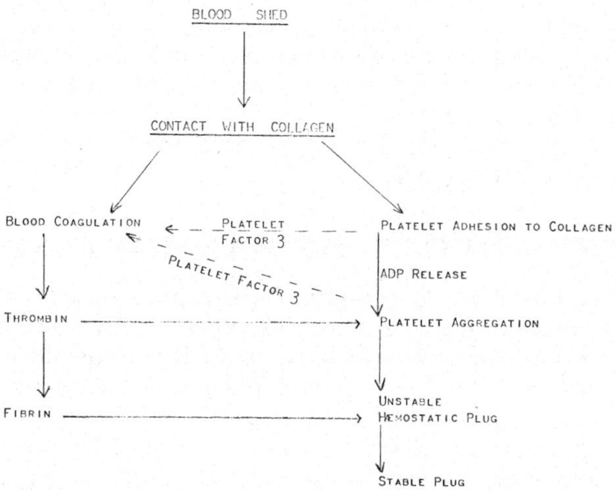

FIG. 30 Normal haemostatic mechanism

BLOOD COAGULATION

The process of blood coagulation occurs as a series of complex steps which terminate in the formation of a fibrin clot. Blood coagulation occurs either by activation of the intrinsic pathway, which is a relatively slow process, or by activation of the extrinsic pathway, a faster process.

The Intrinsic System

The coagulation factors circulate in the form of inactive precursors, some of which are pro-enzymes and some substrates. Each clotting factor is converted into an active form, which in turn activates the next factor in the clotting sequence. This concept has been likened to a 'cascade' or 'waterfall'. A scheme of clotting by the intrinsic pathway is shown in Fig. 31 (to the right and above the diagonal line).

Clotting by the intrinsic pathway begins with activation of factor XII when this coagulation factor comes in contact with a 'foreign surface'. This activating surface is usually glass in in-vitro test systems, but may be collagen, skin or other tissues when coagulation is initiated in vivo. The active factor XII in turn activates factor XI to form contact product. This step is independent of calcium, but all of the subsequent steps in the activation of the intrinsic pathway are calcium dependent. The contact product activates factor IX and this in turn activates factor VIII. The activation of factor VIII is accelerated by the presence of platelet factor 3 and by thrombin. The activated factor VIII in turn activates factor X and this forms a complex with factor V and platelet factor 3, which affects the enzymatic conversion of prothrombin to thrombin. Thrombin then converts the soluble protein fibrinogen into an insoluble gel, fibrin. Thrombin also activates factor XIII, which in the presence of calcium stabilizes the fibrin gel.

The Extrinsic System

When extracts of various tissue, such as brain or lung, are added to blood a number of the early time-consuming steps in the intrinsic clotting pathway are bypassed and coagulation occurs more rapidly through activation of the extrinsic clotting system. A scheme of clotting by the extrinsic system is shown in Fig. 31 (to the left and below the diagonal line). The tissue factor reacts with factor VII and the complex so formed functions as an enzyme to activate factor X. Beyond this point clotting proceeds along the common pathway with the intrinsic system. That is, the active factor X in the presence of factor V converts prothrombin to thrombin, and thrombin then converts fibrinogen to fibrin.

Interaction of Intrinsic and Extrinsic Pathways

During blood coagulation in vivo the intrinsic and extrinsic pathways are activated as soon as blood is shed. Both pathways appear to be necessary for normal haemostasis, but the intrinsic pathway is the more important. Thrombin is a key factor in the interaction of the extrinsic and intrinsic system. Thus thrombin, which is formed rapidly by activation of the extrinsic system, not only produces fibrin but accelerates clotting through the intrinsic pathway by activating factor VIII and possibly also factor V. It is probable that only small amounts of thrombin and fibrin are produced by the extrinsic pathway and that stabilization of the haemostatic plug is delayed until sufficient amounts of thrombin and fibrin are formed by activation of the intrinsic pathway. The main role of the extrinsic pathway may then be to produce rapidly small amounts of thrombin which then accelerates clotting by the intrinsic pathway.

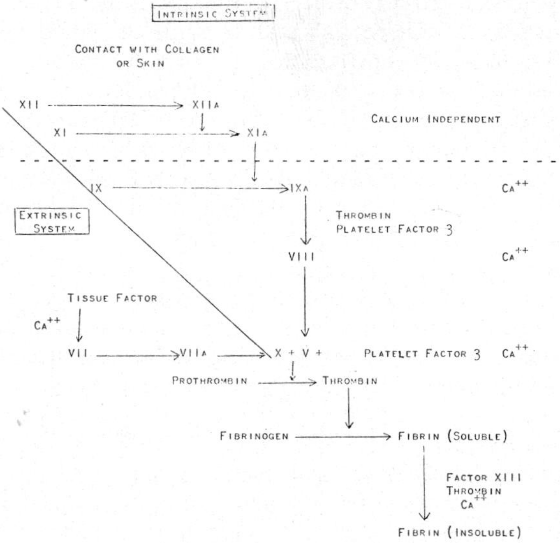

FIG. 31 Extrinsic system of blood clotting

THE CLINICAL AND LABORATORY DIAGNOSIS OF BLEEDING DISORDERS

The majority of patients who present clinically with significant bleeding do not have a generalized defect of haemostasis but bleed from local causes. Defective haemostasis leading to abnormal bleeding may be caused by a vascular defect, thrombocytopenia, abnormalities of platelet function, defects in blood coagulation or by excessive fibrinolytic activity. In patients with a severe haemostatic defect a diagnosis of a generalized bleeding disorder can usually be made from the history of bleeding. The diagnosis is then confirmed and the precise nature of the haemostatic defect determined by laboratory tests. On the other hand, in patients with a mild haemostatic defect bleeding symptoms are less severe and often the generalized haemostatic abnormality is unmasked by local factors or by trauma, and laboratory tests are required both to confirm the diagnosis and to determine the nature of the defect.

The approach to the investigation of patients with bleeding disorders varies according to the clinical circumstances. In every case the clinical history is of utmost importance in diagnosis. In obtaining a history answers to the following four questions should be sought:

1. Has the patient a generalized haemostatic defect?
2. Is this defect inherited or acquired?
3. Is the defect likely to be due to a vascular or platelet abnormality, a coagulation abnormality, or a mixture of the two?
4. What is the precise nature and extent of the haemostatic abnormality?

The answers to the first three questions can often be obtained by careful evaluation of the patient's bleeding symptoms but the answer to the fourth question can only be provided by special tests. Although these four questions are closely interconnected it is useful to consider them separately.

1. *Is the patient suffering from a generalized haemostatic defect?* A generalized bleeding disorder is likely to be present if there is a history of bleeding from multiple sites, particularly if bleeding occurs spontaneously and if the manifestations include petechiae, large superficial bruises, haemarthroses and large haemotomas. It should be noted that epistaxes, uterine bleeding and gastro-intestinal bleeding are frequently caused by local lesions and even when they occur in combination they may not be caused by a generalized bleeding disorder. Spontaneous bruising of the legs is a common symptom, particularly in females. It is usually a benign condition and is not associated with any detectable haemostatic defect. It is thought to be due to a mild increase in vascular fragility. In some of these patients the bleeding symptoms are aggravated by aspirin ingestion and the possibility of aspirin ingestion should be excluded in all patients who present with superficial bruising. The haemostatic defect produced by aspirin will be considered in more detail below.

2. *Is the disorder inherited or acquired?* Patients with an inherited bleeding disorder usually present in infancy or childhood if the underlying defect is severe but may not show manifestations of abnormal bleeding until adult life if the defect is mild. When a patient with a mild bleeding disorder presents for the first time in adult life, with either post-operative or post-traumatic haemorrhage, it may be difficult to decide whether the patient has a mild life-long bleeding disorder or if the disorder has been recently acquired. Differentiation between these two possibilities may sometimes be

obtained from detailed enquiry into the family history and from the patient's response to previous operations or trauma. A detailed family history may also establish the mode of inheritance and so narrow down the diagnostic possibilities. A positive family history of bleeding is of great value in diagnosis but a negative history does not exclude the possibility of an inherited bleeding disorder, particularly if the patient is an unreliable witness or if the number of members in the family is small. In addition it should be noted that approximately 30 per cent of patients with life-long bleeding disorders such as haemophilia do not have a family history of bleeding.

Specific enquiry should always be made about tooth extraction, circumcisions and tonsillectomy, because these operations are often overlooked by the patient. If tonsillectomy or abdominal operations have been tolerated without excessive blood loss, it is unlikely that the patient is suffering from a severe or even moderately severe inherited bleeding disorder. The importance of these aspects of the history cannot be stressed too greatly. Most patients who are referred for coagulation tests do not have a generalized bleeding disorder and in the majority this possibility could have been excluded by careful history.

3. *Is the disorder due to a platelet abnormality, vascular abnormality or a coagulation defect?* The bleeding manifestations of patients with vascular disorders, thrombocytopenia and defects in platelet function are similar and include spontaneous skin and mucous membrane bleeding, petechiae and superficial bruises. Bleeding usually starts within seconds of injury and continues for hours, but once it stops it usually does not recur. In contrast, patients with coagulation defects develop deep spreading haematomas, bleeding into joints, haematuria and retroperitoneal bleeding. Post-traumatic bleeding tends to be delayed sometimes for hours after the traumatic episode and may then recur on a number of occasions after a number of days.

4. *The precise nature of the haemostatic abnormality.* The laboratory tests used to investigate a patient with a suspected bleeding disorder can be most conveniently divided into (1) screening tests for vascular and platelet disorders, (2) screening tests for coagulation disorders, (3) special investigations for platelet disorders and (4) special tests of coagulation and fibrinolysis.

The tests used in any individual patient are determined by the nature of the bleeding manifestation and by the clinical circumstances. The screening tests for vascular, platelet and coagulation disorders are listed in Table 1.

TABLE 1

Investigation of bleeding disorders

Screening tests

Test	*Platelet-vascular disorder*	*Coagulation defect*
Vascular fragility	Often abnormal	Normal
Bleeding time	Usually long	Normal
Platelet count	Normal in vascular disorders and platelet function defects	Normal (low in consumption coagulopathy)
Thrombin time	Normal	May be long
Prothrombin time	Normal	May be long
Partial thrombo-plastin time	Normal (except in von Willebrand's disease)	May be long

1. **Screening Tests for Vascular and Platelet Disorders**

These include a capillary fragility test, bleeding time, inspection of the blood film for platelet numbers and size and platelet count.

Capillary Fragility Test. An increase in capillary fragility is characteristically seen in patients who have thrombocytopenia, vascular disorders and defects of platelet function. However, the test is relatively non-specific and may be positive as an isolated finding in patients without other bleeding manifestations.

Bleeding Time. The bleeding time is measured by determining the time required for bleeding to stop after a small incision is made in the skin. Of the number of different techniques used the Ivy bleeding time or its modifications appear to be most reliable. The bleeding time is an index of the early stages of haemostatic plug formation, i.e. vessel contraction, platelet adhesion and aggregation. It is therefore characteristically prolonged in patients with vascular defects, thrombocytopenic purpura and thrombocytopathic purpura. It is usually normal in patients with coagulation disorders, presumably because the arrest of bleeding from the small vessels punctured in this test occurs independently of rapid fibrin formation. The bleeding time is a fairly crude and non-specific test. Nevertheless it is simple and provides a fairly reliable indication of the overall severity of the haemostatic defect in patients with vascular and platelet disorders. The normal range for the Ivy bleeding time is 3 to 7 minutes.

Platelet Count and Platelet Size. Careful inspection of the blood film may reveal the presence of the underlying cause of the thrombocytopenia, e.g. leukaemia; it also gives an indication of the platelet count, and may reveal the presence of large platelets which are sometimes present in patients with thrombocytopathic purpura and are characteristically seen when there is an increase in platelet turnover. The platelet count is prone to error. Abnormal results should therefore be confirmed by a second count and by inspection of the blood film. The normal range of the platelet count is 150,000–400,000 per cubic millimeter.

Serious skin or mucous membrane bleeding associated with a normal platelet count and a long bleeding time suggests a diagnosis of either von Willebrand's disease or of a platelet function disorder and these possibilities should be investigated by performing the appropriate special investigations (see below). If the platelet count is low appropriate investigation should be performed to determine the cause.

2. **Screening tests for coagulation abnormalities**

Relatively simple screening tests are available to investigate abnormalities in both the intrinsic and extrinsic clotting systems. The intrinsic clotting system can be readily assessed by the partial thromboplastin time and the extrinsic system by the one-stage prothrombin time. In addition the conversion of fibrinogen to fibrin, which is common to both pathways, can be assessed by the thrombin time test. Although not highly specific these tests are sufficiently sensitive to be abnormal in the large majority of patients with clinically significant coagulation defects.

One-stage Prothrombin time (PT)

The one-stage prothrombin time is performed by adding tissue extract or tissue thromboplastin to plasma. The pathway involved is shown below in Fig. 32. It can be seen that this test is sensitive to deficiencies of factors VII, X, V, prothrombin and fibrinogen.

Activated partial thromboplastin time (PTT)

The activated partial thromboplastin time is performed in two steps. First the citrated plasma is incubated with a surface active agent such as kaolin or celite to produce activated factor XI. (Fig. 33 step 1.) Platelet phospholipid and calcium are then added to the activated plasma so that coagulation by the intrinsic pathway can proceed to fibrin formation. (Fig. 33 steps 2, 3.) This test is therefore sensitive to deficiencies in the factors leading to the production of activated factor XI (factors XII and XI, step 1); to factors necessary for the activation of factor X (i.e. factors IX and VIII step 2) and to the factors common to both the intrinsic and extrinsic pathway, i.e. factors X, V, prothrombin and fibrinogen (step 3). It should be

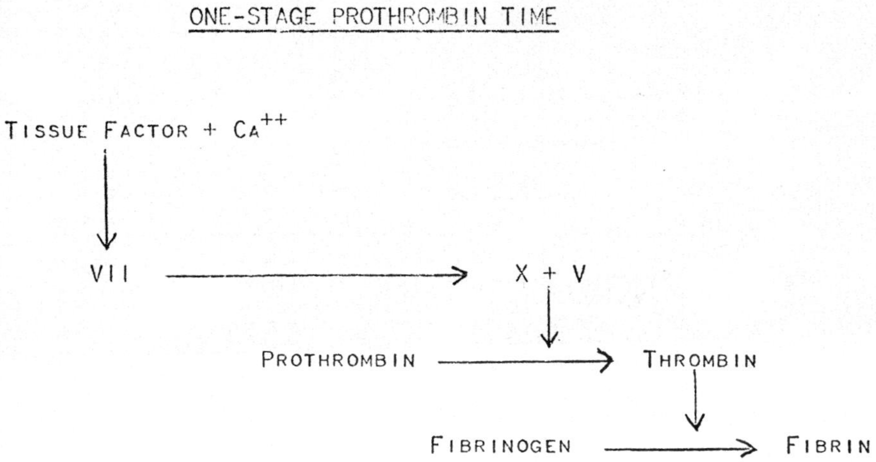

FIG. 32 Pathway of one-stage prothrombin time

noted that this test is insensitive to factor VII deficiency and is uninfluenced by platelet concentration or platelet function since platelet phospholipid is added to the test system.

Thrombin time (TT)

The thrombin time is performed by adding thrombin to plasma. This test is influenced by the fibrinogen level and by inhibitors of the fibrinogen to fibrin conversion reaction, the most important of which are heparin and the breakdown products of fibrinogen and fibrin. This test is frequently abnormal in patients with consumption coagulopathy and primary pathological fibrinolysis.

Interpretation and Significance of Abnormalities of the One-stage Prothombin Time, Partial Thromboplastin Time and Thrombin Time

Five possible combinations of results may be obtained (Table 2).

1. *All tests normal.* For practical purposes this result excludes the presence of any significant coagulation disorder. However, all three tests are normal in patients with factor XIII deficiency and may be normal in patients with mild factor VIII or factor IX deficiencies, particularly if one of these deficiencies is associated with abnormally high levels of other clotting factors.

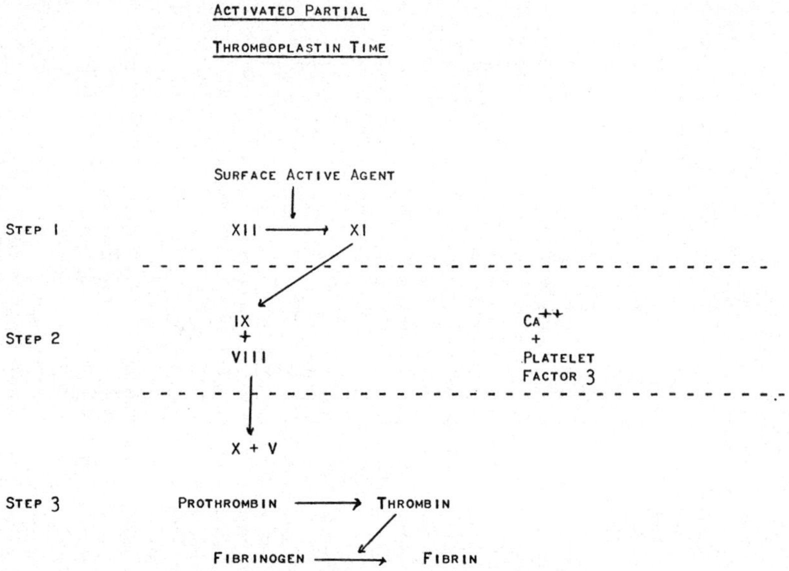

FIG. 33 The estimated partial thromboplastin time

2. *Partial Thromboplastin Time Long, Prothrombin Time Normal, Thrombin Time Normal.* This combination of results if found in patients with single inherited deficiencies of factors VIII, IX, XI or XII, or when there is an inhibitor of factor VIII.

3. *Partial Thromboplastin Time Long, Prothrombin Time Long, Thrombin Time Normal.* This combination of results is found in patients with inherited (congenital) deficiencies of factors II, V or X (these disorders are very uncommon), and much more commonly as an acquired coagulation disorder in liver disease, Vitamin K deficiency and during treatment with oral anticoagulants. In addition it may occasionally occur in patients with disseminated lupus

TABLE 2

	Tests: PTT	Tests: PT	Tests: TT	Inherited (Congenital)	Acquired Disorder	Defect
1.	Normal	Normal	Normal	Factor XIII deficiency Mild factor VIII or IX deficiency		
2.	Long	Normal	Normal	Deficiencies of factors VIII, IX, XI, XII	Inhibitor of factor VIII	Factor VIII
3.	Long	Long	Normal	Deficiencies of factors II, V, X	Liver disease Vitamin K deficiency Oral Anticoagulants Inhibitor in DLE	Factors II, VII, IX, X (V) Factors II, VII, IX, X Factors II, VII, IX, X Prothrombin activation
4.	Normal	Long	Normal	Deficiency of factor VII		
5.	Long	Long	Long	Hypofibrinogenemia	Consumption coagulopathy Primary pathological fibrinolysis Severe liver disease Heparin therapy	Factors V, VIII, fibrinogen, FPP,* platelets Factors V, VIII, fibrinogen, FPP,* Clot lysis Factors II, VII, IX, X, V, fibrinogen, antithrombin, thromboplastin formation

*FPP = Split Products of Fibrin or Fibrinogen

erythematosis who develop an inhibitor. The nature of the defect found in these conditions is shown in Table 2.

4. *Partial Thromboplastin Time Normal, Prothrombin Time Long, Thrombin Time Normal.* This combination is found in patients with an inherited deficiency of factor VII (a very rare condition).

5. *Partial Thromboplastin Time Long, Prothrombin Time Long, Thrombin Time Long.* These results are found in patients with congenital (inherited) hypofibrinogenaemia, a rare condition, and

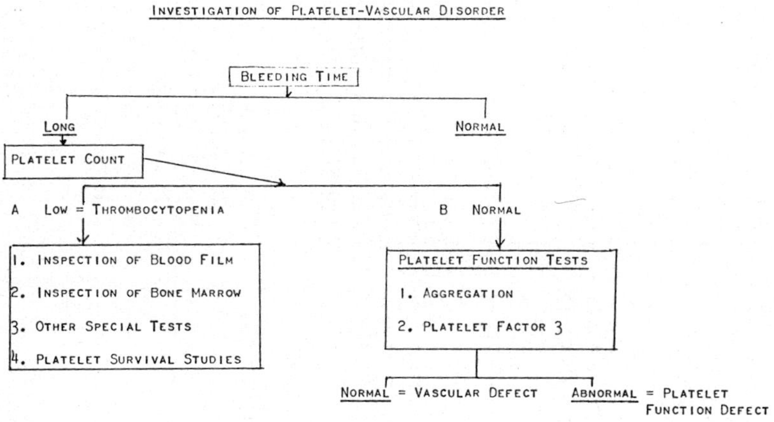

FIG. 34 Scheme of investigation for platelet and vascular disorders

more commonly in patients with consumption coagulopathy, severe liver disease, primary pathological fibrinolysis and in patients receiving treatment with heparin. The nature of the defect found in these conditions is shown in Table 2.

3. Special tests to investigate platelet and vascular disorders

A simplified scheme for the investigation of platelet and vascular disorders is set out in Fig. 34 and the causes of these disorders in Fig. 35. The following combination of screening tests may occur.

(a) *Long bleeding time, low platelet count*

1. *Inspection of Blood Film*

This may reveal the presence of the underlying cause of thrombocytopenia, e.g. leukaemia.

2. *Inspection of bone marrow aspiration*

Inspection of the bone marrow aspiration may give an indication of megakaryocyte numbers and may reveal the primary cause of thrombocytopenia, e.g. leukaemia, multiple myeloma, aplastic anaemia, megaloblastic anaemia. In addition it may provide a clue to the mechanism of thrombocytopenia. In general, the presence

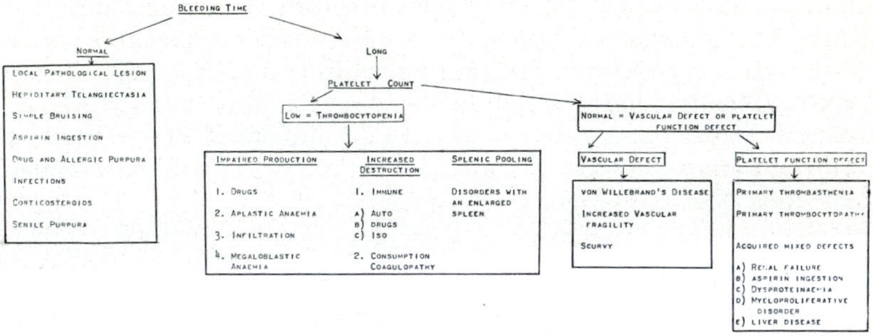

FIG. 35 Causes of platelet and vascular disorders

of normal or increased numbers of megakaryocytes suggests that thrombocytopenia is caused by either an increased rate of destruction or a combination of increased destruction and increased splenic pooling. A decreased number of megakaryocytes suggests that the thrombocytopenia is due to impaired production. However, there are exceptions: for example, in megaloblastic anaemia thrombocytopenia is associated with normal numbers of megakaryocytes but survival is normal and thrombocytopenia is thought to be due to ineffective thrombopoiesis.

3. *Other investigations*

These include a search for LE cells and antinuclear factor, special tests to exclude drug-induced thrombocytopenia if there is a history drug ingestion, and tests to exclude associated haemolytic anaemia.

4. *Platelet survival studies*

Platelet survival studies are only indicated if the cause of thrombocytopenia is uncertain after the above investigations have been performed. This test makes it possible to differentiate between thrombocytopenia caused by impaired production and that caused by an increased rate of destruction.

(b) *Long bleeding time, platelet count normal*

If the platelet count is normal and the bleeding time long, platelet function tests should be performed to differentiate between a platelet function abnormality and a vascular cause for the prolonged bleeding time. The platelet function tests include platelet aggregation after exposure of platelet-rich plasma to adenosine diphosphate, collagen and adrenalin, and platelet factor 3 availability tests. Tests of platelet glass adhesiveness are less specific and are of limited value in differentiating between a platelet function defect and a vascular disorder.

Vascular Disorders

Long bleeding time, normal platelet count, normal platelet function tests.

This combination is seen most commonly in von Willebrand's disease. Patients with von Willebrand's disease also have a low factor VIII level. Other features of this disorder are discussed in more detail below.

4. Special Tests for Coagulation Disorders

1. *Thromboplastin Generation Test.* This test is more difficult to perform than the partial thromboplastin time but has the advantage that it is able to differentiate between a factor VIII and a factor IX deficiency.
2. Coagulation factor assays
3. Tests for inhibitors
4. Tests for fibrin and fibrinogen split products
5. Tests of fibrinolysis

Details of these tests are beyond the scope of this discussion.

Abnormalities of Platelet function (Thrombocytopathic Purpura)

1. *Thrombasthenia*

This is a rare disorder characterized by the failure of platelets to aggregate with ADP. Since collagen and adrenalin induced aggregation is mediated by release of ADP, aggregation with these agents is also defective. Platelet factor 3 availability is affected to a variable extent.

2. *Thrombocytopathy*

This is a platelet defect characterized by a failure of platelet factor 3 availability. A number of these patients have also been shown to have defective platelet aggregation with collagen and adrenalin but normal primary aggregation with adenosine diphosphate.

3. *Acquired Platelet Function Disorders*

In these disorders, listed in Fig. 35, there is a variable defect in platelet aggregation and platelet factor 3 availability. The nature of the defect in these conditions is discussed in more detail below.

THE VASCULAR DISORDERS

Vascular defects are the commonest cause of bleeding disorders seen in clinical practice. These disorders constitute a heterogeneous group of conditions which are characterized by easy bruising and spontaneous bleeding from small vessels. The underlying abnormality is often uncertain but it is thought to be either in the vessels or in the perivascular connective tissue. There is a considerable variation in the severity of bleeding manifestations. In most cases bleeding is not severe and is limited to the skin, causing bruising and petechiae.

In these patients the bleeding time is often normal and the tourniquet test may or may not be positive. However, in some vascular disorders bleeding is more severe and occurs from mucous membranes as well as from the skin. In these patients the bleeding time is usually long and the tourniquet test is positive.

The diagnosis of a vascular defect is usually made after thrombocytopenia and a qualitative platelet defect have been excluded. An abnormality in platelet function has been reported in some of these vascular disorders, e.g. von Williebrand's disease and scurvy, but it is uncertain to what extent the platelet defect contributes to the overall bleeding tendency in these conditions. On the other hand it is now recognized that the bleeding that occurs in renal failure, dysproteinaemias and following large doses of aspirin is due mainly to defective platelet function and these latter three conditions will be considered in the section on bleeding due to platelet function defects.

The Inherited Vascular Disorders

Von Willebrand's disease. The pathogenesis and classification of this disorder has been the subject of considerable confusion. It is now generally accepted that von Willebrand's disease is a hereditary disorder which is transmitted as an autosomal dominant trait, characterized by prolonged bleeding time, a normal platelet count and a low factor VIII level. Platelet adhesiveness to glass is reduced in a large percentage of patients when this test is performed using either native blood or heparinized blood, but it is uncertain whether this abnormality contributes in any way to the haemorrhagic manifestations or to the prolonged bleeding time. Unlike most other inherited bleeding disorders the severity of the defect observed clinically or measured in the laboratory varies among individuals within a given family. In addition, the bleeding time may fluctuate widely in individual patients so that the finding of a normal bleeding time in a single examination does not necessarily exclude this diagnosis. The factor VIII concentration, on the other hand, tends to remain more constant in individual patients. Studies of a large number of related patients with von Willebrand's disease has revealed that although most of the patients have both a low factor VIII level and a long bleeding time, a small percentage only have one or the other defect. It is possible, however, that in these subjects the second defect would have been revealed by repeated examinations. Both the low factor VIII concentration and the long bleeding time can be corrected by intravenous administration of normal plasma or of a fresh haemophilic plasma. This suggests that in von Willebrand's disease there is a deficiency of one or perhaps even two plasma factors which are present in the haemophilic blood and which are necessary for the synthesis of factor VIII and for the control of bleeding from small vessels. It has also been claimed by some that infusion of fresh plasma corrects the defect in platelet adhesiveness, but others have failed to demonstrate such an effect.

The bleeding manifestations are chiefly those of a vascular disorder. Thus patients complain of easy bruising and excessive postoperative bleeding. They bleed from superficial cuts and abrasions and from mucous membranes, and females may suffer from menorrhagia and post-partum haemorrhage. Haemarthroses are uncommon and only occur in patients with very low factor VIII levels.

Fresh plasma is effective in controlling bleeding in von Willebrand's disease. It produces an increase in factor VIII because it contains the clotting factor and because it induces synthesis. Following transfusion even with factor VIII deficient plasma, there is a slow rise in factor VIII concentration which reaches a maximum in 6–12 hours and falls to pre-treatment levels in approximately 48 hours.

The bleeding time is also sometimes shortened following transfusion of fresh plasma but the effect on the bleeding time is not as consistent and is relatively short-lived. It is important to exclude the diagnosis of von Willebrand's disease in patients with symptoms of vascular bleeding before surgery is attempted. This is because severe postoperative bleeding, preventable by appropriate replacement therapy, may occur even though the symptoms of spontaneous skin and mucous membrane bleeding are mild.

Increased Vascular Fragility with normal Factor VIII level (*Hereditary Capillary Fragility*). This is a disorder of uncertain pathogenesis characterized by abnormal bleeding following trauma or surgery and occasionally by spontaneous skin and mucous membrane bleeding. There is often a family history of bleeding affecting both sexes equally, but it has also been reported to occur sporadically. The characteristic feature on investigation is a prolonged bleeding time. Like von Willebrand's disease, the bleeding time often fluctuates in individual patients and may be normal on occasions. However, unlike von Willebrand's disease the factor VIII level is normal.

It is possible that the reported cases of increased vascular fragility represent a heterogeneous group of disorders which include defects in platelet function and von Willebrand's disease.

Hereditary Haemorrhagic Telangiectasia. This is an uncommon disorder transmitted as an autosomal dominant trait. It is characterized by telangiectases in the skin and mucous membranes and less commonly at other sites.

The skin lesions are mainly seen on the face, the tips of the fingers and the feet, and the mucous membrane lesions are seen mainly on the lips and in the mouth, and they commonly affect the nasal mucosa. The lesions blanch on pressure and become more numerous and more prominent with advancing age. The bleeding usually first occurs during early adult life and is characterized by recurrent epistaxes and less commonly by bleeding from the telangiectases in the skin. Iron deficiency anaemia, due to recurrent blood loss, is a relatively common complication. The tourniquet test and bleeding time are characteristically normal.

Epistaxis is the most troublesome symptom and at times it is severe and intractable. Long term benefit may be obtained from treatment by systemic oestrogen therapy, which in large doses produces squamous metaplasia of the nasal mucosa, or by excision and grafting of the affected area.

Acquired Vascular Defect

Simple easy bruising. This is a benign disorder which occurs predominantly in otherwise healthy women. It is probably the commonest cause of referral of patients for diagnosis and assessment of unexplained skin bruising. Onset of bleeding usually begins in early adult life and is characterized by recurrent small bruises, either occurring spontaneously or after minor trauma, on the legs, the forearms and less commonly on the trunk. The bruises are occasionally preceded by pain, which is thought to be due to the rupture of a small blood vessel. There is sometimes a family history of bleeding but this is by no means clear cut. Petechiae do not occur. The cause of the disorder is unknown. Aspirin ingestion, even in low doses, may aggravate bruising in patients with simple bruising. These patients may first seek medical advice when the mild bruising which they have tolerated for years is aggravated by aspirin ingestion. In the uncomplicated case, the special tests related to bleeding disorders, including the bleeding time and tourniquet test, are normal. In the cases complicated by aspirin ingestion, the bleeding time is usually normal or borderline, the tourniquet test is variable and platelet aggregation studies show a defect characteristic of that produced by aspirin (see below).

Simple easy bruising is a benign disorder and is only of importance because of its cosmetic significance. Although aspirin ingestion in low therapeutic doses may increase the severity of the skin bleeding, it is improbable that it ever leads to serious spontaneous bleeding. However, the patient should be discouraged from taking aspirin, particularly if skin bleeding is troublesome or if there is associated menorrhagia. The disorder does not cause excessive bleeding at operation, but it is possible that abnormal operative and post-operative bleeding might occur if the patient takes aspirin.

Senile Purpura. Senile purpura is a form of purpura which commonly occurs in elderly subjects. It mainly affects the extensor aspects of the forearms and hands and is due to loss of subcutaneous fat and connective tissue which results in the skin being freely movable over the deeper tissues. The small vessels passing through to the skin are therefore easily torn.

Infections. Purpura may occur in patients with septicaemia, particularly meningococcal septicaemia, bacterial endocarditis and typhoid fever, and more commonly when septicaemia occurs in infancy and childhood. Biopsy of the purpuric lesions sometimes reveals thrombi and micro-organisms in the microcirculation and the purpura is believed to be due to vascular damage produced either by the microthrombi or bacterial toxins. In some of these patients there is co-existing thrombocytopenia due to consumption coagulopathy;

however, thrombocytopenia does not occur in all cases of purpura associated with septicaemia.

Drugs. Non-thrombocytopenic purpura occasionally occurs as a manifestation of a drug or chemical toxicity; however, other types of skin rash are more common. The purpura, which is thought to be due to endothelial damage, disappears within a few days of stopping the drug. Some of the drugs which cause vascular purpura also cause thrombocytopenic purpura.

Henoch Schönlein Syndrome. This disorder is caused by a hypersensitivity reaction which results in widespread vasculitis. The onset may follow an upper respiratory tract infection, often with a group A beta haemolytic strepococcus, or it may follow the ingestion of certain drugs or foods. It is characterized clinically by the acute onset of some or all of the following symptoms: a macular rash, purpura, joint pains, abdominal pain, gastrointestinal bleeding and haematuria. The condition occurs most commonly in children but may occur in adults. It is usually self-limiting and may recur for a period of up to two or three months. The purpuric rash occurs most commonly on the buttocks, on the backs of the elbows and extensor surfaces of the arms, on the extensor surfaces of the lower legs, the ankle and the foot. It is usually bilateral and may occur on the face, but the trunk is usually spared. The rash tends to occur in crops which progressively fade over two weeks. Occasionally frankly haemorrhagic lesions become bullous and may go on to local necrosis.

Treatment of this disorder includes antibiotics, if a pathogenic organism is isolated from the nose, throat or sputum, and analgesics for the relief of joint pain or abdominal pain. Aspirin, because of its effect on platelet function, should be avoided as an analgesic. Corticosteroids, which may relieve joint and abdominal pains, should only be given if symptoms are severe.

Scurvy. Bleeding into skin and mucous membranes is a common feature of scurvy, particularly in adults. A defect in platelet function has been reported in both experimental and clinical scurvy, and this may be an additional contributing factor to bleeding. Bleeding may occur anywhere in the skin but is particularly common in the legs and at sites of trauma. Petechiae are commonly peri-follicular. The bleeding time is usually prolonged when there is overt skin bleeding and the tourniquet test is usually positive.

Cortico-steroid administration. Bruising is not uncommon in Cushing's disease and in patients who are treated with large doses of steroids.

The cause of the skin bleeding is uncertain but it may be due to alterations in the subcutaneous connective tissue. The bleeding is usually not a serious problem and in the few patients investigated has not been associated with a long bleeding time or with a defect in platelet function.

PLATELET DISORDERS

Platelet function may be impaired because there is a low concentration of circulating platelets (thrombocytopenia) or because there is impaired platelet function. In general, clinically significant platelet abnormalities either quantitative or qualitative are associated with prolongation of the bleeding time.

Platelet Production, Circulation and Destruction

Platelets are anuclear 'cells' which are produced in the marrow from multinuclear cells, the megakaryocytes. Megakaryocytes undergo nuclear replication without cytoplasmic replication. As the nuclear material increases in amount so too does the cytoplasm and in the mature megakaryocyte the amount of cytoplasm is roughly proportional to the amount of nuclear material. Platelet formation occurs in the cytoplasm of the mature megakaryocyte and is indicated by light microscopy by the appearance of cytoplasmic granules. In the normal marrow about 25 per cent of megakaryocytes have no apparent granules; these are the most immature cells, and the other 75 per cent have variable degrees of granulation. When maturation is studied by electron microscopy it is seen that during maturation membranes form and demarcate the cytoplasm into platelet subunits which mature and are released into the circulation. The production of platelets in the marrow is regulated by a humoral factor which is known as thrombopoietin. The mode of action of thrombopoietin has not yet been fully elucidated but it probably acts to increase the number of megakaryocytes formed from precursor cells and also to increase the rate of platelet production and release.

Platelets are disc-shaped particles which circulate in the blood stream in a concentration of 150,000 to 400,000 per cu. cm. The platelet volume diminishes as the platelets age, so that in states of increased platelet turnover platelets which are larger than normal may appear in the circulation. The young platelets are thought to be functionally more active and to contain higher concentrations of platelet glycogen, ATP and a number of glycolytic enzymes.

About two-thirds of the body platelets circulate within the blood stream and one-third resides in the spleen. This phenomenon is known as splenic pooling. There is free exchange between the circulating and splenic platelets. Splenomegaly is associated with an increase in splenic pooling, so that in massive splenomegaly up to 90 per cent of the body platelets may be pooled in the spleen. Platelets survive in the circulation for approximately 10 days and under normal circumstances when they end their lifespan they are destroyed in the reticulo-endothelial system, particularly in the spleen and liver.

Thrombocytopenia

A classification of the causes of thrombocytopenia is listed in Fig. 35. Thrombocytopenia may occur because platelet production is impaired, platelet survival diminished or because there is increased splenic pooling.

There is no absolute relationship between the platelet count and incidence and severity of bleeding. However, spontaneous bleeding is uncommon when the platelet count is above 50,000 per cu. mm., and serious bleeding usually occurs only after trauma or when a local lesion is present. Bleeding is common but not always present when the platelet count is below 50,000 per cu. mm, but is the rule, and usually severe, when the platelet count is less than 10,000 per cu. mm. If severe spontaneous bleeding occurs when the platelet count is above 50,000 per cu. mm. the possibility of an associated platelet function defect or coagulation abnormality should be considered. It should be noted that some patients with chronic thrombocytopenia, even of a severe degree, may have little in the way of bleeding manifestations for months or even years, whereas others with comparable degrees of thrombocytopenia have frequent and severe bleeding manifestations. The reason for this difference is uncertain; however, it may be related to the functional capacity of the platelets.

Thrombocytopenia due to Impaired Platelet Production. In thrombocytopenia due to impaired production there is usually a decreased megakaryocyte mass and platelet survival is normal or only slightly reduced. Occasionally, however, the megakaryocyte mass is normal and impaired production occurs as a result of ineffective thrombopoiesis. Thrombocytopenia due to impaired production associated with a decreased megakaryocyte mass may be caused by radiation, chemicals or drug toxicity, and it occurs in aplastic anaemia and infiltrative disorders of the bone marrow such as leukaemia, myeloscleroisis, multiple myeloma and secondary carcinoma. It also occurs in some cases of congenital thrombocytopenia. Thrombocytopenia due to ineffective platelet production is seen in megaloblastic anaemias and in erythremic myelosis.

Thrombocytopenia due to an increased rate of destruction. Thrombocytopenia due to reduced platelet survival is characteristically seen in disseminated intravascular thrombosis and in the immune thrombocytopenias. The bone marrow is able to compensate by increasing the rate of platelet production three to four-fold in acute thrombocytopenia, and by increasing production up to eight-fold in chronic thrombocytopenia due to reduction in platelet survival.

Thrombocytopenia due to disseminated intravascular thrombosis. The subject of disseminated intravascular thrombosis will be considered more fully later. Thrombocytopenia is the major or even the only manifestation of disseminated intravascular thrombosis when there is direct consumption of platelets at sites of damaged or altered endothelium and when there is direct interaction of platelets with circulating particles such as viruses, bacteria and immune complexes (Table 3).

TABLE 3

Conditions in which Thrombocytopenia is the Major Manifestation of Disseminated Intravascular Thrombosis

1. *Due to interaction with vessel wall*
   (a) Thrombotic thrombocytopenic purpura
   (b) Prosthetic cardiovascular devices
   (c) Immune vasculitis

2. *Due to interaction with abnormal particles in the circulation*
   (a) Viruses
   (b) Bacteria
   (c) Immune complexes

This latter mechanism may be responsible for some cases of acute idiopathic thrombocytopenia.

Acute Idiopathic Thrombocytopenic Purpura. This more commonly occurs in children and is usually self-limiting. Acute idiopathic thrombocytopenia often occurs during, or more commonly two to three weeks after, an infection. The mechanism of thrombocytopenia is uncertain but it is possible that in many cases it is due to direct interaction of platelets with the infecting micro-organism (either virus or bacteria) or with circulating immune complexes.

Immune Thrombocytopenia. Platelet antibodies may interact with platelets and sensitize them so that they are destroyed in reticulo-endothelial tissues. With moderate sensitization removal occurs primarily in the spleen but with marked sensitization platelets are destroyed diffusely throughout the reticulo-endothelial system but predominantly in the liver. The causes of immune thrombocytopenia are listed in Table 4.

Chronic Immune Thrombocytopenia

Thrombocytopenia is classified as being chronic if the patient has had documented thrombocytopenia for at least three months. There is usually no evidence of underlying disease. However, chronic immune thrombocytopenia may occur as a complication of a lymphoma, chronic lymphocytic leukaemia or systemic lupus erythematosus. Patients with chronic immune thrombocytopenia of the idiopathic type occasionally have auto-antibodies directed against red cells and thyroid gland.

In chronic immune thrombocytopenia the auto-antibodies in the patient's serum coat the platelets and sensitize them so that they are destroyed in the reticulo-endothelial tissues. The evidence that thrombocytopenia in this condition is due to an auto-antibody can be summarized as follows.

1. The transfusion of plasma from a patient with idiopathic thrombocytopenic purpura has been shown to cause thrombocytopenia in the recipient.

2. The survival of normal platelets is reduced when normal platelet-rich plasma is incubated in vitro with plasma from a patient with chronic immune thrombocytopenia or with a gammaglobulin fraction of this plasma.

3. This thrombocytopenic factor is a gammaglobulin and can be absorbed from the patient's plasma by passage of normal platelets through the plasma.

4. Transient thrombocytopenia occurs in approximately 50 per cent of infants born to mothers with chronic immune thrombocytopenic purpura, suggesting the occurrence of transplacental passage of the factor from mother to foetus.

5. Platelet antibodies have been demonstrated in the plasma by in vitro tests but the incidence of positive results has varied widely depending on the tests used and the laboratories in which the tests have been performed.

Diagnosis of Chronic Immune Thrombocytopenia

The diagnosis of chronic immune thrombocytopenia is made from the clinical features, blood and bone marrow findings and occasionally, when indicated, from the results of platelet survival studies.

TABLE 4

Causes of Immune Thrombocytopenia

1. *Auto-immune*
   - (a) Primary { Acute / Chronic
   - (b) Secondary
     - (i) Systemic lupus erythematosus
     - (ii) Lymphoma
2. *Drug-induced immune thrombocytopenia*
   - Quinine
   - Quinidine
   - Sedormid
   - Digitoxin
3. *Iso-immune thrombocytopenia*

A diagnosis can only be made after careful investigation has excluded the possibility of a secondary thrombocytopenia. The clinical features include recurrent petechiae, ecchymoses and mucous membrane bleeding in a patient without other abnormal physical findings. In particular there is no bone tenderness, no hepatomegaly and the spleen is not usually palpable. The blood findings show thrombocytopenia as the only abnormality although occasionally there may be a mild leukopenia or a haemolytic anaemia. Anaemia when present is usually due to chronic blood loss and is often hypochromic and microcytic. The bone marrow typically shows normal or increased numbers of megakaryocytes, often with an increase in the percentage of immature cells. Platelet survival is reduced, usually to a degree which is proportional to the severity of thrombocytopenia. Thus, patients with chronic immune thrombocytopenia who have only a mild thrombocytopenia have a moderately reduced platelet survival whereas in those with severe thrombocytopenia (e.g. with a platelet count of 10,000 per cu. mm. or less) the platelet half life may be an hour or less. Although differentiation from other causes of thrombocytopenia can usually be made from the clinical features and blood and bone marrow examination, it should be noted that chronic thrombocytopenia, which is otherwise identical with primary auto-immune thrombocytopenic purpura, may be the first manifestation of systemic lupus erythematosus or occasionally of a lymphoma.

Treatment of Chronic Immune Thrombocytopenia

The choice of treatment of chronic immune thrombocytopenia is influenced by the age of the patient, the duration of symptoms and the degree of spontaneous bleeding. The age of the patient is important. This is because spontaneous remissions may occur in children after they have been thrombocytopenic for up to a year or even more, while this is very uncommon in adults. Patients with mild asymptomatic thrombocytopenia, e.g. platelet counts of 50,000 per cu. mm. or more, frequently require no treatment. If there are bleeding symptoms or if the thrombocytopenia is severe, treatment with adrenocorticosteroids is commenced in high doses with the aim of reducing the dose when symptoms come under control. In general, if a patient is given 60 mg. of prednisolone or its equivalent, bleeding manifestations usually come under control within a few days, the bleeding time returns to normal and the tourniquet test becomes negative. The effect on the platelet count is more variable and a number of patterns of response may occur. The first is that the bleeding manifestations rapidly disappear and the platelet count increases during treatment with high doses of corticosteroids but falls when the dose is reduced. Spontaneous bleeding may then recur when the dose is reduced further or remain under control with low doses of corticosteroids. The second type of response is that the bleeding manifestations rapidly disappear on high doses of steroids but there is no effect on the platelet count. Bleeding then recurs when the dose of corticosteroids is reduced. Other types of response such as the failure of bleeding manifestations to be controlled by corticosteroids or the maintenance of a platelet count at normal levels when corticosteroids have been stopped are uncommon in patients with chronic immune thrombocytopenia.

Splenectomy. Splenectomy is indicated in adults when chronic immune thrombocytopenia has been present for six months unless symptoms of bleeding can be controlled by acceptably low doses of corticosteroids. In general splenectomy should be delayed for one or two years or even longer in children with chronic thrombocytopenia. It is important to exclude other causes of thrombocytopenia and if possible to confirm that there is a significant reduction in platelet life span with platelet survival studies before splenectomy is carried out. The reported remission rate after splenectomy has varied from series to series and depends to a large extent on the method of selection. However it is probably about 70 per cent in adults and 90 per cent in children. Occasionally remission is followed by a relapse. Najean, in a comprehensive review of his experience with splenectomy in chronic immune thrombocytopenia, suggested that the following factors are of predictive value.

1. Platelet survival studies and surface scanning. Splenectomy is more likely to produce benefit if uptake of radioactive labelled platelets occurs predominantly in the spleen.

2. The age of the patient. Children with immune thrombocytopenia are more likely to respond to splenectomy.

3. Response to corticosteroids. Patients who show a rise in platelet count following the administration of corticosteroids are more likely to respond to splenectomy than those who show no effect with corticosteroids.

4. The immediate platelet count response to splenectomy. A long term remission is more likely when the immediate post-splenectomy platelet count is greater than 500,000 per cu. mm. On the other hand, contrary to common belief there appeared to be no relationship between the length of time that the patient had had thrombocytopenia and the chances of response to splenectomy. Other investigators, on the basis of experience with much smaller series, have questioned the value of surface scans in predicting the outcome of splenectomy, but Najean's data appears convincing.

Immunosuppressive Therapy. Treatment with immunosuppressive drugs such as azathioprine and cyclophosphamide has recently been reported to be of value in patients with chronic immune thrombocytopenic purpura. In most cases the patients treated with immunosuppressive therapy had failed to respond to a combination of corticosteroids and splenectomy. It is of interest that in some of these the favourable platelet count response to therapy was sustained for up to 6–12 months after the drug had been stopped. Immunosuppressive therapy may in future be used in selected patients with chronic immune thrombocytopenia before splenectomy is undertaken. However, at present these drugs are usually limited to patients who have failed to respond to splenectomy.

Congenital, Neonatal and Inherited Thrombocytopenias

Thrombocytopenia in the neonatal period may be inherited or acquired. Inherited disorders may not present clinically for months or even years after birth and they usually remain a problem throughout life.

Immune Neonatal Thrombocytopenia. This may occur in neonates of mothers who have idiopathic thrombocytopenia, or as an isoimmune phenomenon due to the passage of a platelet antigen, which is present in the foetus but lacking in the mother, across the placenta and inducing antibody formation in the mother. The antibody then passes across the placenta from mother to foetus and induces thrombocytopenia in the infant.

Infection. Thrombocytopenia may occur at birth or in the neonatal period as a result of infection. The mechanism of thrombocytopenia has not been fully elucidated. In some cases it may be due to a consumption coagulopathy while in others it may be due to depression of platelet production.

Drug Ingestion by the Mother. Neonatal thrombocytopenia may be produced as a result of passage of a drug across the placenta which has been administered to the mother. The drugs most commonly implicated are the thiazide drugs.

Giant Haemangioma. Thrombocytopenia due to giant haemangioma may be evident in the first few months of life or may first appear after a number of years. Although the haemangioma is usually clinically obvious it may occasionally be localized to an internal organ such as the liver and when this occurs it may produce a diagnostic problem. The thrombocytopenia is occasionally, but not invariably, associated with other evidence of a consumption coagulopathy.

Thrombocytopenia associated with Splenomegaly

Thrombocytopenia in patients with splenomegaly may be caused by a combination of factors. Excessive pooling of platelets in the spleen almost invariably occurs. This is usually associated with normal or moderately reduced platelet survival; occasionally platelet survival is severely reduced. In addition, in some diseases (e.g. leukaemia or myelofibrosis) thrombocytopenia is caused by a combination of increased splenic pooling and reduced platelet production.

The causes of hypersplenic thrombocytopenia include congestive splenomegaly, rheumatoid arthritis, Gaucher's disease, lymphoma and the chronic leukaemias. Bleeding is often mild and treatment is of the underlying disorder. Adrenocorticosteroids may be helpful during periods of severe haemorrhage. Platelet transfusions are only of limited value because the platelets rapidly pool in the enlarged spleen. Splenectomy will often produce some improvement in the platelet count, but the decision to perform splenectomy is as much influenced by the nature of the underlying disorder as by the severity of the bleeding manifestations.

QUALITATIVE PLATELET DISORDERS

The diagnosis of a qualitative disorder is made when a patient with abnormal bleeding has a prolonged bleeding time, a normal platelet count and an abnormality of either platelet aggregation or platelet factor 3 availability.

Primary Qualitative Platelet Defects

Thrombasthenia

This disorder was originally described by Glanzman in 1918 as a bleeding disorder associated with a normal platelet count and defective clot retraction. It is now recognized that thrombasthenia is a rare inherited disorder, transmitted as an autosomal recessive trait in which the major abnormality is a failure of the platelets to aggregate with adenosine diphosphate. The platelets undergo the usual morphological changes and release ADP when exposed to agents such as collagen and thrombin, but fail to aggregate with these agents, presumably because they are unable to aggregate with the released ADP. In addition, they fail to adhere to glass, show decreased platelet factor 3 availability and defective clot retraction and often have a low content intracellular fibrinogen.

Clinically the disorder is characterized by bruising and petechiae, excessive bleeding after cuts and abrasions, epistaxis and menorrhagia. The bleeding time is long and the tourniquet test is usually positive.

Thrombocytopathy.

Thrombocytopathy is a haemorrhagic disorder caused by a failure of platelet factor 3 availability. The disorder may be inherited or acquired. Characteristically the bleeding time is prolonged although sometimes the prolongation is only marginal, the platelet count is usually normal but may be moderately decreased in the inherited group and in some cases the platelets are abnormally large. The tourniquet test may be positive and the prothrombin consumption test and other tests of platelet factor 3 availability are abnormal. It has recently become apparent that many if not most of these patients also have a defect in ADP release when their platelets are exposed to aggregating agents such as collagen and adrenalin and it may be that both failure of ADP release and failure of availability of platelet factor 3 are due to a common defect.

The condition is relatively uncommon but more common than thrombasthenia. The patients complain of superficial bruising, petechiae and excessive bleeding after trauma. Those with the acquired disorder may present for the first time in adult life with abnormal postoperative bleeding.

Secondary Qualitative Platelet Defects

Combined defects of platelet aggregation, adhesion and platelet factor 3 availability may complicate a number of clinical disorders.

Renal Failure. Bleeding is a relatively common symptom of advanced renal failure and is usually manifested by epistaxis, bleeding into the skin and gastrointestinal tract, and by renal tract bleeding. A number of haemostatic defects have been described in renal failure but it is now recognized that the most important factor is an abnormality in platelet function which may or may not be associated with a mild to moderate thrombocytopenia. Characteristically patients with renal failure and abnormal bleeding have a prolonged Ivy bleeding time, an abnormal prothrombin consumption test, an abnormality of platelet adhesiveness and aggregation and a variable abnormality of other tests of platelet factor 3 availability. The factor responsible for bleeding and the abnormal tests appears to be dialyzable and the abnormalities in bleeding time and tests of platelet function may be improved by dialysis. It has been suggested that this dialyzable factor is guanidino-succinic which is a metabolite of urea.

Aspirin Ingestion. The ingestion of aspirin, even in small doses, has been shown to produce an abnormality in platelet function which is characterized by defective release of adenosine diphosphate when platelets are exposed to aggregating agents such as collagen, adrenalin and adenosine diphosphate itself. The defect in platelet function may be present for up to 7 days after a small therapeutic dose of aspirin. When aspirin is given to normal control subjects it leads to a slight prolongation of the bleeding time but this test usually remains within the normal range and there is no associated generalized bleeding tendency. Aspirin ingestion may, however, produce a mild generalized bleeding tendency if taken in high doses by normal subjects and it has been reported to aggravate post-tonsillectomy bleeding. In contrast to its effects in normal subjects aspirin may produce a marked prolongation of the bleeding time and aggravate the bleeding tendency in patients with established vascular, platelet or coagulation defects, even when it is given in therapeutic doses. It is therefore advisable to avoid the use of aspirin in patients with known bleeding disorders.

In addition to the effect on platelets aspirin is a weak vitamin K antagonist and is a common cause of superficial gastritis with gastric erosions.

Myeloproliferative Disorders. Bleeding associated with a high platelet count may occur in patients with myeloproliferative disorders. Bleeding is uncommon when the platelet count is less than

1,000,000 per cu. mm. but is relatively common and may be severe when the platelet count exceeds this figure. The underlying mechanism of bleeding in thrombocythemia is uncertain; however, some of these patients have been shown to have a defect in platelet function. When the platelet count is over 1,000,000 per cu. mm. and bleeding is present the manifestations may be controlled by decreasing the platelet count. In an emergency situation this can be achieved by platelet-phoresis or by treatment with uracil mustard or nitrogen mustard. In most cases, however, rapid reduction is not indicated and the platelet count can be reduced either by treatment with radioactive phosphorus or busulfan.

Defective platelet function associated with a normal platelet count has also been reported in patients with polycythaemia vera, myelofibrosis and leukaemia.

Hypergammaglobulinaemia. Bleeding due to hypergammaglobulinaemia is seen in patients with macroglobulinaemia, benign hypergammaglobulinaemic purpura and less commonly in multiple myeloma and in secondary hypergammaglobulinaemia. A number of factors may contribute to the bleeding tendency in these conditions but defective platelet aggregation, adhesion and platelet factor 3 availability have been described in these disorders. The defect in platelet function is presumed to be due to coating of platelets with gammaglobulin.

Cirrhosis. There are multiple causes for bleeding in patients with liver disease. Defective platelet function, both aggregation and platelet factor 3 availability, have been described but these defects are probably not important contributing factors to the overall bleeding tendency.

THE LIFE-LONG COAGULATION DEFECTS

Hereditary deficiencies of each of the 10 plasma clotting factors have been described. Although it has been generally considered in the past that these disorders are primarily deficiency states, caused by failure of synthesis, recent evidence suggests that in some cases of fibrinogen, factor VIII, factor IX and factor X deficiency the clotting factor is synthesized but is functionally abnormal.

In general there is a fairly good correlation between the intensity of the patient's symptoms and the severity of the coagulation deficiency as measured by in vitro tests. There are, however, exceptions. Patients with a factor XII deficiency are nearly always asymptomatic and those with factor VII or XI deficiencies often only have a mild bleeding tendency. All of the inherited coagulation deficiencies are uncommon and all except haemophilia (factor VIII deficiency) and Christmas disease (factor IX deficiency) are rare. Haemophilia occurs about five times more commonly than Christmas disease.

Haemophilia

This disorder is transmitted as a sex-linked recessive trait so that bleeding only occurs in affected males. Females carry the trait but do not, with rare exceptions, have a significant factor VIII deficiency. Various grades of severity of haemophilia are recognized on clinical and laboratory grounds. Severely affected patients usually have less than 1 per cent of factor VIII activity, the moderately affected have between 1 and 5 per cent factor VIII activity and the mildly affected have more than 5 per cent factor VIII activity. Bleeding manifestations in the severely affected are usually obvious in early childhood, are severe, and occur both spontaneously and after trauma. In contrast, mildly affected patients do not usually bleed spontaneously unless they have an underlying local lesion and they may have their first clinically significant bleed in adult life after operative trauma. Spontaneous bleeding characteristically affects joints and muscles and may lead to permanent crippling unless treated promptly and adequately. The severely affected patients may also bleed spontaneously into the kidney and into the retroperitoneal tissues. Haemophiliacs may not bleed excessively after superficial abrasions but deep injuries can produce dangerous bleeding which may continue for days. Large haematomata can produce pressure on nerves and vessels, and trivial injuries such as a bite on the tongue or cheek or a torn frenum can produce oropharyngeal bleeding with serious obstruction.

Treatment of Haemophilia

Recent advances in the treatment of haemophilia have markedly improved the outlook of this condition, even in the most severely affected patients. When considering therapy it is useful to divide haemophiliac bleeding into spontaneous and post-traumatic. As a general rule spontaneous bleeding can be controlled if the patient's factor VIII level is increased above 20 per cent of normal. On the other hand the factor VIII level should be increased to 50–60 per cent of normal in cases of post-traumatic bleeding or if major surgery is contemplated.

Treatment of Bleeding. The principles of treating bleeding episodes include (1) the application of local measures to the site of bleeding, (2) the correction of the coagulation defect by replacement therapy.

Local measures should never be considered as a substitute for replacement therapy but merely as an adjunct. It is much more difficult to treat haemorrhage once a large haematoma has developed than to prevent it or treat it at an early stage.

Local Measures. The affected part should be rested and protected from further trauma. It is important not to apply prolonged heavy pressure because this leads to necrosis and further bleeding. If the bleeding site is obscured by blood clot, as often occurs with mouth bleeding and particularly after tooth extraction, the clot should be gently removed after replacement therapy has been given and gauze soaked in bovine thrombin or Russell's viper venom applied to the area. Suture of wounds should be avoided if at all possible and if required should only be carried out after the patient has been given adequate replacement therapy.

Replacement Therapy. Factor VIII has an in vivo half life of approximately 10 hours. It is relatively unstable in vitro and disappears rapidly from stored blood. Therefore bank blood is unsatisfactory for replacement therapy. Factor VIII is available as fresh frozen plasma, as antihaemophiliac globulin concentrate (AHG concentrate) and as animal AHG concentrate.

Fresh frozen plasma is adequate for the treatment of spontaneous bleeding and for maintaining the factor VIII level at about 20 per cent during the healing period after surgery; however, this is inadequate for the control of bleeding if major surgery is contemplated; if serious post-traumatic bleeding has occurred; if spontaneous bleeding has produced serious pressure symptoms. In these circumstances human AHG concentrate should be used. The recent introduction of cryoprecipitate has made it possible to prepare human AHG concentrate in routine blood transfusion centres and has greatly simplified the treatment of serious haemophiliac bleeding. In severe haemophiliacs approximately 4–8 ml. per kg. of cyroprecipitate is required to elevate the factor VIII level to approximately 60 per cent of normal. Animal AHG concentrate is only indicated in the treatment of serious bleeding in a patient who has a factor VIII inhibitor. The value of animal AHG lies in the fact that it can be obtained in very high concentrations and that it is less susceptible to inactivation by some of the acquired inhibitors.

Christmas Disease

This disorder, like haemophilia, is transmitted as a sex-linked recessive trait. There is a similar relationship between the level of factor IX and the severity of bleeding. Factor IX is much more stable in vitro than factor VIII and has a longer survival in vivo.

Because of its stability in vitro, stored plasma can be used for replacement therapy. Factor IX concentrate is now also available.

THE ACQUIRED COAGULATION DISORDERS

The acquired coagulation disorders are seen more commonly in clinical practice than the inherited disorders. These disorders may be caused by defective synthesis, increased utilization or by inhibitors of coagulation factors. Unlike the inherited coagulation disorders, the acquired disorders are usually associated with multiple coagulation deficiencies. The underlying cause of the acquired coagulation disorder is often suggested by associated clinical circumstances, but occasionally bleeding may be the first manifestation. The diagnosis is often obvious after the screening tests, prothrombin time, thrombin time, partial thromboplastin time and platelet count have been performed.

The acquired coagulation disorders that will be considered here are vitamin K deficiency, liver disease, disseminated intravascular thrombosis (consumption coagulopathy) and massive transfusion syndrome. Primary pathological fibrinolysis will be discussed in the section on fibrinolysis.

Vitamin K Deficiency

Vitamin K is a fat-soluble vitamin which is necessary for hepatic synthesis of factors II, VII, IX and X. Vitamin K is obtained in part from food, especially green vegetables, and in part from synthesis by bacterial flora in the bowel. Either source can compensate for the deficiency of the other. It appears unlikely that a vitamin K deficiency severe enough to produce a haemorrhagic disorder is ever caused by simple dietary deficiency. Clinically significant vitamin K deficiency occurs most commonly in disorders which impair fat absorption; these include obstructive jaundice, idiopathic steatorrhoea, localized small bowel disease and pancreatic disease. In almost all cases the underlying disorder is clinically evident but on rare occasions bleeding, particularly postoperative bleeding, may be the presenting manifestation of these disorders.

Haemorrhagic Disease of the Newborn

This disorder, which occurs in the first few days of life, is due to a defect in the synthesis of vitamin K dependent clotting factors. It results from a combination of reduced stores of vitamin K, functional immaturity of the liver, and lack of bacterial synthesis of vitamin K. It may also occur as a consequence of the administration of certain drugs to the mother; these include oral anticoagulants, large doses of aspirin and anticonvulsant drugs.

The principles of treatment of vitamin K deficiency include correction of the cause of the disorder (e.g., biliary obstruction by surgery, or idiopathic steatorrhoea by a gluten-free diet) administration of vitamin K and replacement therapy by transfusion if bleeding is severe. Haemorrhagic disease of the newborn is treated in most centres with prophylactic vitamin K_1 given to the infant at birth.

Liver Disease

A mild haemorrhagic defect is not uncommonly seen in patients with liver disease. Severe bleeding is relatively uncommon but may occur under the following circumstances.

(1) When there is associated trauma, e.g. liver biopsy, (2) when there is a local lesion, e.g. oesophageal varices or peptic ulcer, (3) in patients with cirrhosis during and after porta-caval shunt operations, (4) in acute fulminating hepatitis or in the terminal stages of cirrhosis. In most cases of bleeding due to liver disease the patient is jaundiced and the underlying disorder is clinically obvious. However, the bleeding may occasionally be the presenting manifestation of anicteric liver disease.

Theoretically, a number of factors could contribute to the haemostatic defect in liver disease. These include (1) defective synthesis of clotting factors, (2) thrombocytopenia, (3) increased fibrinolytic activity, (4) defective platelet function and (5) consumption coagulopathy. Although the contribution of each of these factors differs in different clinical circumstances, defective synthesis is usually the most important. When this is the main factor both the prothrombin time and the partial thromboplastin time are prolonged and the defect is not completely reversed by the administration of vitamin K.

1. *Defective Synthesis of Coagulation Factors.* The coagulation factors I (fibrinogen), II (prothrombin), V, VII, IX and X are synthesized in the liver. The synthesis of the vitamin K dependent clotting factors II, VII, IX and X are first to be affected in liver disease; with more severe disease there is depression of factor V and in very severe liver disease there is hypofibrinogenaemia. The defective synthesis of the vitamin K dependent clotting factors may be partly due to malabsorption of vitamin K which occurs in some patients with parenchymatous liver disease as a result of impairment of bile salt synthesis.

2. *Thrombocytopenia.* Thrombocytopenia in liver disease is usually seen in patients with portal hypertension and congestive splenomegaly and is due to increased splenic pooling, often with an

associated mild to moderate reduction in platelet survival. Thrombocytopenia may also occur in patients with acute alcoholic liver disease and in patients with fulminating hepatitis. Both depression of platelet production and a reduction in platelet survival have been reported in patients with alcoholic liver disease and it is likely that the thrombocytopenia in these patients is due to a combination of these two factors. The pathogenesis of thrombocytopenia in fulminating hepatitis is uncertain but it may be due to consumption coagulopathy (see below).

3. *Increased Fibrinolytic Activity.* The liver is the site of the inactivation and clearance of plasminogen activator and the site of synthesis of the antiplasmins. Increased fibrinolytic activity may therefore occur in liver disease as a result of delayed inactivation of plasminogen activator and decreased levels of circulating antiplasmins. In practice increased fibrinolytic activity is not an important contributing factor to bleeding in liver disease except in patients with cirrhosis when they are subjected to surgery, particularly porta-caval shunt surgery.

4. *Defective Platelet Function.* Defective platelet factor 3 availability and decreased platelet adhesiveness have been reported in patients with cirrhosis but it is unlikely to be a significant contributing factor to bleeding in liver disease.

5. *Consumption Coagulopathy.* The liver is an important site of inactivation of thrombin and other activated clotting factors. It is also a site of clearance of insoluble fibrin monomer complexes. Theoretically, impairment of clearance of these 'clot promoting factors' could lead to consumption coagulopathy. However, in practice consumption coagulopathy appears to be an important contributing factor to the coagulation defect only in fulminant liver disease or following hepatic transplantation.

Clinical Considerations

Patients with acute infectious hepatitis do not usually bleed abnormally and often have a mild or insignificant coagulation defect even though other tests of liver function are abnormal. In contrast, patients with severe acute hepatitis, either infective or drug induced, and patients with acute liver damage due to hepatic congestion, hypotension or septicaemia, usually have a prolonged one-stage prothrombin time and a long activated partial thromboplastin time which may or may not be associated with a significant bleeding tendency. As a rule, these abnormal screening tests are not corrected by vitamin K_1. Patients with acute fulminating hepatitis usually have a marked coagulation defect, often with a severe factor V deficiency, hypofibrinogenaemia and sometimes with severe thrombocytopenia. Diffuse bleeding from skin, mucous membranes and gastrointestinal tract and large hematomata frequently occur.

Patients with chronic hepatitis often have only a mild to moderate coagulation defect which is manifested as a prolonged prothrombin time and mild to moderate thrombocytopenia. However, even the mild defect may aggravate bleeding from a local lesion, such as oesophageal varices or a peptic ulcer, or it may predispose to surgical and post-surgical bleeding.

Prophylaxis and Treatment

The nature and severity of the haemostatic defect should be assessed in all patients with liver disease before liver biopsy or surgery is contemplated. The defect should be investigated by performing a prothrombin time, an activated partial thromboplastin time, a bleeding time and a platelet count. If the prothrombin time is less than 60 per cent, the partial thromboplastin time prolonged, the platelet count less than 100,000 per cu. mm. and the bleeding time prolonged, an attempt should be made to correct the defect before liver biopsy or surgery is performed.

Specific Treatment

Vitamin K. A slow response may be obtained after the intravenous administration of 50 mg. of vitamin K_1 for 4–5 days.

Replacement Therapy. A number of different blood products are available for replacement therapy. Fresh frozen plasma contains factor V as well as the vitamin K dependent clotting factor but is of limited value because large volumes are required to produce a significant improvement in the coagulation defect. Concentrates containing factors II, VII, IX and X are now available and should prove useful for the treatment of the coagulation defect of liver disease. Platelet-rich plasma or platelet concentrates can be used to treat patients with severe thrombocytopenia but recovery of transfused platelets is often poor because the platelets are rapidly sequestered in the enlarged spleen. If increased fibrinolytic activity is demonstrated by laboratory tests epsilon-amino-caproic acid (EACA) should be administered intravenously in a dose of 5 g. in the first hour and 1 g. per hour thereafter until bleeding has stopped.

Haemorrhage Following Massive Transfusion of Stored Blood

Thrombocytopenia and deficiencies of factors V and VIII may occur when a patient's blood volume is replaced by large amounts of stored blood. This is because platelets and these clotting factors are unstable in blood which is stored at 4°C. Thrombocytopenia regularly occurs when more than 10 units (5,000 ml.) of stored blood is administered over a 48 hour period. The platelets return to normal approximately 3–6 days after transfusion. The levels of factors V and VIII are variably depressed and usually contribute less to the overall haemostatic defect than thrombocytopenia. The circumstances requiring blood transfusion are important. The severity of the haemostatic defect is more marked when the capacity to produce platelets or clotting factors is impaired or when the rate of consumption of the platelets and clotting factors is increased. Thus transfusion with large volumes of stored blood is most likely to aggravate bleeding (1) in mild haemophiliacs who bleed excessively during or after surgery, (2) in patients with liver disease with bleeding oesophageal varices or with serious postoperative bleeding and (3) in consumption coagulopathy states, particularly when they complicate surgery or childbirth.

Citrate overdosage with consequent hypocalcaemia may occur as a rare complication of massive blood transfusion. Although in most patients the heart is affected by hypocalcaemia before the coagulation process, abnormal in vitro clotting tests corrected by the addition of extra calcium has been reported in patients who have bled abnormally after transfusion with large volumes of blood. Patients with liver disease are especially vulnerable to the hypocalcaemic effect of transfusion with citrated blood because citrate is normally metabolized in the liver.

Treatment

The haemostatic defect produced by large volumes of stored blood can be prevented or minimized by including fresh blood when large volumes of blood are required rapidly. As a rule, 2 units of fresh blood or blood that is less than 12–24 hours old should be given with every 10 units of blood that is rapidly transfused. In addition, hypocalcaemia can be prevented by giving calcium gluconate, 10 ml. of a 10 per cent solution with every 2–4 units of citrated blood. Bleeding caused by transfusion with large volumes of bank blood is treated with fresh blood, platelet transfusion or fresh frozen plasma.

Consumption Coagulopathy (Disseminated Intravascular Thrombosis, Defibrination Syndrome)

Consumption coagulopathy is a disorder in which diffuse thrombosis in the microcirculation causes a haemostatic defect which results from the utilization of clotting factors and platelets in the thrombotic process. Consumption coagulopathy may complicate a variety of clinical conditions but serious bleeding occurs most frequently after surgery or childbirth. Disseminated intravascular thrombosis may be produced by any one of three interrelated factors. (1) The sudden release or entry into the blood stream of tissue factors which act as coagulants. This occurs following trauma, e.g. obstetrical accidents or surgical trauma, during the acute haemolytic episodes or when there is breakdown of neoplastic tissue. (2) The appearance of factors in the blood stream which induce platelet aggregation. Such factors include endotoxin, which is released in gram negative septicaemia; ADP, which is released during intravascular haemolysis; and circulating viruses, bacteria and immune complexes, which are phagocytosed by platelets. (3) When there is extensive endothelial damage. This occurs in patients subjected to severe trauma or burns, and in patients with vasculitis and purpura fulminans.

Experimental Induction of Disseminated Intravascular Thrombosis.

The mechanism and consequences of disseminated intravascular thrombosis can best be understood by considering the changes which occur during the experimental induction of the process. Disseminated intravascular thrombosis can be produced experimentally by infusing thrombin, tissue extracts, endotoxin, or red cell lysate into experimental animals. These substances either initiate the clotting process, induce platelet aggregation or do both. When thrombin or tissue extract is infused there is initial shortening of the coagulation time, but as the process continues the blood becomes incoagulable because platelets, fibrinogen, prothrombin and factors V and VIII are consumed during the coagulation process. The fibrin and platelet aggregates which are formed are deposited diffusely throughout the microcirculation. Widespread intravascular thrombi can usually be demonstrated in animals soon after the process is induced. However these deposits are no longer evident hours or days after their induction because they are digested by local fibrinolytic mechanisms. This increase in local fibrinolytic activity occurs as a result of the release of tissue activator from endothelial cells at the site of disseminated intravascular thrombosis; the stimulus to this release is thought to be the anoxia produced by the microthrombi. If the fibrinolytic process is blocked by an inhibitor such as epsilon-amino-caproic acid, widespread thrombosis with infarction of many organs may occur, a process which resembles the generalized Schwartzman reaction. This observation suggests that the activation of fibrinolysis locally may be an important protective mechanism. The local breakdown of fibrin results in the formation of fibrin split products which circulate in the blood stream and may contribute to the coagulation defect. The diagnostic significance and mechanism of action of fibrin split products is discussed in more detail in the section on fibrinolysis.

Manifestations of Consumption Coagulopathy

1. *Laboratory defect only.* In the majority of patients the process of disseminated intravascular thrombosis produces no symptoms, but evidence of a coagulation defect can be demonstrated by laboratory tests.

2. *Bleeding.* Bleeding may occur as a consequence of consumption of platelets and labile coagulation factors; this is particularly severe when associated with surgical trauma or childbirth.

3. *Vessel Obstruction.* Disseminated intravascular thrombosis may produce (a) organ damage due to ischaemia, (b) red cell fragmentation due to mechanical trauma and (c) acute pulmonary hypertension due to obstruction to pulmonary vasculature.

Organ Damage. The kidney is commonly involved in severe cases of disseminated intravascular thrombosis. Renal involvement is usually manifested as proteinuria, haematuria and oliguric renal failure. There may also be evidence of ischaemic damage to brain, liver and heart.

Red Cell Fragmentation. Red cells may be markedly distorted as they are forced through vessels which are partly blocked with fibrin deposits. This leads to a haemolytic anaemia characterized by marked red cell fragmentation and known as microangiopathic haemolytic anaemia.

Pulmonary Vascular Obstruction. The pulmonary vascular bed is able to tolerate a considerable degree of obstruction without significant elevation of pulmonary arterial pressure. Acute cor pulmonale, due to obstruction of the pulmonary microcirculation, and perhaps contributed to by pulmonary vascular spasm, which occurs as a consequence of microthrombosis, occurs in amniotic fluid embolism and may be an important manifestation of disseminated intravascular thrombosis complicating gram negative septicaemia.

4. *Shock.* Shock may occur as a complication of disseminated intravascular thrombosis. This is a serious consequence and it is sometimes difficult to determine whether the shocked state is due to the underlying disorder, such as septicaemia, burns or trauma, due to the effects of severe blood loss, or whether it is due to the process of disseminated intravascular thrombosis itself.

Laboratory Features

The diagnosis of consumption coagulopathy is confirmed by demonstrating evidence of depletion of platelets and labile clotting factors. Thus there may be hypofibrinogenaemia, thrombocytopenia and a decreased level of prothrombin, factor V and factor VIII. In addition, there is usually an increased level of circulating fibrin split products which occurs as a consequence of local fibrinolytic activity. These abnormalities are reflected by the presence of a prolonged thrombin time, prothrombin time, partial thromboplastin time, by thrombocytopenia, and by the presence of fibrin split products in the serum. It should be noted that not all of the coagulation factors which are normally consumed during coagulation are necessarily depressed in individual patients with a consumption coagulopathy state.

Aetiology. Disseminated intravascular thrombosis may complicate a number of clinical disorders; these are summarized in Table 5. In some of these conditions, e.g. post-surgical and post partum states, bleeding is the most significant manifestation and is sometimes catastrophic. In others, such as thrombotic thrombocytopenic purpura, there may be a combination of renal damage, red cell damage and haemorrhagic manifestations, while in patients with Gram negative septicaemia the first manifestation of disseminated intravascular thrombosis may be shock.

Treatment of Consumption Coagulopathy

The principles of treatment are: (1) eliminate the precipitating factor if possible, (2) replacement of coagulation factors and platelets if these are depleted and there is overt or threatened bleeding and (3) interrupt the thrombotic process with heparin, particularly if there is evidence of organ damage or shock.

1. *Eliminate the precipitating factor.* The precipitating cause is usually self-limiting in cases of disseminated intravascular thrombosis which complicate surgery and haemolytic transfusion reactions. Underlying causes requiring specific treatment include septicaemia, carcinoma of the prostate, snake bite, foetal death in utero, acute leukaemia and giant haemangioma.

2. *Replacement of coagulation factors and platelets.* Replacement therapy should be used in patients with evidence of significant depletion of coagulation factors and platelets who show evidence of overt bleeding or are in danger of serious bleeding (e.g. post-operative or post partum). On the other hand, replacement therapy should be used with caution and probably in association with heparin

therapy if the manifestations of the disseminated intravascular thrombotic state are those of organ or tissue damage or shock.

Patients requiring replacement therapy should be treated with fresh blood, both to replace blood loss and to replace coagulation factors and platelets. Alternatively platelet-rich plasma, platelet

TABLE 5

Causes of the disseminated intravascular thrombosis

Acute

Obstetrical accidents
- (a) abruptio placentae
- (b) aminotic fluid embolism
- (c) abortion

Surgery, especially of the heart and lung
Haemolytic transfusion reaction
Septicaemia, especially gram-negative but also gram-positive
Viraemia
Pulmonary embolism
Fat embolism
Snake bite
Drug reactions
Burns

Sub-acute or chronic

Carcinoma
Acute leukaemia
Foetal death in utero
Thrombotic thrombocytopenic purpura
Purpura fulminans
Giant haemangioma
Vasculitis
Haemolytic uraemic syndrome

concentrates, fresh frozen plasma, or fibrinogen may be preferable, depending on the availability of these blood products and on the factors which are depressed. Stored blood should be avoided if possible because it not only lacks platelets but is also relatively deficient in factors V and VIII. If bleeding is severe and there is a delay in obtaining fresh blood, treatment should be with fresh frozen plasma. If the latter is not available, fibrinogen should be given since many commercial fibrinogen preparations not only contain fibrinogen but also contain factor VIII. However, it should be noted that there is a significant incidence of hepatitis following fibrinogen administration.

3. *Inhibition of the clotting process with heparin.* Treatment with heparin is rarely required in disseminated intravascular thrombotic states which complicate abruptio placentae or surgery. However, this form of treatment is indicated in addition to replacement therapy when there is evidence that the intravascular thrombosis is causing damage to vital organs, such as kidney, liver, brain or heart; or if there is evidence of significant micro-angiopathic haemolytic anaemia; if the patient is shocked or when there is evidence that the consumption coagulopathy is continuing and producing bleeding despite adequate replacement therapy.

Treatment with heparin is potentially dangerous and should be carefully monitored. Patients with hepatic or renal insufficiency or those in circulatory failure are often sensitive to heparin and should be treated initially with a single intravenous dose of heparin of 0·5 to 1 mg. (50–100 units) per kg., and the effect of treatment monitored by the activated partial thromboplastin time. Further treatment with heparin may not be necessary if the underlying cause of the disseminated intravascular thrombosis is self-limiting or if it is brought under control (e.g. by antibiotics in patients with septicaemia). However, if the process continues, as evidenced by the clinical state and the results of laboratory tests (e.g. persisting thrombocytopenia, persisting prolongation of the thrombin time, prothrombin time and partial thromboplastin time in the presence of added protamine), the patient should be treated with heparin given by continuous intravenous infusion.

The required dose of heparin is usually less than that necessary to treat patients with overt thrombosis, although occasionally the requirement may be extremely high, especially in patients with microangiopathic haemolytic anaemia (haemolytic uraemic syndrome, purpura fulminans, thrombotic thrombocytopenic purpura, disseminated carcinoma). When heparin is given by continuous intravenous infusion it should be monitored to prolong the activated partial thromboplastin time by 50–100 per cent of the normal value, i.e. by 20–40 seconds.

If bleeding continues in spite of adequate replacement therapy and heparin administration, tests of fibrinolytic activity should be repeated and if there is evidence of increased fibrinolytic activity, the inhibitor epsilon-amino-caproic acid should be given intravenously in addition to heparin and replacement therapy. However, EACA should not be given unless there is definite evidence of systemic fibrinolytic activity as this may aggravate the thrombotic tendency.

THE FIBRINOLYTIC SYSTEM

The fibrinolytic system will be considered under the following headings:

1. Physiological fibrinolysis
2. Pathological fibrinolysis
3. Impaired fibrinolytic activity
4. Fibrinolytic therapy.

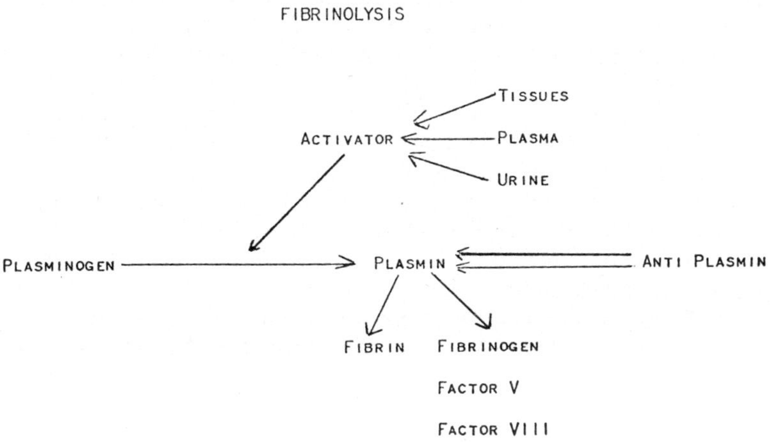

FIG. 36 Scheme of fibrinolysis

Physiological fibrinolysis

A simplified scheme of physiological fibrinolysis is shown in Fig. 36. Plasminogen, a beta globulin, is a pro-enzyme which is normally present in the blood stream and body fluids and is converted into the active enzyme plasmin by plasminogen activators. Plasmin digests fibrin, which is the desired physiological effect; in addition, it digests certain clotting factors including fibrinogen, factor V and factor VIII. Circulating plasmin is rapidly inactivated by antiplasmins which are present in the blood stream in about 10 times the concentration of plasminogen. This high level of antiplasmin protects the plasma clotting factors from digestion by plasmin.

The plasminogen activators are present in tissues, plasma and in urine. *Tissue activator* is present in endothelial cells where it exists in a readily diffusible form, and in the particulate fraction of cells where it is less available. The endothelial activator is released into the blood stream by a number of stimuli. These include anoxia, vaso-active agents such as adrenaline, hyperpyrexia and exercise. The tissue activator derived from the particulate fraction does not normally diffuse into the blood stream but may be released following extensive trauma. The *plasma activator* is thought to be released tissue activator. This is labile and is inactivated by circulating inhibitors (which are as yet poorly characterized) and by the liver. For this reason enhanced fibrinolytic activity is sometimes seen in patients with chronic liver disease. The *urinary activator* is known as urokinase. This is antigenically distinct from tissue activator and plasma activator; it is synthesized in the kidney and excreted in the urine where it may be important in maintaining the patency of the renal tract.

The fibrinolytic system is stimulated during blood coagulation. This is because both active factor XII and thrombin have a weak activating effect on plasminogen, converting it to plasmin.

When a thrombus or a haemostatic plug forms, plasminogen is trapped in the fibrin mesh. Diffusible tissue activator is released from the endothelial cells and converts plasminogen to plasmin close to its substrate fibrin. The fibrin is then hydrolyzed into soluble split products and the thrombus or haemostatic plug undergoes dissolution. Any plasmin that escapes from the thrombus into the blood stream is rapidly inactivated by antiplasmins which protect the circulating clotting factors from digestion by plasmin.

Pathological Fibrinolysis

In certain conditions, known as pathological fibrinolytic states, large concentrations of plasminogen activator are released into the blood stream and may induce a bleeding tendency. Tissue activator may be released into the blood stream in large amounts as a result of extensive trauma to tissues, such as follows burns, surgery, childbirth, or in patients with neoplasms as a result of breakdown of the tumour tissue. In addition, in chronic liver disease large amounts of activator may persist in the blood stream following mild stimuli because there is impaired inactivation of plasminogen activator.

A number of factors contribute to the haemostatic defect in pathological fibrinolytic states. These include: (1) Digestion of fibrin which is present in haemostatic plugs. (2) Interference with normal fibrin clot formation by the presence of split products of fibrinogen or fibrin digestion. (3) Digestion of fibrinogen, factor V and factor VIII by circulating plasmin. Of these three, digestion of fibrin in haemostatic plugs appears to be the most important and digestion of fibrinogen factor V and factor VIII the least important.

Impaired Fibrinolysis

The large majority of patients who develop thrombosis have no demonstrable impairment of fibrinolytic activity. However, high levels of anti-activators and antiplasmins have been described in a small percentage of patients with thrombotic tendencies. In some cases this has been familial and in others it has been sporadic. In addition, high levels of anti-activators have been described in patients with carcinoma and in patients following renal transplantation, particularly during rejection. This may be of some significance, since thrombosis is a recognized complication of carcinoma and since small vessel thrombosis has been shown to occur during the rejection phenomenon and is thought to be an important contributing factor to the pathology of rejection. Impaired fibrinolytic activity due to poor release of activator has also been described in obesity. Again this may be of some importance since it is known that obese individuals are particularly susceptible to postoperative and post partum thrombosis. Finally, it has been shown that leg veins have less available activator than the upper limb veins and that the release of activator from leg veins is impaired in some patients who develop postoperative venous thrombosis. It is possible therefore that impaired local fibrinolytic activity may be an important contributing factor to the development of venous thrombosis in the postoperative period.

Fibrinolytic Therapy (Thrombolytic Therapy)

The fibrinolytic enzymes have now been purified and used in the treatment of thrombosis. There is now good experimental and clinical evidence that fibrinolytic agents can produce dissolution of thrombi in veins and arteries and dissolution of emboli in pulmonary arteries. To date, the most effective thrombolytic agents have been the activators of plasminogen, streptokinase and urokinase. Streptokinase is prepared from cell-free filtrates of streptococci and is antigenic to man. Urokinase is prepared from human urine and has the advantage of being non-antigenic, but it is relatively unavailable and very expensive.

Most clinical experience has been obtained with streptokinase, which is now available in a highly purified form and which no longer produces the troublesome allergic reactions which complicated the earlier preparations of streptokinase. The aim of thrombolytic therapy, with either streptokinase or urokinase, is to deliver the plasminogen activator into the blood stream where it diffuses into the thrombus and converts plasminogen to plasmin and hence produces thrombus dissolution.

As might be expected from the foregoing discussion, the major complication of thrombolytic therapy is bleeding. Local bleeding may occur in patients who have undergone recent surgery or in patients with a local lesion, such as peptic ulcer, because of lysis of fibrin in the wounds or haemostatic plugs. A generalized bleeding tendency may result if treatment is poorly controlled and if a prolonged hyperplasminaemic state is obtained with the infusion of activator. This generalized bleeding tendency results from the presence of circulating fibrinogen and fibrin breakdown products and from deficiencies of fibrinogen, factor V and factor VIII as a result of plasmin digestion. Thrombolytic therapy is contraindicated (1) in cerebrovascular thrombosis because cerebrovascular thrombosis is often associated with a haemorrhagic infarct, (2) in patients with local lesions (e.g., peptic ulcer), (3) in the early postoperative period, and (4) if there is a generalized haemostatic defect.

Induction of Increased Fibrinolytic Activity by Pharmacological Means

A number of drugs and agents are able to induce a moderate increase in fibrinolytic activity. These include adrenaline, nicotinic acid, drugs which interfere with carbohydrate metabolism and steroid hormones. Of these drugs the biguanides and steroid hormones have proved most promising. Resistance to the fibrinolytic effects of these agents occurs when they are used alone. However, a combination of the biguanides (either metformin or phenformin) with the steroid ethyloestrenol have been shown to produce a sustained, moderate increase in fibrinolytic activity. This approach might prove useful in the management of thrombo-embolic disease.

Selected Bibliography

BIGGS, R. and MacFARLANE, R. G. (1962) *Human Blood Coagulation and its Disorders.* 3rd Ed. Blackwell, Oxford.

HARDISTY, R. M. and INGRAM, G. I. C. (1972) Bleeding Disorders. *Investigation and Management.* 2nd Ed. Blackwell, Oxford.

MARCUS, A. J. and ZUCKER, M. B. (1965) *The Physiology of Blood Platelets.* Grune and Stratton, New York.

POLLER, L. (Editor) (1969) *Recent Advances in Blood Coagulation.* Churchill, London.

RATNOFF, O. D. (1968) *Treatment of Haemorrhagic Disorders.* Harper and Row, London.

SPAET, T. H. (1966) Haemostatic Homeostasis. *Blood* 28, 112.

XV

Computer-Assisted Medicine

INTRODUCTION

A NEW FORM OF MACHINE POWER

Although computers are machines, much the same as motor cars and refrigerators are machines, there is one important difference: no simple answer exists to the question 'What do they do?' A good analogy is electricity, whose function is likewise undifferentiated. In order to answer the question in this case one might adopt one of two extreme forms of answer. One is to say that electricity by itself can do absolutely nothing; it is only potentially useful; is only when somebody has decided in precise terms what they want to do with it and has then proceeded to build a corresponding electrical apparatus that electricity becomes useful. The other alternative is to say that there is no limit to the number of things that electricity can do; this is also a true statement. The limit at any given stage is only set by man's ingenuity to think up new forms of electrical apparatus that will enable new uses to be made of it.

In a similar sense the same situation is true of computer power. One view is to say that by itself it can do absolutely nothing, which is quite true. The other view, particularly evident in the press and elsewhere over the last twenty years, is that there is no limit to the number of things that computer power can do—which is also a true statement. In order to realize computer power it is only necessary to decide precisely what one wants to do with it and then to design and construct a computer program which is the counterpart of an electrical apparatus. Once the computer program exists, a computer can perform the particular task required.

Beyond all this, however, there is an even more fundamental difference between computing machines and the many thousands of machines that are a familiar part of our lives. In order to see precisely what this difference is it is useful in the first instance to review some of the characteristics of familiar machines. Machines throughout the ages, and particularly during the past 200 years since the advent of automatic power in the form of the steam engine, have largely been used to *deploy muscle power more effectively*: typewriter plus muscle is more effective than muscle alone; bicycle plus muscle is more effective than muscle alone, and so on. In both these cases, and in many more that might be mentioned, the machine actually *assists* muscle power, but there are a correspondingly large number of machines which actually *replace* muscle power, as for example the automatic dishwasher, the thermostat, and so on. So familiar are machines that either assist or replace muscle power that it does not upset human vanity to acknowledge that machines can now do what only humans could previously do. Even so, machines that merely assist or replace human muscle, that is, which only enable us to do what we could do before (perhaps a little more cheaply, quickly and precisely) are in many ways the least important consequence of machine power. The main feature of machine power (which has changed the manner and organization of our whole existence in the past 200 years) is its ability to extend or augment human muscle power, to enable tasks to be accomplished which no amount of muscle power alone, however combined, could possibly achieve at all. Obvious examples are the aero engine, which can lift tens of tons and propel it at hundreds of knots; or the button-making, screw-making, knife-making machine systems that turn out thousands of items an hour cheaply and precisely; or the distillation columns, tyre extruders or automatic baking ovens that process material by the ton. Take away all this and much else that machine systems do for us, and no amount of human muscle could possibly make up for it. The main impact of machine power therefore has been to extend human capability in terms of what can be physically accomplished, and as a direct consequence, to alter the basic character of how man's physical activity is organized and employed.

Before machine power it will be recalled that productive enterprise depended entirely on the manual craftsman. He it was in whom both design and making were inextricably interwoven. Ask him to spell out precisely how he achieved his results and he could not say other than that it was the product of a long apprenticeship and a lifetime's experience, and that if another wished to acquire his skills he too would have to submit himself to the same long apprenticeship and experience. (Much the same, of course, is true of medicine today, but of that more in due course.) The key change from the regime of the manual craftsman induced by machine power is the *separation of design and making*: those with any creative abilities to design do, and those who cannot (machine-assisted) make. What the designers produce are not goods but jigs and tools and machine systems, and when these exist, human operators, usually without any great skill or training, produce items by the hundred and thousand. A characteristic feature therefor of the system is that it makes *the largely unskilled and largely untrained* (indeed in many cases unskillable and untrainable) *physically productive*. Moreover, the goods they produce are not produced according to some personal subjective standard as were those of the manual craftsman, but according to a known specification. And when a known specification exists for anything it is possible for others remote in time and place to add their own distinctive contributions. For example, the modern typewriter, the modern refrigerator and the modern radio, or the modern anything, represent not one man's skills and ideas but the contributions of many. And thus it is that the standard of goods produced by largely unskilled operators (machine-assisted) corresponds in a very real sense to the *aggregate* knowledge and experience of many. An important feature of machine power therefore is that it enables us to consolidate knowledge and experience which would otherwise be lost, as it was in the age of the manual craftsman and as it is today in medical practice. Another important feature about machines that must be mentioned before we come to address ourselves to the corresponding features of computers, is the way their objective is achieved. Man did not have to invent muscle to exceed human physical performance. It all started with the incredibly simple action of the steam engine, consisting essentially of a reciprocating piston moving up and down a cylinder, and it is interesting to contemplate a conversation that might well have taken place between James Watt and the manual craftsman:

Watt: 'I have here a machine a thousand times more powerful than human muscle which will eventually completely displace the need for your skills.'

Craftsman (singularly unimpressed): 'My dear James, you may well have a device there a thousand times more powerful than human muscle, but until you show me something with the dexterity and subtlety of these fingers coupled with a lifetime's experience, then your machine is hardly likely to displace the needs for my skills. *No machine can possibly do what I do*!'

Quite true: no machine has ever successfully simulated the behaviour of a manual craftsman. But equally, quite wrong: the point is that machines which exceed human physical performance do not do so by emulating human physical function. No machine has ever done what a manual craftsman did *the way he did it*. In order to get a machine to make tumblers, ash trays or whatever, the last thing one tries to do is to mimic the motions of the human craftsman. Instead one *analyzes* the object to be produced to see what *system* of physical movements would effect it, and when the 'systems analysis' (design) is complete, one then gets an engineer to 'program' the system of movements using basic machine operations: levers, gears, linkages, differentials and so on. When he has finished and when the machine system exists then, as is well-known, it can *in its own way* greatly exceed human performance. Given that machine power is the largest single determinant of the way in which we now live then not surprisingly engineering is by far and away the biggest single activity of the advanced industrial nations. Before machine power it barely existed.

Now the point of this long preamble about machine power is this: what has been achieved and accepted in relation to machine power and muscle can now (is now) be achieved, if less readily accepted, in relation to computer power and cerebral activity. Whereas almost all machines prior to the computer could be classed as *energy machines*, the computer, though still very much a machine, is uniquely different in that it is essentially an *information machine*. Before the computer all trained cerebral activity was carried out by what might be called *mental craftsmen* (professional and white collar workers who comprise more than one half of the entire work force): the persons in whom both knowing what to do and doing it is inextricably interwoven. Ask them how they do it and generally speaking they cannot say, other than that it is art, hunch, feel and intuition, generated by a thorough apprenticeship and a lifelong's experience. Their minds in exercising a particular cerebral skill work as spontaneously towards effecting the 'right' decisions and actions as a manual craftsman's hands work towards achieving a particular product. Their standards are personal. It is a feature of human physical and cerebral skills that once acquired, the rationale of why and how has long since been forgotten, if indeed it was ever consciously formulated.

The key feature of the computer age is *the separation of knowing what to do and doing it*. Those who can design management control and decision-making information systems will; those who cannot will (computer-assisted) provide the services: calculational and clerical, of course, but also surveillance, assessment, evaluation, decision-making and control. Designing procedures, thinking what to do, will become a full-time professional activity; such an activity will not directly produce any service at all. What the designers produce will be information systems expressed in the form of computer programs (the counterpart of jigs and tools), and once these 'cerebral jigs' exist (as they already do for radiation treatment planning, dietetic analysis, cardiovascular monitoring, and so on) then people without any cerebral skill at doing these things, people very often without the ability to acquire such skills (namely the computer operators), will with the assistance of computers perform the services quickly, cheaply and accurately. Computer power, in other words, makes the *cerebrally unskilled cerebrally productive*. The services that can be supplied will no longer be directly related to the cerebral skills available, but to the number of suitably programmed computer systems. Furthermore, the standard of these services (calculational, clerical, analytical, diagnostic) provided by computer-assisted operators will conform to a *known specification* rather than their personal subjective best. This in turn will enable others remote in time and place to add their own improvements, so that the standards of performance of the operators will approximate to the best that is known at any given time; they will always be improving and not fluctuating with the life and death cycle as do those of the single individual.

But most revealing of all is the way it is achieved. It is no more necessary to invent cerebral activity to exceed human cerebral performance than it was necessary to invent muscle to exceed human physical performance; indeed, a computer is as simple a device in relation to the cerebral cortex as the steam engine is to human muscle. Mental craftsmen with a lifetime's experience, able to virtually intuit decisions and judgements, can be forgiven therefore for exclaiming, 'No machine can possibly do what I do!' Quite true, but equally quite wrong. In order to get a machine to extract relevant information, to monitor the occurrence of extrasystoles or arrythmias, to cytologically screen a cervical smear, to produce a differential diagnosis, to suggest an appropriate drug, the last thing one tries to do is mimic the cerebral actions of the mental craftsman (even if we knew what they were). Instead one *analyzes* the *system* of information (rules, criteria, and so on) that will enable a consistently correct result to be reached, and when this *systems analysis* is complete it can be programmed into the basic machine operations of the computer, a process which is facilitated by using specially structured computer languages such as COBOL and FORTRAN. When this has been done then a computer can (and does) *in its own way* exceed human performance. As professional and white collar workers comprise about one-half the entire working population, then information engineering (systems analysis and programming skills) is likely to become as extensive in size, scope and variety as physical engineering. Indeed, it is already happening at quite a pace when one considers that reliable, fully engineered, reasonably priced computing machines have existed for little more than five years. Its pervasiveness should surprise no one.

The National Health Service, costing some £1,900 m. per annum, disburses about 70 per cent of its monies on (inadequate) wages and salaries: it is highly cerebrally dependent. Not all of the 700,000 people employed are particularly highly trained and qualified; nor are all of them making critical or complex decisions all the time. There is a hierarchy of ability, widest at the bottom. The advent of the computer enables us to gear technology to much of this activity, especially as the costs of cerebral units, even the humblest, are increasing whilst those of the new technology are decreasing, and especially as the fund of experience for applying it grows steadily.

THE CONCEPT AND SCOPE OF DATA PROCESSING

Basically, an information machine, that is a computer, has only four attributes, three of which are quite unsurprising. First, information (or data, as it is often called) can be inserted or 'input' into the machine; second, such information can actually be stored inside the machine; third, the machine can actually operate on the stored data to carry out a specified procedure; and fourth, the information can be 'output' (usually printed or transmitted) from the machine. Only the third of these attributes, namely the ability to carry out a data procedure, is at all exceptional; moreover it is exceptional to the extent that the computer is the first machine in history to be able to do this. Previously only the cerebral cortex has possessed this ability. Carrying out a data procedure (or 'data processing') is all that any computer can do, and in order to do it it needs to be provided with both the data and the procedure in a suitably acceptable form. Once the data and the procedure relating to a particular problem or activity are inserted into the computer, then pressing the starter button causes the procedure to act upon the data thereby giving rise to a certain action on the part of the computer.

And this in effect explains all there is to explain about a computer, but since the ability to carry out a data procedure does not obviously equate to the many different kinds of cerebral activity which it is claimed computers can replace, a few words of explanation about different kinds of data procedure (see Table 1) may be in order. If, for example, the data supplied to a computer is numerical and the procedure is arithmetical, then the computer's action in applying the one to the other will be to calculate. Thus computers, as is well known, have a considerable role to play in carrying out a host of arithmetical procedures such as arise in clerical and administrative work, scientific calculations, clinical trials and health statistics, epidemiological work, molecular biology and so on. One example in this category which is already widely operational arises in the context of radiotherapy. In applying a lethal dose of radiation to malignant tissue a great deal of careful calculation is required to prepare a suitable radiation treatment plan, a task which clearly requires trained and experienced cerebral activity. The existence of computer procedures embodying the relevant calculations, however, now enable computer operators unskilled in radiation treatment planning to carry out this task. Moreover, as a result of conferences, articles and other ways of communicating experience, the computer programs for the planning of radiation treatment are all tending to incorporate aggregate ideas so that the standard of the treatment

TABLE 1

Data	*Program*	*Action*
Numerical	Arithmetic	Calculation
Dictionaries	Syntax	Translation
Chess positions	Rules	Play
Traffic densities	Rules	Traffic Control
Electrocardiographic	Rules	Pattern Recognition
etc.	etc.	etc.

plans produced by the computer-assisted operators tend towards the highest known possible standard, as distinct from the personal standards of individuals.

The role of computers, however, is by no means confined to calculation; the latter simply being one particular kind of data-procedure. It is worth pointing out that only a tiny part, probably less than one per cent, of our total universe of experience can be described in terms of formulae and hence rendered susceptible to calculation. By contrast, most of what most of us do most of the time falls under the heading of rational procedures rather than calculations, and the outstanding merit of the computer is that it enables us to render machine assistance in this wider context. In fact the word computer is a complete misnomer: the thing computers do least is compute! Computers have in effect liberated us from mathematics and statistics and all we need do now to take advantage of their versatility is to liberate computers from mathematicians. This is especially true in medicine.

In order to demonstrate this, consider an entirely different example (see Table 1). If the data supplied to a computer is that contained in the English and Russian dictionaries and if the computer procedure embodies the rules of syntax in these two languages, then the effect of the procedure acting on the data will be to translate. The standard of translation, of course, will depend entirely on how well the rules have been formulated, and this in turn will depend on the linguistic understanding employed. Computer skills will certainly be required to implement the procedure in detail, but they have little bearing on the quality of the translation produced. This is a point worth emphasizing since it is a common practice to rely too heavily on computer specialists in the actual formulation of computer procedures. If computers are to be used effectively in psychiatry, cardiology, obstetrics and so on, then the detailed knowledge of the procedures in these specialties must obviously be incorporated in the specification of the computer procedures. And whilst it will certainly be necessary to involve computer skills in the design of the procedures, the responsibility for the *specification* of the procedures must remain that of the *medical* specialists involved. Reverting then to the case of computer translation we therefore observe that the machine can no more be blamed for a bad translation than it can be applauded for a good one. It, the machine, is neither intelligent nor stupid; it has no more idea of the procedure it is performing than a washing machine has that it is handling coloureds or whites: both are carrying out a prescribed sequence of operations.

Yet another example (that of chess playing) enables us to consider a quite different type of data procedure that has its relevance in the medical context (no knowledge of chess is required by the reader). It is a straightforward matter to supply a computer with data indicating the positions of each chess piece: BK (5, 4) for example would amply indicate that black knight is at five across and four down. In addition we could supply the computer with a 'directory' listing for each possible configuration of the chess pieces the moves that a first class chess player would consider. Such a directory would be extensive, and would doubtless take many years to compile; in paper form it would certainly occupy thousands of cubic feet, but stored in a computer (see below) it would be very compact indeed. Given the existence of the directory, then a possible computer procedure could be as follows:

(a) Scan the directory to ascertain what moves are possible.

(b) Select one of these moves at random (random selection procedures are quite straightforward to devise).

Since a computer could accomplish this procedure in a matter of seconds, and since it would consist of playing first class moves at random, it would clearly be a very effective player. The *effectiveness*, however, *does not depend on intelligence*, but on the ability to store millions of first class moves (which the cerebral cortex cannot) and access them incredibly quickly (which the cerebral cortex cannot). It is a fact well worth pondering that given adequate good quality information, more effective action is possible without intelligence than will result from considerable intelligence acting on inadequate information.

Such an approach underlies most of the attempts at computer-assisted diagnosis. Medical diagnosis and treatment essentially rest on the ability of clinicians to identify a patient as belonging to

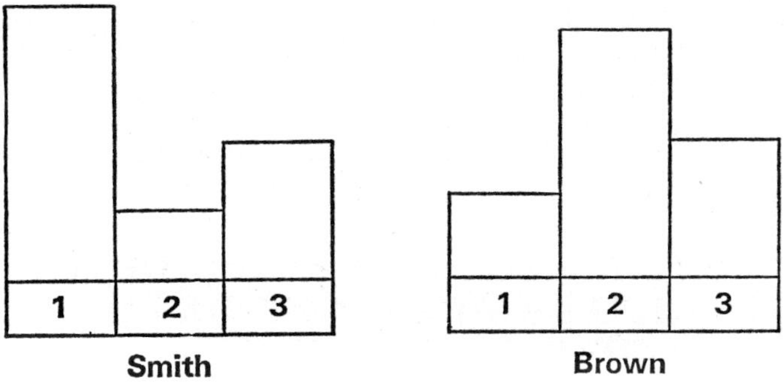

FIG. 37 Weighting factors

one or other of upwards of 30,000 treatable categories continually being refined and extended. An updated directory of such categories (listing for each defining characteristics in terms of symptoms, signs, test results, age, sex and so on, together with associated treatments and prognoses) which could be quickly accessed by telephone to extract relevant possibilities could be a useful adjunct to any single clinical memory in deciding what 'moves' are possible. There are a variety of ways by which this can be achieved.

Still on basic principles, the chess playing example enables another important point to be illustrated. Any chess player quickly learns which particular moves are most effective against particular opponents. Some of this 'learning' ability can be incorporated into data procedures. All one needs to do is to insert into the computer additional data pertaining to the relative success of particular moves against particular players. What this may consist of is shown in Fig. 37.

The computer procedure is then modified as follows:

(a) Scan the directory to ascertain what moves are possible.

(b) Select one of these at random taking account of the weighting factors.

If such a procedure were designed in detail it would clearly be possible for the designer of the program to say, 'although I designed the computer procedure I do not know which move the computer will select; I only know that it will be a first class move, taking into account what has happened in previous games against this particular player.'

Computers, then, are machines for carrying out rational procedures *once they have been adequately formulated.* Calculation simply happens to be one particular class of rational procedure. Since rational procedures are always to a degree intelligent or stupid, depending upon how they are formulated, then so are computers' actions to a degree intelligent or stupid, though the machine is neither. And since rational procedures are a significant part of all human activity, then the scope for using computers is very wide indeed.

THE BASIC MECHANICS OF A GENERAL-PURPOSE DATA-PROCESSING SYSTEM

We have seen that the raw material, as it were, that has to be supplied to a computer for it to undertake any particular task consists of the data and the procedure in some suitable form. But since a computer is a machine it has no capacity to understand meaning, which is what the cerebral cortex principally relies upon to interpret information presented to it. *Meaning*, in fact, *has to be replaced by structure*, in which position and sequence play the key roles. An item is interpreted as age, sex, address, disease category and so on by virtue of its *position* on a particular document, or by virtue of its *sequence*, the order in which it is presented to the machine. What this means in practice, for example, is that medical record data must be set out tidily according to some pre-arranged format or sequence. Any format or sequence is possible—the computer as such imposes no constraint—but once a particular format or sequence is chosen, then it must be maintained if a particular computer procedure is to be applied to it, for how else could the machine 'know' what data was on a particular document?

Although data format is the principal way in which using a computer affects a particular user, generally speaking a further stage (binary conversion) is necessary before the data can be inserted directly into a computer. This is because computers work in a 2 symbol alphabet as compared with the familiar 26 letter and 10 digit alphabets; a feature which considerably simplifies the engineering. Binary conversion is most commonly effected by punching and verifying. A data sheet, such as a medical record, is handed to a girl called a punch operator, who types out the information on a keyboard with a punch attachment (Fig. 38). As each symbol (numeral, letter, space and so on) is typed it produces a coded row of holes in a paper tape or card. The punched paper tape or card is handed to a second girl called a verifier, who inserts it into her keyboard punch and independently retypes the data sheet. Should she type out a symbol at any stage different from the punch operator the keyboard jams, and she can then decide whether a correction is

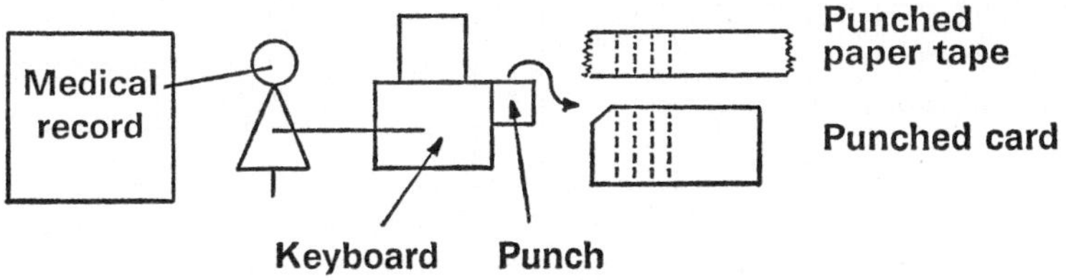

FIG. 38 Punching: a common method of binary conversion

required. Punching and verifying reduces errors of transcription to a low level, and the punched paper tapes and cards that it produces enable data to be inserted directly into a computer.

Although punching and verifying adequately copes with data that is originally handwritten or typed, it cannot deal with data generated by instruments such as blood pressure recorders, temperature recorders, auto-analysers, electrocardiographs. The procedure in this case is to attach a small piece of equipment called an analogue-to-digital converter to the instrument, as shown in Fig. 39. The analogue-to-digital converter in effect samples the height of recorded

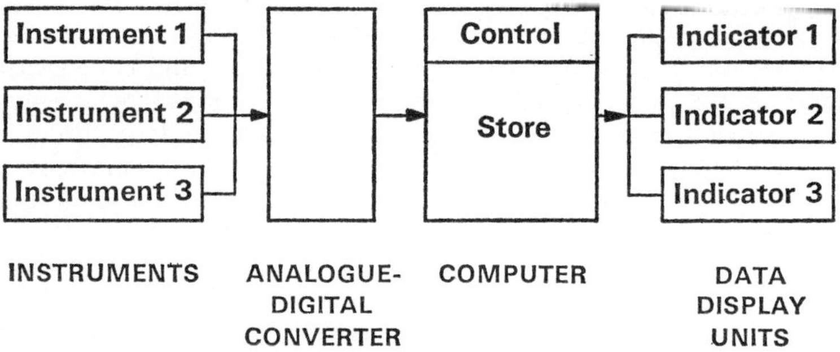

FIG. 39 Analogue-to-digital conversion

data at frequent and regular intervals, and encodes each separate height as a row of holes on punched paper tape. Thus any continuously recorded signal can be converted into a form suitable for direct insertion into a computer. In practice a single analogue-to-digital converter can be used to 'digitize' data from several instruments. (Fig. 40.) In some situations, such as might arise in laboratory data processing or patient monitoring, it may be advantageous or even necessary to communicate data directly ('on-line') from instruments to the computer without going through the punched paper tape stage. In this case, of course, the computer procedure must be

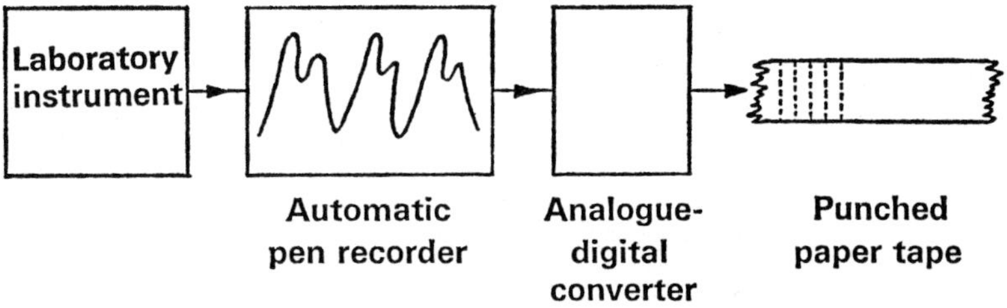

FIG. 40 Data processing system suitable for dealing with data from instruments

designed to cope with the data at the rate at which it is actually being produced: this is what is meant by 'real time' data processing.

Yet another category of data that is sometimes transferred to computers for processing is two-dimensional or pictorial data, such as radiographs and microphotographs of cervical smears. The drocess of binary conversion in this case involves a flying spot scanner as well as an analogue-to-digital converter. The flying spot scanner scans the picture line by line (television-wise) and passes the linear signal into the analogue-to-digital converter; the latter samples the linear signal frequently and regularly and encodes the contrast level at each point as a row of holes. 'Digitized' pictures can be inserted directly into computers or transmitted over large distances by teleprinter/telegraph systems. It might be worth mentioning at this point that although some useful progress has been made into the development of computer procedures for cytologically examining cervical smears, two-dimensional 'pattern recognition' procedures are intrinsically more difficult to design than one-dimensional pattern recognition procedures (such as those for classifying electrocardiograms, which have been most successful).

One way or another, therefore (and by no means every way has been mentioned), it is possible to structure any sort of data into binary form for direct insertion into a computer or for remote transmission over teleprinter/telegraph/telephone systems for remote insertion.

So much for data. Procedures likewise cannot be communicated to a computer in familiar everyday language. This is because each of us has, to a degree, his own turn of phrase and syntax, his own vocabulary and dialect, and although the cerebral cortex can usually assign meaning to the rich variety of ways of saying the same thing,

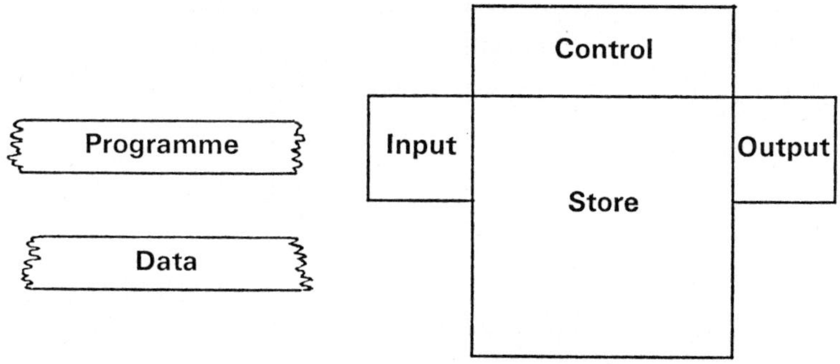

FIG. 41 Basic plan of a computer

no machine per se has any such virtue. Procedures therefore must be set down systematically, structured and then translated step by step into a special computer language such as COBOL, FORTRAN or ALGOL. Computer languages employ a well-defined vocabulary and a strictly logical syntax which enables them to be translated into basic machine operations by the computer itself. A procedure duly structured and translated into a computer language so that it can be inserted (after binary conversion) directly into a computer is called a *program*, and the process involved is called *programming*. Unfortunately, it is not possible within the scope of a single chapter to describe in any detail what is involved. Suffice it to say that once a program exists it can then be typed out by a punch operator and so converted into either a piece of punched paper tape or a set of punched cards. Thus we have seen how both the data and the program can be converted to punched form.

The basic configuration of any computer consists of a store, a suitable input and output device and a control mechanism. (Fig. 41.) The program tape is inserted into the input device and at the press of a button the program is transferred to the store; the data is then inserted and similarly transferred to the store. At the press of the start button the control unit causes the programmed procedure to operate on the data, and any results are presented via the output unit, which might be an automatic typewriter or a graph plotter (if graphic results are wanted).

Because the store in which these operations take place (usually a ferrite core store) is expensive, 'back-up' storage for retaining file data (directories, records, non-active programs and so on) is pro-

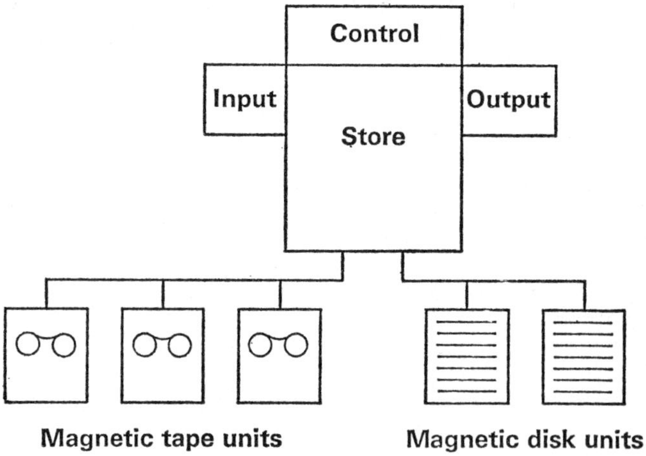

FIG. 42 A general purpose data-processing system

vided by either magnetic tape units or magnetic disc units. A typical data processing system is illustrated in Fig. 42. Magnetic tapes, usually about as big as a reel of cinematograph film and similar in appearance to tapes used on ordinary tape recorders, store symbols in a similar way to paper tape, except that magnetic marks of two polarities are used instead of holes and not-holes. The most important difference is that whereas paper tape only stores about ten symbols to the inch, magnetic tape stores many hundreds of symbols to the inch. In fact a single reel of magnetic tape usually has a capacity of several tens of millions of characters—equivalent to a few thousand records each containing a few hundred facts. Magnetic tapes can be detached when they are not in active use. Because magnetic tape is a serial device with information distributed over a length of some 2,400 feet, it can on occasions take several minutes to retrieve a particular item of information stored on it. The magnetic disc unit is a device invented to overcome this. It consists essentially of a number of discs on a common axis, with information stored in concentric circular tracks on each side of each disc. Since there is independent access electrically to each disc, any particular item can be retrieved in a fraction of a second. Improved access time is purchased at somewhat greater expense, but both magnetic tapes and magnetic discs have their place in practical data processing systems. So do magnetic drum units and magnetic card units, on occasions, but these will not be described here. One might also mention the existence of other kinds of input devices besides punched paper tape readers and punched card readers, such as optical character readers which read specialized print directly, magnetic character readers used widely by the banks, mark-sensing devices and analogue-to-digital converters. There are also output devices other than automatic typewriters, such as tape punches, card punches, line-at-a-time printers, graph plotters, and digital-to-analogue converters for reconstructing control signals, for example to activate traffic lights, drip feeds, intravenous injections, levels of anaesthesia and so on.

Such is the essential character of what is often called a general-purpose data processing system; general-purpose because it can accept data in a variety of forms, store an extensive variety of files, operate on the data of files according to any prescribed procedure and 'output' the results in a variety of ways according to what is required.

A WIDE VARIETY OF MEDICAL APPLICATIONS

Many medical uses can be made of a general-purpose data processing system. One in common use will be described sufficiently to show the modus operandi that generally applies: it concerns a vaccination and immunization procedure pioneered in the county of West Sussex as far back as 1963, and which with extensions has been operational ever since.

On the birth of each child a pattern of vaccination and immunization is agreed by the parents who signing a form which describes what has been agreed. In addition the form contains details of the child's address, age, and the clinic or general practitioner's surgery where the parents wish the child to be treated. These forms, numbering tens of thousands, are punched onto paper tape and thus transferred into the computer store, where under program control they are transferred to magnetic tape reels which can be detached. These reels of magnetic tape constitute in modern form the filing system. Once a fortnight the magnetic tapes (in effect the 'data') are fitted to the magnetic tape unit of a computer and the vaccination and immunization program is inserted into the store. At the pressing of a button the computer carries out the procedure entirely automatically and incredibly quickly. For each and every one of the thousands of records (transferred from the magnetic tape to the computer store in turn) it subtracts the current date from the date on which the child had its last particular dose. If the interval of time is sufficient the computer works out a suitable appointment and prints out an appointment card (postage prepaid) with the appropriate address so that it can be posted directly. In arranging the appointment the computer procedure will have 'looked up' and updated the appointments record for the relevant practitioner or clinic; it is thus able to print out for each doctor and clinic the list of appointments made for it, containing the names of who will be attending, what they are attending for, and the time they are invited to attend. The third list which the computer prints out specifies the 'kit' that each clinic or doctor will require at their vaccination and immunization sessions. All this is reliably carried out in a few hours without any human effort.

In due course the appointments are (or are not) kept. The general practitioner completes the attendance information and returns the sheet to the computer centre. There it is punched out and inserted into the computer together with an updating program. This causes each record on the magnetic tape file to be appropriately updated; it also causes the appropriate item-by-item fees to be worked out for each general practitioner, for the accounts to be generated and the cheques to be printed for remittance. Once again no human effort is required. In the cases where appointments are not kept, the attendance is not registered by the general practitioner and thus the child's record is not updated. Consequently, at the next fortnightly run an even greater interval of time will have elapsed since the child was vaccinated and so automatically another appointment is arranged. The number of appointments, however, is scored and a printout given of those who have ignored successive appointments, so that the Medical Officer of Health can at his discretion decide whether a visit by a health visitor would be useful.

Apart from the virtual elimination of clerical effort required to service 100,000 records in this way, the routine thoroughness of this procedure has upgraded the population immunity to the exceptionally high level of over 90 per cent. Economy and effectiveness therefore go hand in hand. A similar procedure has also been in operation for some time dealing with call-up of women for cervical and breast cancer screening. But the technique—essentially one of keeping records on magnetic tape files that can be scanned, searched, updated and modified by computer program—is perfectly general. Automated followup registers, cancer, perinatal, orthopaedic and psychiatric registers are also serviced in this way; so are hopsital admissions and discharges, out-patient appointments and bed state control procedures, as well as such things as age-sex registers in general practice. Nor need the use of such methods be confined to situations involving large numbers of records. Particular specialists with particular interests who assiduously collect a relatively large amount of information on relatively few patients may also find these methods useful: for example, a paediatrician interested in the specific diagnostic profiles of dyslexics; a cardiac surgeon wishing to examine the postoperative morbidity of his atrial septal defect manoeuvres in relation to different methods of management; a urologist interested in the histological classification of testicular tumours, and so on. In effect any rational procedure for dealing with record data, whether for administrative or clinical purposes, may benefit from computer-assisted methods of record keeping.

Laboratories, too, whose work loads grow steadily (almost doubling every five years) as medicine depends increasingly on measurement, can and do take advantage of such methods to sort test requests into order; to prepare work sheets for technicians; to prepare the day sheet setting out the total daily work load; to analyze the digitized output of instruments and to combine this with patient data to prepare test reports; to retrieve past test measurements on patients from previous records; to maintain quality control procedures and to produce any statistical returns that may be required. This latter takes us into the familiar area of calculation which features in many types of biomedical research as well as in day-to-day requirements for dietetic analysis, radiation treatment planning (mentioned earlier), survey work, epidemiological studies and so on. Pattern recognition procedures of blood pressure recordings, E.C.G. tracings and other continuously recorded physical signs (particularly in the patient monitoring environment) are also numbered amongst the many tasks carried out by general-purpose data processing systems.

THE EVOLUTION OF REAL TIME SYSTEMS AND PORTABLE COMPUTER POWER

Despite the astonishing progress already made in computer development the pace continues, and perhaps the best way of indicating present trends is to review what has happened in the short span of one generation.

It all started in 1946 when the first electronic digital computer ever, the ENIAC, was invented at the Moore School of Engineering in Pennsylvania. It weighed 30 tons, contained some 18,000 thermionic valves generating between them as much heat as 150 one-bar electric fires, and it was thoroughly unreliable! Nevertheless it was the first information machine in history capable of performing data processing, and moreover it could carry out such procedures (when it worked) at a thousand operations a second. Thus it was that each brief utterance by the machine sent banner headlines round the world, since it could in a few minutes accomplish tasks which hitherto had required several man-weeks of trained cerebral effort. Following a report by John von Neumann of Princeton in 1947, the concept of binary logic was widely applied to all engineering aspects of computers, to enable a reduction in equipment of about one-sixth of what was originally required. The first 'Princeton-type' machines appeared at English and American universities during 1949/50.

Early in the 1950s the manufacturers plucked up sufficient courage to produce the so-called first-generation computers. Like the ENIAC their design was based on the thermionic valve, but despite the application of the Princeton philosophy they were still bulky, expensive and pretty unreliable. Nevertheless the so-called 'giant brains' accomplished prodigious feats of calculation and were widely used in universities and research establishments, where their unreliability (still probably more than 50 per cent) was unimportant compared with the fact that during the time they did work they saved many weeks or months of calculation. Then, with the advent of the transistor (which displaced the thermionic valve and thereby considerably reduced both volume and heat generation) the second generation computers emerged around 1959/60. These machines were much more reliable (about 90 per cent at the start), considerably more compact, and although costing roughly the same price were up to 100 times faster, thereby greatly reducing the unit cost of data processing. The changed economics allowed much more complicated computer procedures to be run, and in particular facilitated the development of 'high level' computer languages which the computer itself translates into its basic operations.

Thus 1960 in effect marks the take-off point for computer application. The computer's wider role as a data processing machine rather than as simply a fast calculator was quickly appreciated and many different kinds of organization began enlisting its services: banks and government departments as well as aviation and industry;

insurance companies and mail order firms as well as traffic controllers and printers; though not yet the medical profession. As the information needs of each of these quite different organizations were as different as the nature of the organizations themselves, the computer manufacturers quickly found themselves having to provide in effect 'tailor-made' computing systems. Hence, in 1965/66 they brought out what were called the third generation computers, whose main feature was their modularity. Fully engineered and highly reliable production modules could be interconnected with sufficient flexibility to meet the diversity of different requirements.

Accompanying the third generation computers was a much more crucial development: they were capable of operating at as much as a million operations a second, that is 1,000 times faster than ENIAC. This very fact provided a new and remarkable opportunity, the full implications of which have yet to be worked out; whereas the first generation machines could perform a thousand operations a second for one user, the fast third generation machines could in principle provide a thousand operations a second for up to 1,000 users! This is the concept of 'time-sharing' or 'multi-access' computer systems. Evidently such an arrangement allows no time for manual insertion of each user's data and program; instead two things are necessary:

(a) Each user must be directly connected (usually electrically over a telephone system) to the computer (i.e. be 'on-line').

(b) Some arrangement must be made inside the computer for it to switch rapidly from one user's program to another.

This then is the stage now emerging: that of a computer utility to which users with 'data-terminals' only are remotely connected via the telephone system or some private communication system. The data terminal may simply consist of a teleprinter arrangement (for typing in data and program, and printing out results), but in a more advanced form consists of a video display unit (VDU), in effect the combination of a television-like display tube with a keyboard. In this way information in the computer files (perhaps many miles away) can, on request, be instantly displayed. Furthermore, since the computer is performing about a thousand operations a second for each and every user every second, each user gets the impression that the computer is keeping up with him at his own rate (in his own real time). Hence the phrase 'real-time data terminal systems'.

Real-time data terminal systems which in effect constitute a communication system not simply for message transfer (as does the telephone system) but also for interacting with the information in a dynamic way, are becoming known as the fourth generation computer systems. During 1968/69, in the United Kingdom, the Department of Health and Social Security has sponsored a number of major projects, essentially experimental in nature, to explore the application of fourth generation computer systems in both hospital work and general practice. Each system envisages a 'data bank' that is a central computerized filing system (either in a hospital or in a community) that can be 'accessed' via data terminals by doctors, nurses and others to call up individual patient records; by administrators, epidemiologists or research workers for their respective needs (due care being taken to guard confidentiality as required). General practitioners, it is thought, may have prescriptions and test request forms printed out for them, may make out-patient appointments or arrange hospital admissions; may arrange their own appointment systems, and even perhaps request advice on possible treatments or differential diagnoses. In 1972, then, this is where experiment stands in computer-assisted medicine; now that many valuable uses have been demonstrated for off-line general-purpose data processing systems, experiment is towards assessing the feasibility and practicality of on-line systems.

Beyond all this the advent of micro-electronics (which facilitates a degree of miniaturisation well beyond that already accomplished by transistorisation) is having an equally profound effect on the application of computer power. Computers more powerful than the original ENIAC are now available for a few thousand pounds, weighing less than 30 lbs and requiring as little electric power as an ordinary lamp. This portable computer power is finding its way into laboratories, intensive-care units and the like. Where a given number of routine tasks need to be performed on a fairly continual basis, a small computer may be entirely committed to carrying out any one of up to perhaps a dozen programs that constitute a useful part of the activity which would otherwise have to be carried out by trained technicians or nurses. Such a computer is said to be used in a 'dedicated' role, as distinct from a general-purpose role.

Thus the astonishing capability created in 1946, but only available in a reasonably engineered form since 1960, is already being widely applied to many aspects of medical practice. Now that a fair number of officially financed projects are at last under way, the breadth of application is likely to grow steadily. The bottleneck which can be expected to persist for some years is in the education and training of those whose activities can benefit from its effective use, for the task of computer-assisted medicine cannot conceivably be left to the computer scientists themselves.

Selected Bibliography

ATKINS, H. (Editor) (1965) *Progress in Medical Computing*. Blackwell, Oxford.

BOWDEN, B. V. (Editor) (1968) *Faster than Thought: A Symposium on Digital Computing Machines*. Pitman, London.

BOYLE, J. A., GREIG, W. R., FRANKLIN, D. A., HARDEN, R. M., BUCHANAN, W. W. and MCGIRR, E. M. (1966) Construction of a Model for Computer-Assisted Diagnosis: Application to the Problem of Non-Toxic Goitre. *Quart. J. Med.* 35, 565.

HOLLINGDALE, S. H. and TOOTHILL, G. C. (1970) *Electronic Computers*. Penguin Books, Harmondsworth.

PAYNE, L. C. (1966) *An Introduction to Medical Automation*. Pitman, London.

TAYLOR, S. H., MACDONALD, H. R., ROBINSON, M. C. and SAPRU, R. P. (1967) Computers in Cardiovascular Investigation. *Brit. Heart J.* 29, 352.

Index

313